Recent Results in Cancer Research 131

W.-D. Ludwig E. Thiel (Eds.)

Recent Advances in Cell Biology of Acute Leukemia

Impact on Clinical Diagnosis and Therapy

With 98 Figures and 79 Tables

Springer-Verlag
Berlin Heidelberg New York
London Paris Tokyo
Hong Kong Barcelona
Budapest

Priv.-Doz. Dr. Wolf-Dieter Ludwig
Universitätsklinikum Steglitz
Abt. Hämatologie/Onkologie
Hindenburgdamm 30
W-1000 Berlin 45, Germany

Prof. Dr. Eckhard Thiel
Universitätsklinikum Steglitz
Abt. Hämatologie/Onkologie
Hindenburgdamm 30
W-1000 Berlin 45, Germany

ISBN-13:978-3-642-84897-1 e-ISBN-13:978-3-642-84895-7
DOI: 10.1007/978-3-642-84895-7

Library of Congress Cataloging-in-Publication Data. Recent advances in cell biology of acute leukemia : impact on clinical diagnosis and therapy / [edited by] W.-D. Ludwig, E. Thiel. p. cm.—(Recent results in cancer research ; v. 131) Includes bibliographical references and index. ISBN-13:978-3-642-84897-1
1. Leukemia. 2. Cancer cells. 3. Leukemia—Molecular aspects. 4. Leukemia—Immunological aspects. I. Ludwig, W.-D. (Wolf-Dieter), 1952- II. Thiel, Eckhard, 1944- . III. Series. [DNLM: 1. Leukemia—genetics—congresses. 2. Leukemia—therapy—congresses. 3. Chromosome Aberrations—congresses. 4. Immunotherapy—congresses. W1 RE106P v. 131 1993 / QZ 350 R295 1993] RC261.R35 vol. 131 [RC643] 616.99'4 s—dc20 [616.99'419] DNLM/DLC for Library of Congress 93-16157

Typesetting by Best-set Typesetter Ltd., Hong Kong
19/3130/SPS-5 4 3 2 1 0 – Printed on acid-free paper

Preface

The development of new techniques such as immunophenotyping, cytogenetic investigations and, more recently, molecular studies has considerably increased our diagnostic repertoire and broadened our ideas about the biology of acute leukemias. While immunophenotyping with monoclonal antibodies has yielded increased diagnostic precision and made it possible to develop a highly reproducible classification of acute leukemias based on cell-biological features, further insights have been gained into the pathogenetic mechanisms involved in leukemogenesis by means of cytogenetic detection of acquired structural chromosomal abnormalities. Analysis of the leukemia-associated chromosomal breakpoints using molecular techniques can now pinpoint many genomic sites essential for normal development and maturation of hematopoietic cells but functionally disrupted in leukemic cells.

The main goal of the international workshop that we held in Berlin with a select group of scientists and clinicians involved in leukemia research was to describe the state of the art and new developments in the immunologic, cytogenetic, and molecular characterization of acute leukemias and to discuss the clinical importance of cell-biological features. After introductory survey lectures dealing with the immunological and molecular-biological characteristics of normal vs. malignant lymphatic and myeloid progenitor cells, the workshop centered on contributions characterizing the immunophenotype and both numerical and structural chromosomal abnormalities in acute leukemias. The results presented from European and American multicenter therapy studies have revealed in part characteristic correlations between the morphological subtype, the immunophenotype, the karyotype, and the clinical features, and have clearly shown that combined immunologic and cytogenetic analyses are particularly suitable for identifying prognostically relevant subtypes that can be used to supplement the known clinical risk factors for a risk-adjusted therapeutic strategy.

The workshop also featured lectures on new methods for recognizing residual leukemia cells not eliminated by chemotherapeutic treatment or bone marrow transplantation. In a comparison with conventional hematological diagnostics, special attention was called to the high sensitivity of the immunological (e.g., double color immunofluorescence analysis, multiparameter flow cytometry) and molecular-biological (e.g., polymerase chain reaction) techniques, with a critical discussion of both their possibilities and limitations in detecting minimal residual disease. (MRD) The clinical importance of immunological and molecular-biological MRD detection in acute leukemia is now being prospectively analyzed in multicenter studies. The evaluation of these studies will hopefully answer the important question of whether various subtypes of acute leukemias differ with respect to MRD so that clinical consequences may be drawn in tailoring the therapeutic intensity and possibly also immunotherapeutic strategies.

The constructive and often lively exchange of experience and ideas at this workshop successfully illuminated the essential aspects of the topics discussed and pointed to important questions for future investigations. Decisive for the success of the workshop were the outstanding contributions of the invited scientists, now published in this book. These studies elucidate with numerous illustrations the possibilities of modern immunological, cytogenetic, and molecular-biological diagnostics and give a very up-to-date overview of the pathophysiological and clinical relevance of the phenotypic and genotypic characterization of acute leukemias.

Our gratitude is due to numerous coworkers, including Ms. Barbara Komischke, Dr. Michael Notter, and Dr. Christian Sperling, members of the local organizing committee, for their exceptional dedication and valuable support in preparing and organizing this workshop.

Berlin, January 1993

W.-D. Ludwig
E. Thiel

Contents

*List of Contributors**

* The address of the principal author is given on the first page of each contribution.
[1] Page on which contribution begins.

I. Hematopoietic Differentiation

Differentiation of Physiological and Malignant Cells of the B-Cell System

H. Stein

Freie Universität Berlin, Universitätsklinikum Steglitz, Institut für Pathologie, Hindenburgdamm 30, W-1000 Berlin 45, Fed. Rep. of Germany

Major Events and Characteristics of B-Cell Development

The common differentiation pathway in the human body is a one-wave process of proliferation and differentiation. This can be illustrated using granulopoiesis as an example (Fig. 1). In contrast, the development of B and T cells from stem cells to effector or memory cells results from at least a two-wave and usually a multiple-wave pathway of proliferation and differentiation. In the first proliferation and differentiation wave, B or T cell determined stem cells, designated progenitor B or T cells, pass through an intermediate stage to become what are termed precursor B or T cells, which then develop into resting, naive, antigen-reactive, and recirculating B or T lymphocytes. These cells are not the final cells because they can undergo a second wave of proliferation and differentiation by forming proliferating blasts in response to an appropriate antigen. These are called activated lymphoid blasts. These antigen-induced blasts transform into effector cells or memory cells after several rounds of proliferation. Thus the first and second wave of proliferation and differentiation serve different functions, and are regulated differently.

In the first wave of proliferation and differentiation the diversity of antigen receptors is generated, whereas in the second wave a certain antigen receptor specificity is multiplied. Since the generation of the antigen receptor diversity develops due to a random rearrangement of immunoglobulin or T-cell receptor (TCR) genes, there is not only production of receptors that react with foreign antigens, but also of ones that react with self-antigens. However, any cells carrying self-reactive receptors must be eliminated, suppressed, or inactivated so that destructive autoimmunity is avoided. One important mechanism by which self-antigen-reactive B and T cells are eliminated was recently clarified by a series of simple experiments, some results of which are shown in Table 1. It has been known for quite some time that incubation of mature peripheral T cells with

Recent Results in Cancer Research, Vol. 131

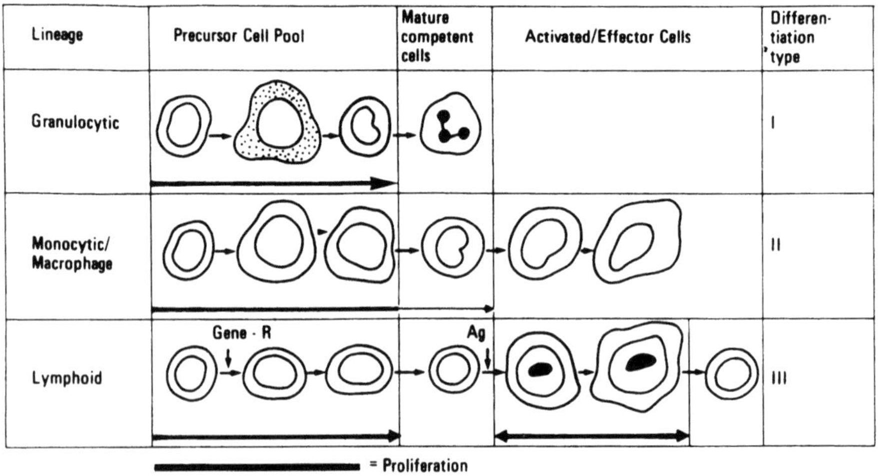

Fig. 1. The uniqueness of proliferation and differentiation of lymphoid cells

Table 1. Clonal deletion of autoreactive thymocytes

Treatment	Immature thymocytes	Mature peripheral T cells
Anti-CD3	100% Apoptosis	Proliferation
Anti-TCR	50% Apoptosis	Proliferation

Conclusion: Binding of the TCR to self-antigens produces clonal deletions and thus contributes to self-tolerance.
Data from Smith et al. (1989); Finkel et al. (1991)

certain antibodies to the CD3 or TCR complex induced proliferation. Smith and colleagues (1989) showed, however, that treatment of thymocytes with antibodies to CD3 or TCR complex has a completely different effect. Instead of induction of proliferation the immature thymocytes die of apoptosis, which is also often referred to as programmed cell death. Apoptosis means an endogenous pathway of DNA degradation. It is detectable in gel electrophoresis analysis as ladders of diffuse bands whose molecular sizes are approximate multiples of 200 base pairs. According to the results of Smith and colleagues, the induction of apoptosis in immature T cells by binding of the TCRs to self-antigens may be the mechanism by which clonal deletion is produced, and consequently self-tolerance by the T-cell system. In B-cell generation and differentiation, there are three major episodes of selection (Gallagher and Osmond 1991): (1) during primary B-cell genesis; (2) during extrafollicular B-cell proliferation; (3) during germinal center reaction.

Primary B-Cell Genesis

In human beings, primary B-cell genesis takes place in the bone marrow. However, there is no exclusive B-cell domain in the bone marrow, but, according to the studies of Gallagher and Osmond (1991), there is an identifiable migration from the edge of the marrow, where precursor B cells are formed, towards the center, where mature B cells congregate. Each single progenitor at the stage of immunoglobulin rearrangement may give rise to as many as 64 progeny. This event is closely associated with intimate cell contact between the precursor B cells and the long dendritic processes extended by the stromal reticular cells. Adhesion molecules and the production of short-range growth factors, for example interleukin-7, by the stromal cells may also be important in B-cell regulation. It is not clear whether positive selection, negative selection, or both are occurring during this stage of B-cell lymphopoiesis. However, there is growing evidence that the loss of cells may be a result of negative selection: Binding of self-reactive newly expressed immunoglobulin molecules on the surface of the developing B cells may be the stimulus for a process which leads to apoptosis, analogous to deletion of self-reactive T cells in the thymus. From the pre-B cells generated in the marrow around 75% are culled. Contact between B cells and macrophages is a prelude to rapid phagocytosis and apoptotic cells. Those cells in the bone marrow that escape deletion home to and accumulate in sinusoidal spaces near the central sinus, from which they are released en masse into the peripheral blood and into extrafollicular regions of peripheral lymphoid tissue in response to unknown signals.

Extrafollicular B-Cell Proliferation

The second bout of B-cell selection occurs as a result of an encounter with free antigens in extrafollicular areas of peripheral lymphoid tissue. These areas are the first sites at which B-cell proliferation (MacLennan and Gray 1986; MacLennan et al. 1988, 1990) is seen in response to free antigens (Fig. 2). The first blasts appear during the second day of immunization. The B-cell proliferation response only lasts for about 48 h. This extrafollicular response of B cells starts with either memory B cells or newly produced virgin B cells. The B cells that cannot bind to antigens will die after some time, whereas those that bind to antigens transform into either short-lived plasma cells or recirculating memory B cells. The short-lived plasma cells populate medullary cords of the same lymph node. In the extrafollicular areas, there is also the antigen-induced T-cell proliferation. The extrafollicular B and T blasts exhibit the activation antigen CD30 that was initially designated Ki-1. It has been suggested that, following malignant transformation, these extrafollicular blasts give rise to CD30-positive anaplastic large cell lymphomas (Stein et al. 1985). This assumption has

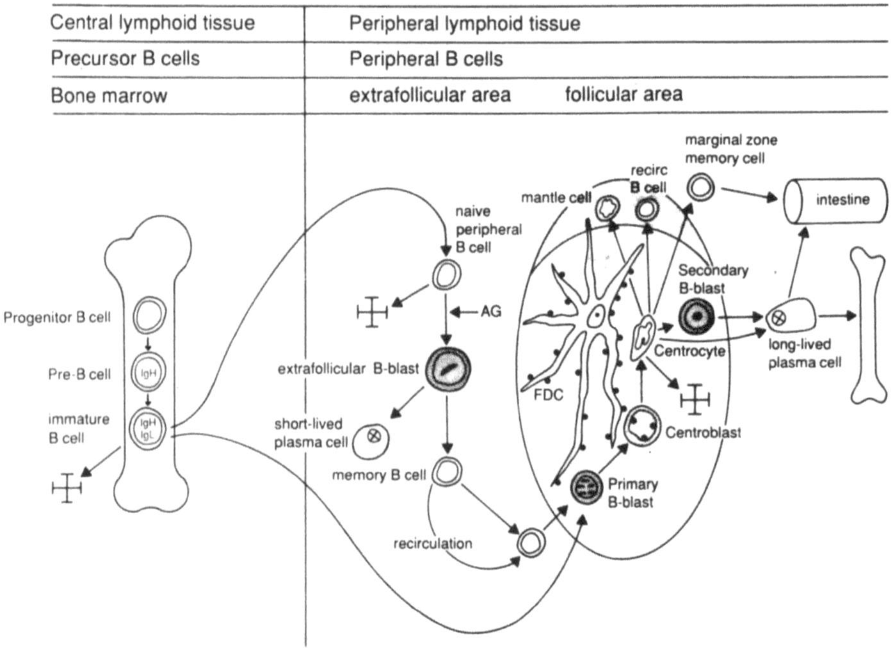

Fig. 2. Schematic representation of B cell development based on animal experimental and immunohistologic data by MacLennan et al. (1988, 1990)

been based on the observation that the first site of involvement of CD30-positive anaplastic large cell lymphomas is the perifollicular region. It might also be of interest that the extrafollicular blasts are the cells in which Epstein-Barr virus is detectable during infectious mononucleosis.

Germinal Center Cell Reaction

The third round of discrimination during B-cell development takes place in the B-cell follicles with their meshwork of follicular dendritic cells (FDC). Resting or primary follicles consist of a collection of FDC which form a dense meshwork throughout the follicle. The primary follicles are the structures where the germinal center reaction starts. The sequence of the germinal center reaction can be subdivided into four stages based on immunohistochemical studies of the follicular response to two haptens conjugated to the same carrier protein (MacLennan et al. 1990). First, 72 h after immunization follicles are colonized by fewer than five primary B blasts, which proliferate rapidly to fill the spaces in the FDC meshwork and expand to total about 10000 cells within 3 days. Secondly, by around day 4 after antigenic challenge the primary B-cell blasts metamorphose into centroblasts which lack surface immunoglobulin (i.e., immunoglobulin-type antigen receptors) and migrate to one pole of the FDC meshwork, forming the dark zone. The centroblasts within it are a self-renewing, although nonexpanding population that gives rise to centrocytes. The centroblasts as well as the centrocytes are *bcl-2*-negative and thus, are very susceptible to apoptosis. The differentiation of centroblasts into centrocytes is associated with hypermutation of the *V* region and of the heavy chain class switch of the immunoglobulin-type antigen receptors. Mutations can increase, decrease, or fail to modify the affinity of antigen receptors of centrocytes. The centrocytes with low affinity for antigen cannot interact with the antigen presented by FDC, and thus die of apoptosis. In contrast, the centrocytes with high-affinity receptors can interact with the antigen expressed on the surface of FDC, and are therefore rescued from dying of apoptosis. The surviving centrocytes then proceed into the fourth stage of development. In this stage these centrocytes transform either directly or via secondary follicular B blasts into memory cells and migrant long-living plasma cells. The signals which rescue the centrocytes from apoptosis and which direct their following differentiation are provided by antigens immobilized on the surface of FDC, by CD23, interleukin-1α (IL-1α), and the CD40 molecule (Gray 1988; Rocha et al. 1990). In the presence of CD23 and IL-1α a centrocyte is directed to transform into a plasma cell while rescue via CD40 results in a memory cell formation. There is evidence that at least three subtypes or sublineages of memory cells exist: two of them reside in the follicular mantle and one in the marginal zones. One follicular mantle cell type memory cell recirculates whereas the other is more sessile and has intimate contact with the tender processes of FDC which extend into the follicular mantle.

How Does the Scenario of B-Cell Differentiation Relate to Some of the B-Cell Neoplasias?

The extrafollicular CD30-positive blasts of B-cell as well as T-cell origin appear to give rise to extrafollicular Hodgkin's disease and to what we described several years ago as CD30-positive anaplastic large cell (ALC) lymphomas. This concept is supported by the observation that the neoplastic cells of Hodgkin's disease and ALC lymphoma resemble in cytology and in their perifollicular distribution the physiologic extrafollicular lymphoid blasts. Like the latter, Hodgkin's disease and ALC lymphoma can be of either B-cell or T-cell type, with the B-cell type being more common in the former and the T-cell type more common in the latter.

Malignant transformation of germinal center B cells can result in three types of lymphomas: follicular centroblastic-centrocytic (CB-CC) lymphomas, centroblastic (CB) lymphomas, and probably Burkitt's lymphoma.

In CB-CC lymphoma there is an accumulation of slow-dividing centrocytes. This might result from failure of the apoptotic mechanism. As discussed earlier, centrocytes which are the progeny of centroblasts kill themselves by apoptosis if not selected by antigens presented on the FDC. It is likely that this mechanism fails to work in CB-CC lymphoma. There are lines of evidence for this assumption: first, apoptotic cells are missing in CB-CC lymphoma; and second, CB-CC lymphomas express the bcl-2 protein, unlike normal germinal center cells. The bcl-2 protein blocks apoptosis, thus prolonging cell survival. Accordingly, the CB-CC lymphoma appears to be a neoplasm due to bcl-2 protein-induced generation of atypically long-living germinal center cells. The cause of the bcl-2 protein expression by the neoplastic germinal center cells has been identified. It is the translocation t(14;18), which causes the *bcl-2* gene, due to its juxtaposition to the immunoglobulin heavy chain gene, to come under the influence of the strong enhancer of the latter mentioned gene. In CB lymphomas and Burkitt's lymphomas the defect must be different. Both lymphomas show rapid proliferation of the tumor cells and a high rate of apoptosis, this being especially pronounced in Burkitt's lymphomas. In CB lymphoma there is nearly total block of the capacity of centroblasts to differentiate into centrocytes. The problem in Burkitt's lymphoma seems to be the complete lack of capacity of primary B blasts to differentiate into centroblasts. The underlying molecular mechanism is still totally obscure in CB lymphoma, whereas in Burkitt's lymphomas a deregulated c-*myc* gene is involved. This deregulation is caused by the translocation t(8;14) which is constantly encountered in Burkitt's lymphomas.

References

Finkel TH, Kubo RT, Cambier JC (1991) T-cell development and transmembrane signaling: changing biological responses through an unchanging receptor. Immunol Today 12:79–85

Gallagher RB, Osmond DG (1991) To B, or not to B: that is the question. Immunol Today 12:1–3

Gray D (1988) Population kinetics of rat peripheral B cells. J Exp Med 167:805–816

MacLennan ICM, Gray D (1986) Antigen-driven selection of virgin and memory B cells. Immunol Rev 91:61–85

MacLennan ICM, Liu YL, Ling NR (1988) B cell proliferation in follicles, germinal center formation and the site of neoplastic transformation in Burkitt's lymphoma. Curr Top Microbiol Immunol 141:138–148

MacLennan ICM, Liu YJ, Oldfield S, Zhang J, Lane PJL (1990) The evolution of B cell clones. Curr Top Microbiol Immunol 159:37–63

Rocha B, Penit C, Baron C, Vasseur F, Dautigny N, Freitas AA (1990) Accumulation of bromodeoxyuridine-labeled cells in central and peripheral lymphoid organs: minimal estimates of production and urnover rates of mature lymphocytes. Eur J Immunol 20:1697–1708

Smith CA, Williams GT, Kingston R, Jenkinson EJ, Owen JJT (1989) Antibodies to CD3/T-cell receptor complex induce death by apoptosis in immature T cells in thymic cultures. Nature 337:181–184

Stein H, Mason DY, Gerdes J, O'Connor N, Wainscoat J, Pallesen G, Gatter K, Falini B, Delsol G, Lemke H, Schwarting R, Lennert K (1985) The expression of the Hodgkin's disease-associated antigen Ki-1 in reactive and neoplastic lymphoid tissue. Evidence that Reed-Sternberg cells and histiocytic malignancies are derived from activated lymphoid cells. Blood 66:848–858

Expression of B-Cell-Associated Antigens During B-Cell Ontogeny

B. Dörken

Dep. of Medical Oncology and Tumor Immunology, URKV, Free University of Berlin, O-1115 Berlin, Fed. Rep. of Germany

Introduction

The development of the B-cell lineage from stem cells to mature B lymphocytes and antibody-secreting plasma cells is a multistep process of differentiation. Stages of B-cell maturation have been characterized by the rearrangement and expression of the immunoglobulin (Ig) genes, by surface markers, and by susceptibilities to growth and differentiation factors (Tonegawa 1983; Alt et al. 1986; Campana et al. 1985; Loken et al. 1987; Kishimoto 1987; Cooper 1987). B-lineage acute lymphoblastic leukemias are presumed to result from leukemogenic events that occur in progenitor B cells during early phases of B-cell ontogeny and lead to a maturational arrest at discrete stages of early B-cell differentiation (Greaves 1986). Recently published data on molecular components of the B-cell antigen receptor complex, molecules selectively expressed in pre-B cells, and B-lineage-associated differentiation antigens have provided a new insight into early B-cell development, and this will contribute to a better understanding of the cell biology of B-lineage acute lymphoblastic leukemias.

Molecular Components of the B-Cell Antigen Receptor Complex

Membrane Ig serves as the surface receptor by which B lymphocytes recognize antigen and are activated (Kishimoto 1987; Cooper 1987). The intracytoplasmic portion of surface IgM (sIgM) contains only three amino acids, suggesting a need for associated proteins that can transduce the receptor signal. First in the mouse a protein complex has been found which is associated with sIgM, analogous to the CD3 complex in T cells: IgM molecules are noncovalently associated with a disulfide-linked heterodimer of two transmembrane proteins, designated IgM-α and Ig-β (Hombach et al. 1990a). IgM-α, a 34-kDa glycoprotein, is encoded by the *mb-1* gene while

Ig-β, a 39-kDa glycoprotein, is encoded by the *B29* gene (Hombach et al. 1990b). These genes are B-lineage specific and are co-expressed in pre-B and B cells (Sakaguchi et al. 1988; Kashiwamura et al. 1990; Hermanson et al. 1988). Both IgM-α and Ig-β proteins are transmembrane glycoproteins with extracellular Ig-like domains and cytoplasmic tails with overall structural similarities to CD3 components of the T-cell receptor complex. The B-cell antigen receptor of the IgM class comes on the cell surface only as a complex including the IgM molecule and the IgM-α/Ig-β heterodimer (Hombach et al. 1990a). It is likely that the IgM-α and Ig-β molecules function not only in surface deposition but also in signal transduction of the B-cell antigen receptor. Recent studies of Yamanishi et al. (1991) suggest that the complex is associated with the tyrosine kinase Lyn. The protein encoded by the *mb-1* gene is already expressed on $sIgM^-$ pre-B lymphoma cells (Matsuo et al. 1991; Nomura et al. 1991), suggesting that IgM-α can be transported on the B-cell surface without the complete IgM molecule (see below).

The human homolog of the *mb-1* gene was isolated from a complementary (c)DNA library of the Daudi cell line (Sakaguchi et al. 1988). In human B cells, a disulfide-linked heterodimer of 47- and 37-kDa proteins have been described to be non-covalently associated with sIgM, indicating that molecules similar to IgM-α and Ig-β exist on human B cells (van Noessel et al. 1990). Recently, Mason et al. (1991) have described the generation of monoclonal and polyclonal antibodies directed against a peptide sequence from the cytoplasmic tail of human MB-1. By immunocytochemical staining of normal and neoplastic B cells, the human MB-1 protein was shown to appear early in B-cell differentiation, before expression of cytoplasmic μ chain: of the progenitor B-cell leukemias, 74% were $MB\text{-}1^+$.

Molecules Selectively Expressed in Pre-B Cells

The mature B cell which is capable of responding to an antigen is the result of a multistep process of differentiation. The development of B cells from stem cells to mature sIg^+ B cells can be classified by the rearrangement and expression of Ig H- and L-chain genes. Gene segments of the Ig gene loci are rearranged in an ordered fashion so that first D_H segments are rearranged to J_H segments, followed by V_H to *DJ* (Tonegawa 1983; Alt et al. 1986). The diversity of Ig H-chain genes is generated by both the differential usage of the several *V*, *D*, and *J* gene segments available and by junctional changes, including N region nucleotide addition, catalyzed by the enzyme terminal deoxynucleotidyl transferase, TdT (Desiderio et al. 1984; Blackwell and Alt 1989). This enzyme is exclusively found in early lymphoid progenitors (Janossy et al. 1979). During further B-cell differentiation, the genes encoding L chains are assembled by sequential rearrangements. First, V_κ segments are joined to J_κ, and finally V_λ to J_λ segments (Tonegawa 1983;

Alt et al. 1986). Ig H chains synthesized in pre-B cells are in general believed not to be expressed on the cell surface unless they are associated with L chains. Therefore, the finding that certain human and murine pre-B-cell leukemias express small amounts of surface μ chains in the absence of conventional light chain expression (Vogler et al. 1978; Paige et al. 1981; Gordon et al. 1981; Hendershot and Levitt 1984) has always been an enigma. The first clue to the resolution of this apparent paradox was the demonstration that the λ5 and $V_{\text{pre-B}}$ genes are specifically expressed in murine pre-B cells and that these genes have strong homology to the *C* and *V* regions of the λ L-chain genes (Sakaguchi and Melchers 1986; Kudo and Melchers 1987) and thus are likely to encode μ binding proteins. It was then shown that in pre-B cells μ chains were associated with a 18-kDa protein termed ω and a 14-kDa protein termed ι (Pillai and Baltimore 1987, 1988). It is now clear that these "surrogate" light chains are encoded by the λ5 and $V_{\text{pre-B}}$ genes (Karasuyama et al. 1990; Tsubata and Reth 1990; Cherayil and Pillai 1991; Rolink and Melchers 1991). The λ5 (ω) and $V_{\text{pre-B}}$ (ι) proteins derived from unrearranged genes bind to μ chains (Karasuyama et al. 1990) and have the same capacity as conventional λ chains to allow surface expression of μ chains (Tsubata and Reth 1990). The μ heavy chain and λ5 form a disulfide-linked complex to which $V_{\text{pre-B}}$ is non-covalently attached (Karasuyama et al. 1990; Tsubata and Reth 1990).

Both, $V_{\text{pre-B}}$ and λ5 genes are expressed at the earliest stages of Ig rearrangements (Sakaguchi and Melchers 1986; Rolink et al. 1991). Certain pre-B cell lines which have partially rearranged their Ig heavy chain genes, synthesize a truncated μ chain, the so-called D_μ protein from a D_HJ_H transcript (Reth and Alt 1985; Gu et al. 1991). Recent experiments have shown that the D_μ protein can also be expressed on the pre-B cell surface together with the "surrogate" light chain molecules λ5 and $V_{\text{pre-B}}$ (Tsubata et al. 1991; Rolink and Melchers 1991). At the transition from a pre-B cell to a surface Ig^+ B cell, both, λ5/$V_{\text{pre-B}}$ and conventional κ L-chains are expressed on the cell surface, indicating that the activation of the κ locus precedes the inactivation of λ5 gene expression (Cherayil and Pillai 1991). It is likely that the D_μ chain and later $V_HD_HJ_HC_\mu$ chains are anchored in the surface membrane by the IgM-α/Ig-β protein complex (see above). The various hypothetical steps of early B-cell differentiation are schematically depicted in Fig. 1.

Genes specifically expressed in pre-B cells have also been identified in humans: the human $V_{\text{pre-B}}$ homolog (Bauer et al. 1988) and the Ig λ light-chain-related gene *14.1* (Evans and Hollis 1991; Mattei et al. 1991; Hollis et al. 1989; Schiff et al. 1990), which is the human homolog of the mouse *λ5* gene. In human pre-B cell lines several polypeptides have been found associated with μ H chains. Kerr et al. (1989) and Hollis et al. (1989) detected a 22-kDa protein, a candidate for λ5 protein, that forms a disulfide-linked complex with μ H chain. Furthermore, 16–18-kDa proteins which are non-covalently associated with μ H chains were detected as candidates for

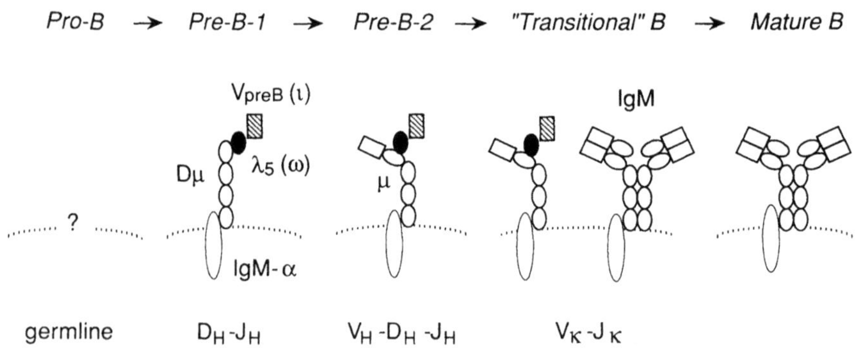

Fig. 1. Hypothetical scheme of early B-cell differentiation. Progenitor B cells (pro-B) differentiate into pre-B-1 cells by rearrangement of the H chain loci from germline to $D_H J_H$. In pre-B-1 cells λ5 and V_{pre-B} gene products associate at the cell surface with D_μ protein. A productively rearranged $V_H D_H J_H$ allele gives rise to μ H chains that can be deposited in the surface membrane of pre-B-2 cells together with the "surrogate" light chain molecules λ5 and V_{pre-B}. A productively rearranged κ L chain gene leads to expression of κ L chains on the surface of a cell that has a productively rearranged H chain allele. In "transitional" B cells μ-λ5/V_{pre-B} can occur together with Ig. In mature $sIgM^+$ B cells the *λ5* and V_{pre-B} genes are not expressed

V_{pre-B} (Kerr et al. 1989; Hollis et al. 1989). Recently, λ5-like and V_{pre-B} gene expression has been described as a lineage- and stage-restricted marker for B-cell precursor leukemias (Schiff et al. 1991; Bauer et al. 1991). The analysis of the malignant forms of precursor B cells showed that λ5-like and V_{pre-B} RNA expression appears at least as early as cytoplasmic CD22 and surface CD19. Rearrangement of V_κ or V_λ loci correlated with the disappearance of the pre-B gene products (Schiff et al. 1991). V_{pre-B} RNA was absent from malignancies of mature sIg^+ B cells (Bauer et al. 1991; Schiff et al. 1991).

B-Cell-Associated Differentiation Antigens

Eighteen different B-cell-associated antigens have been defined as CD antigens in International Workshops by clustering monoclonal antibodies: CD10, CD19–24, CD37–40, CD72–w78 (Dörken et al. 1989). During recent years the amino acid sequence of most of these antigens have been determined by isolating cDNA clones that encode the cell surface-expressed molecules.

CD19. The CD19 antigen is a member of the Ig supergene family (Stamenkovic and Seed 1988b; Tedder and Isaacs 1989). The extensive length of the intracellular region (242 amino acids) markedly contrasts with other surface structures, suggesting that the CD19 molecule might be involved in the generation of a transmembrane signal through its cytoplasmic tail. Recently, CD21 (CR2), the receptor for C3d and Epstein-Barr virus, has been found to be directly associated with CD19, suggesting that these molecules form a signal transduction complex (Matsumoto et al. 1991). The B-cell-specific antigen CD19 is the most broadly expressed surface marker for B cells, appearing at the earliest stages of B-cell differentiation, presumably prior to the heavy chain gene rearrangement. Surface expression of CD19 is a reliable marker for early B-cell malignancies (Nadler et al. 1984).

CD22. The CD22 molecule is also a member of the Ig supergene family (Stamenkovic and Seed 1990; Wilson et al. 1991). The structural homology of the CD22 antigen, which contains seven Ig-like domains in the extracellular portion, with the myelin-associated glycoprotein (MAG) and N-CAM suggested that CD22 is a cell adhesion molecule. Indeed, recent results indicate that the CD22 molecule is directly involved in the interaction between T and B cells. The T-cell ligand of CD22 is CD45RO, an isoform of the leukocyte common antigen class of phosphotyrosine phosphatases (Stamenkovic et al. 1991). The B-cell-specific CD22 antigen is expressed in the cytoplasm of virtually all B cells, including progenitor B cells, and is present on the cell surface mainly on mature stages of B-cell differentiation (Dörken et al. 1986). Virtually all B-lineage acute lymphoblastic leukemia cases express cytoplasmic CD22 (Dörken et al. 1987). Conflicting results regarding the expression of CD22 on the surface of acute lymphoblastic leukemia cells may be explained by differences in expression between different epitopes (Dörken et al. 1987) or by staining of cytoplasmic CD22 which may become accessible to antibodies in damaged surface CD22-negative cells.

CD72. The CD72 antigen, which has recently been found to be identical with human Lyb-2, is a member of a gene superfamily of lectin-like glycoproteins with inverted orientation including asialoglycoprotein receptors or hepatic lectins and CD23, the low-affinity Fc receptor for IgE (von Hoegen et al. 1990). Recent results indicate that the B-cell surface protein CD72 is the ligand for CD5 expressed on mature T cells, a small proportion of B lymphocytes, and B-cell chronic lymphocytic leukemia cells (van de Velde et al. 1991). The B-cell-associated CD72 antigen is a new pan-B marker which occurs, like CD19, at the earliest stages of B cell differentiation (Dörken et al. 1989). CD72 expression was found in progenitor B- and pre-B-cell leukemias and in normal, immature, TdT-positive, cytoplasmic μ heavy chain-negative B-lineage cells, and pre-B cells in fetal liver and bone marrow.

CD10. The CD10/CALLA antigen is identical to neutral endopeptidase, which cleaves peptides at the amino terminals of the hydrophobic residues and inactivates a variety of peptide hormones (Shipp et al. 1988). CD10 is expressed on early B-progenitor cells and is lost during pre-B-cell differentiation (Nadler et al. 1984; Ryan et al. 1986). While Nadler et al. (1984) proposed that CD19 expression precedes CD10 expression based on the identification of $CD10^-/CD19^+$ B precursor leukemias, multiparameter flow cytometric analyses of normal precursor B cells in fetal liver and bone marrow suggest that CD10 expression appears at least as early as CD19 (Ryan et al. 1986; Loken et al. 1987; Uckun 1990).

CD73. The CD73 antigen is the membrane-associated enzyme ecto-5′-nucleotidase (5′-NT), which catalyzes the dephosphorylation of purine and pyrimidine ribo- and deoxyribonucleoside monophosphates (Thompson et al. 1990). The CD73 molecule appears to be important for the maturation of B cells since 5′-NT activity was found to be markedly reduced in several immunodeficiency diseases, for example, combined variable immunodeficiency or congenital X-linked agammaglobulinemia. CD73 (5′-NT) expression is high in progenitor B- and pre-B-cell leukemias and low in malignancies of mature surface Ig^+ B cells (Pieters et al. 1991).

CD20. The CD20 antigen is a type III integral membrane protein with the carboxy and the amino termini located within the cell (Stamenkovic and Seed 1988a; Einfeld et al. 1988; Tedder et al. 1989). The membrane-embedded CD20 protein with multiple transmembrane domains has similarities to proteins that form transmembrane ion channels. The B-cell-specific CD20 antigen is expressed during pre-B-cell development, pre-

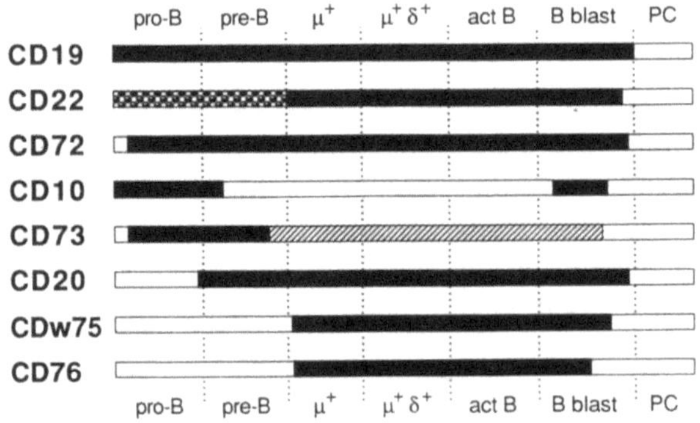

Fig. 2. Sequential expression of B-lineage-associated differentiation antigens during human B-cell ontogeny. Pro-B, pre-B, and B cells are defined by the configuration of their Ig genes and their cytoplasmic/surface Ig expression. Pro-B cells do not express cytoplasmic μ heavy chains or sIgM. Pre-B cells express cytoplasmic μ heavy chains but do not express sIgM. Immature B cells (μ^+) express sIgM but not sIgD. Mature B cells ($\mu^+\delta^+$) co-express sIgM and sIgD. Activated B cells and B blasts are defined by expression of activation antigens and morphology. Plasma cells (PC) express cytoplasmic μ heavy chains but do not express surface Ig

sumably just before the expression of cytoplasmic μ chains: about 50% of cytoplasmic μ chain-negative progenitor B-cell leukemias showing surface expression of the CD19 antigen and cytoplasmic expression of the CD22 antigen are CD20 positive (Nadler et al. 1984).

CDw75 and CD76. The CDw75 and CD76 antigens are expressed only on mature sIg-positive B cells. In contrast to other B-cell-associated CD antigens, both markers are not detectable in sIg-negative B-lineage acute lymphoblastic leukemias (Dörken et al. 1989).

A schematic representation of the sequential expression of B-lineage differentiation antigens is presented in Fig. 2.

References

Alt FW, Blackwell TK, DePinho RA, Reth MG, Yancopoulos GD (1986) Regulation of genome rearrangement events during lymphocyte differentiation. Immunol Rev 89:5–30

Bauer SR, Kudo A, Melchers F (1988) Structure and pre B lymphocyte-restricted expression of the VpreB gene in humans and conservation in other mammalian species. EMBO J 7:111–116

Bauer SR, Kubagawa H, MacLennan I, Melchers F (1991) VpreB gene expression in hematopoietic malignancies: a lineage- and stage-restricted marker for B-cell precursor leukemias. Blood 78:1581–1588

Blackwell TK, Alt FW (1989) Molecular characterization of the lymphoid V (D) J recombination activity. J Biol Chem 264:10327

Campana D, Janossy G, Bofill M, Trejdosievicz LK, Ma D, Hoffbrand AV, Mason DY, Lebacq AM, Forster HK (1985) Human B cell development: I. Phenotypic differences of B lymphocytes in the bone marrow and peripheral lymphoid tissue. J Immunol 134:1524–1530

Cherayil BJ, Pillai S (1991) The ω/λ5 surrogate immunoglobulin light chain is expressed on the surface of transitional B lymphocytes in murine bone marrow. J Exp Med 173:111–116

Cooper MD (1987) Current concepts, B lymphocytes normal development and function. N Engl J Med 317:1452

Desiderio SV, Yancopoulos GD, Paskind M, Thomas E, Boss MA, Landau H, Alt FW, Baltimore D (1984) Insertions of N regions into heavy chains genes is correlated with expression of terminal deoxycotransferase in B cells. Nature 311:752–755

Dörken B, Moldenhauer G, Pezzutto A, Schwartz R, Feller A, Kiesel S, Nadler LM (1986) HD39 (B3), a B lineage-restricted antigen whose cell surface expression is limited to resting and activated human B lymphocytes. J Immunol 136:4470–4479

Dörken B, Pezzutto A, Köhler M, Thiel E, Hunstein W (1987) Expression of cytoplasmic CD22 in B-cell ontogeny. In: McMichael AJ (ed) Leukocyte typing III. Oxford University Press, Oxford, pp 474–476

Dörken B, Möller P, Pezzutto A, Schwartz-Albiez RS, Moldenhauer G (1989) B cell antigens: section report, CD10, CD19–24, CD37–40, CD72–w78, CD45-like group, unclustered antibodies. In: Knapp W, Dörken B, Gilks WR, Rieber EP, Schmidt RE, Stein H, von dem Borne AEGK (eds) Leukocyte typing IV. Oxford University Press, Oxford

Einfeld DA, Brown JP, Valentine MA, Clark EA, Ledbetter JA (1988) Molecular cloning of the human B cell CD20 receptor predicts a hydrophobic protein with multiple transmembrane domains. EMBO J 7:711–718

Evans RJ, Hollis GF (1991) Genomic structure of the human Ig λ gene suggests that it may be expressed as an Ig λ 14.1-like protein or as a canonical B cell Ig λ light chain: implications for Ig λ gene evolution. J Exp Med 173:305–311

Gordon J, Hamblin TJ, Smith JL, Stevenson FK, Stevenson GT (1981) A human B lymphoma synthesizing and expressing surface μ chain in the absence of detectable light chain. Blood 58:552–556

Greaves MF (1986) Differentiation-linked leukemogenesis in lymphocytes. Science 234:697–704

Gu H, Kitamura D, Rajewsky K (1991) B cell development regulated by gene rearrangement: arrest of maturation by membrane-bound Dμ protein and selection of Dμ element reading frames. Cell 65:47–54

Hendershot L, Levitt D (1984) Analysis of surface of μ chain expression in human lymphoblastoid lines that do not produce light chains. J Immunol 132:502–509

Hermanson GG, Eisenberg D, Kincade PW, Wall R (1988) B29: a member of the immunoglobulin gene superfamily exclusively expressed on B lineage cells. Proc Natl Acad Sci USA 85:6890–6894

Hollis GF, Evans RJ, Stafford-Hollis JM, Korsmeyer SJ, McKearn JP (1989) Immunoglobulin λ light-chain-related genes 14.1 and 16.1 are expressed in pre-B cells and may encode the human immunoglobulin ω light-chain protein. Proc Natl Acad Sci USA 86:5552–5556

Hombach J, Tsubata F, Leclercq L, Strappert H, Reth M (1990a) Molecular components of the B cell antigen receptor complex of the IgM class. Nature 343:760–762

Hombach J, Lottspeich F, Reth M (1990b) Identification of the genes encoding the IgM-α and Ig-β components of the IgM antigen receptor complex by amino terminal sequencing. Eur J Immunol 20:2795–2799

Janossy G, Bollum FJ, Bradstock KF, McMichael A, Rapson N, Greaves MF (1979) Terminal transferase-positive human bone marrow cells exhibit the antigenic phenotype of common acute lymphoblastic leukemia. J Immunol 123:1525–1529

Karasuyama H, Kudo A, Melchers F (1990) The proteins encoded by the VpreB and λ5 pre-B cell-specific genes can associate with each other and with μ heavy chains. J Exp Med 172:969–972

Kashiwamura SI, Koyama T, Matsuo T, Steinmetz M, Sakaguchi N (1990) Structure of the murine mb-1 gene encoding a putative surface IgM-associated molecule. J Immunol 145:337–343

Kerr WG, Cooper MD, Feng L, Burrows PD, Hendershot LM (1989) Mu heavy chains can associate with a pseudo-light chain complex (ΨL) in human pre-B cell lines. Int Immunol 4:355–361

Kishimoto T (1987) B-cell stimulatory factors (BSFs) Molecular structure, biological function, and regulation of expression. J Clin Immunol 7:343–348

Kudo A, Melchers F (1987) A second gene, VpreB in the λ5 locus of the mouse, which appears to be selectively expressed in pre-B lymphocytes. EMBO J 6:2267–2272

Loken MD, Shah VO, Dattilio KL, Civin CI (1987) Flow cytometric analysis of human bone marrow: II. Normal B lymphocyte development. Blood 70:1316–1324

Mason DY, Cordell JL, Tse AGD, van Dongen JJM, van Noesel CJM, Micklem K, Pulford KAF, Valenssi F, Comans-Bitter WM, Borst J, Gatter KC (1991) The IgM-associated protein mb-1 as a marker of normal and neoplastic B cells. J Immunol 147:2474–2482

Matsumoto AK, Kopicky-Burd J, Carter RH, Tuveson DA, Tedder TF, Fearon DT (1991) Intersection of the complement and immune systems: a signal transduction complex of the B lymphocyte-containing complement receptor type 2 and CD19. J Exp Med 173:55–64

Matsuo T, Kimoto M, Sakaguchi N (1991) Direct identification of the putative surface IgM receptor-associated molecule encoded by murine B cell-specific mb-1 gene. J Immunol 146:1584–1590

Mattei MG, Fumoux F, Roeckel N, Fougereau M, Schiff C (1991) The human pre-B-specific lambda-like cluster is located in the 22q11.2-22q12.3 region, distal to the Ig C_λ locus. Genomics 9:544–546

Nadler LM, Korsmeyer SJ, Anderson KC, Boyd AW, Slaughenhoupt B, Park E, Jensen J, Coral F, Mayer RJ, Sallan SE, Ritz J, Schlossman SF (1984) B cell origin of non-T cell acute lymphoblastic leukemia. A model for discrete stages of neoplastic and normal pre-B cell differentiation. J Clin Invest 74:332–240

Nomura J, Matsuo T, Kubota E, Kimoto M, Sakaguchi N (1991) Signal transmission through the B cell specific MB-1 molecule at the pre-B cell stage. Int Immunol 3:117–126

Paige CJ, Kincade PW, Ralph P (1981) Independent control of immunoglobulin heavy and light chain expression in a murine pre-B cell line. Nature 292:631–633

Pieters R, Thompson LF, Broekema GJ, Huismans DR, Peters GJ, Pals ST, Horst E, Hählen K, Veerman AJP (1991) Expression of 5′-Nucleotidase (CD73) related to other differentiation antigens in leukemias of B-cell lineage. Blood 78:488–492

Pillai S, Baltimore D (1987) Formation of disulfide-linked μ2ω2 tetramers in pre-B cells by the 18K ω-immunoglobulin light chain. Nature 329:172–174

Pillai S, Baltimore D (1988) The omega and iota surrogate immunoglobulin light chains. Curr Top Microbiol Immunol 137:136–139

Reth M, Alt FW (1984) Novel immunoglobulin heavy chains are produced from DJH gene segment rearrangements in lymphoid cells. Nature 312:418–423

Rolink A, Melchers F (1991) Molecular and cellular origins of B lymphocyte diversity. Cell 66:1081–1094

Rolink A, Kudo A, Karasuyama H, Kikuchi Y, Melchers F (1991) Long-term proliferating early pre-B cell lines and clones with the potential to develop to surface Ig-positive, mitogen-reactive B cells in vitro and in vivo. EMBO J 10:327–336

Ryan D, Kossover S, Mitchell S, Frantz C, Hennessy L, Cohen H (1986) Subpopulation of common acute lymphoblastic leukemia antigen-positive lymphoid cells in normal bone marrow identified by hematopoietic differentiation antigens. Blood 68:417–425

Sakaguchi N, Melchers F (1986) λ5, a new light-chain related locus selectively expressed in pre-B lymphocytes. Nature 324:579–582

Sakaguchi N, Kashiwamura SI, Kimoto M, Thalmann P, Melchers F (1988) B lymphocyte-restricted expression of mb-1, a gene with CD33-like structural properties. EMBO J 7:3457–3464

Schiff C, Bensmana M, Guglielmi P, Millili M, Lefranc MP, Fougereau M (1990) The immunoglobulin λ-like gene cluster (14.1, 16.1 and Fλ1) contains gene(s) selectively expressed in pre-B cells and is the human counterpart of the mouse λ5 gene. Int Immunol 2:201–208

Schiff C, Milili M, Bossy D, Tabilio A, Falzetti F, Gabert J, Mannono P, Fougereau M (1991) Lambda-like and V preB genes expression: an early B-lineage marker of human leukemias. Blood 78:1516–1525

Shipp MA, Richardson NE, Sayre PH, Brown NR, Masteller EL, Clayton LK, Ritz J, Reinherz EL (1988) Molecular cloning of the common acute lymphoblastic leukemia antigen (CALLA) identifies a type II integral membrane protein. Proc Natl Acad Sci USA: 85:4819–4823

Stamenkovic I, Seed B (1988a) Analysis of two cDNA clones encoding the B lymphocyte antigen CD20 (B1, Bp35), a type III integral membrane protein. J Exp Med 167:1975–1981
Stamenkovic I, Seed B (1988b) CD19, the earliest differentiation antigen of the B cell lineage, bears three extracellular immunoglobulin-like domains and an Epstein-Barr virus-related cytoplasmic tail. J Exp Med 168:1205–1210
Stamenkovic I, Seed B (1990) The B-cell antigen CD22 mediates monocyte and erythrocyte adhesion. Nature 345:74–77
Stamenkovic I, Sgroi D, Aruffo A, Sy MS, Anderson T (1991) The B lymphocyte adhesion molecule CD22 interacts with leukocyte common antigen CD45RO on T cells and a 2-6 sialytransferase, CD75, on B cells. Cell 66:1133–1144
Tedder TF, Isaacs CM (1989) Isolation of cDNAs encoding the CD19 antigen for human and mouse B lymphocytes. A new member of the immunolgobulin superfamily. J Immunol 143:712–717
Tedder TF, Klejman G, Schlossman SF, Saito H (1989) Structure of the gene encoding the human B lymphocyte differentiation antigen CD20 (B1). J Immunol 142:2560–3568
Thompson LF, Ruedi JM, Glass A, Moldenhauer G, Moller P, Low MG, Klemens MR, Massaia M, Lucas AH (1990) Production and characterization of monoclonal antibodies to the glycosyl phosphatidylinositol-anchored lymphocyte differentiation antigen ecto-5′-nucleotidase (CD73). Tissue Antigens 35:9–19
Tonegawa S (1983) Somatic generation of antibody diversity. Nature 320:575–581
Tsubata T, Reth M (1990) The products of pre-B cell-specific genes (λ5 and VpreB) and the immunoglobulin μ chain form a complex that is transported onto the cell surface. J Exp Med 172:973–976
Tsubata T, Tsubata R, Reth M (1991) Cell surface expression of the short immunoglobulin μ chain (Dυ protein) in murine pre-B cells is differently regulated from that of the intact υ chain. Eur J Immunol (in press)
Uckun FM (1990) Regulation of human B-cell ontogeny. Blood 76:1908–1923
van de Velde H, von Hoegen I, Luo W, Parnes JR, Thielemans K (1991) The B-cell surface protein CD72/Lyb-2 is the ligand for CD5. Nature 351:662–665
van Noessel CJM, van Borst J, de Vries EFR, van Lier RAW (1990) Identification of two distinct phosphoproteins as components of the human B cell antigen receptor complex. Eur J Immunol 20:2789–2793
Vogler LB, Crist WM, Bockman DE, Pearl ER, Lawton AR, Cooper MD (1978) Pre-B leukemia: a new phenotype of childhood lymphoblast leukemia. N Engl J Med 298:872–878
von Hoegen I, Nakayama E, Parnes JR (1990) Identification of a human protein homologous to the mouse Lyb-2 B cell differentiation antigen and sequence of the corresponding cDNA. J Immunol 144:4870–4877
Wilson GL, Fox CH, Fauci AS, Kehrl JH (1991) cDNA cloning of the B cell membrane protein CD22: A mediator of B-B cell interactions. J Exp Med 173:137–146
Yamanishi Y, Kakiuchi T, Mizugichi J, Yamamoto T, Tyoshima K (1991) Association of B cell antigen receptor with protein tyrosine kinase lyn. Science 251:192–194

Normal and Aberrant T-Cell Receptor Protein Expression in T-Cell Acute Lymphoblastic Leukemia

D. Campana[1], E. Coustan-Smith[1], F.G. Behm[2], and R. Goorha[3]

[1] Division of Bone Marrow Transplantation, Department of Hematology-Oncology, St. Jude Children's Research Hospital, Memphis, TN 38101, USA
[2] Department of Pathology and Laboratory Medicine, St. Jude Children's Research Hospital, Memphis, TN 38101, USA
[3] Department of Virology, St. Jude Children's Research Hospital, Memphis, TN 38101, USA

Introduction

Mature human T lymphocytes recognize self and non-self through two distinct types of T-cell antigen receptors (TCR), TCRαβ and TCRγδ, that are expressed on the cell surface membrane in association with CD3 molecules (reviewed by Davis and Bjorkman 1988; Brenner et al. 1988). Inappropriate pairing of TCR chains, e.g. βδ, or surface expression of single chains apparently does not occur in normal T cells, although such phenomena have been described as rare events in leukemic cell lines (Hochstenbach and Brenner 1989).

During normal T-cell differentiation in the thymus the synthesis and assembly of the CD3/TCR complex occurs gradually. The most immature thymic cells do not have detectable TCR chains but accumulate CD3ε, CD3δ, and possibly CD3γ in the cytoplasm (Furley et al. 1986; Campana et al. 1987, 1989). These CD3 molecules constitute a core onto which TCR proteins are added after the corresponding genes undergo productive rearrangements (Clevers et al. 1988; Klausner et al. 1990).

Most of the understanding of the initial developmental stages of TCR expression derives from studies in rodents, which have shown that TCRγ and TCRδ genes rearrange and are expressed early during embryonic life (Snodgrass et al. 1985; Raulet et al. 1985; Pardoll et al. 1987; reviewed by Strominger 1989). Studies at the protein level in human tissues have failed to convincingly demonstrate an identical sequence of events: TCRαβ-bearing cells usually constitute the majority of TCR-expressing cells, even in fetal tissues collected during early stages of gestation (Campana et al. 1989; Haynes et al. 1989).

Reagents and Methods for Detecting Human TCR Proteins

Several monoclonal antibodies (MAbs) to human TCR proteins have been raised. Technical issues regarding the use of some of these MAbs are as follows. First, MAb WT31 reacts with an epitope of the CD3ε chain (Transy et al. 1989) which is preferentially accessible when the assembled CD3/TCRαβ complex is inserted into the cell membrane (Spits et al. 1985). From a practical point of view this reagent can be used to recognize TCRαβ cells, although it will also weakly react with TCRγδ-bearing cells (Van de Griend et al. 1988). WT31 is not suitable for cytospin staining. Secondly, the epitopes to which βF1 (anti-TCRβ; Brenner et al. 1987), αF1 (anti-TCRα; Henry et al. 1989), and CγM1 (a MAb recognizing TCRγ chains developed by Dr. M.B. Brenner, Boston, MA, USA) bind are not accessible on the surface of intact cells and these MAbs must be used after treating cells with fixatives. The expression of these molecules and of cytoplasmic CD3 can be investigated by staining either permeabilized cells in suspension for flow cytometric analysis, or fixed cytocentrifuge preparations. For the former type of immunolabeling, which has the advantage of allowing a quantitative assessment of the antigen expression, we prefer the method described by Schmid et al. (1991). In this technique, cells are fixed with paraformaldehyde and permeabilized with Tween 20. The treatment is relatively gentle and the light-scattering properties of the cells are not completely destroyed, allowing their morphological recognition. When cytocentrifuge preparations are used the optimal fixative is acetone for 10 min at 20°C. MAbs αF1 and βF1 will also stain well cytospins fixed in acetone: methanol 1:1 at 4°C, whereas CγM1 and TCRδ1 will not work in these conditions. MAb αF1 may react with a nuclear molecule expressed in leukemic blasts and activated T cells. Therefore careful observation of the individual cells is needed: only strong *cytoplasmic* staining in the perinuclear area indicates TCRα expression. For this reason, we do not recommend flow cytometric analysis of αF1 reactivity.

TCR Protein Expression in Human Immature T Cells

T-Cell Development in the Thymus

Human thymocytes express TCR proteins heterogeneously. When unpermeabilized suspensions of infant thymocytes are labeled with MAbs to the CD3ε chain (e.g., UCHT1 or Leu4), three cell subpopulations can be distinguished: $CD3^-$, $CD3^{+/-}$ and $CD3^+$ (Lanier et al. 1986; Fig. 1). Most $CD3^-$ thymocytes, however, express cytoplasmic CD3 molecules (Link et al. 1985; Furley et al. 1986; Campana et al. 1987, 1989; Van Dongen et al. 1987, 1988). By applying a CD3 MAb (UCHT1; gift of Dr. P.C.L.

Beverley, London, UK) to thymocyte suspensions after cell membrane permeabilization we observed that all thymocytes were brightly labeled when analyzed by flow cytometry, suggesting that there is no change in the cytoplasmic amount of CD3ε during thymic differentiation (Fig. 1). Identical semiquantitative methods revealed that the amount of TCRβ chains, detected by βF1 MAb, considerably increases with cell maturation (Fig. 1). By fluorescence microscopy observation, immature, large TdT^+ thymic blasts appear to be mostly TCRβ negative. The next stage of differentiation is probably represented by $\beta F1^+$ thymocytes that are not labeled by αF1 (Campana et al. 1989). Following the synthesis of TCRα chains CD3/TCRαβ complexes are inserted into the cell membrane and thymocytes are subjected to the processes of positive and negative selection.

TCRγδ-bearing cells usually represent <1% of fetal and infant thymocytes (Borst et al. 1988; Campana et al. 1989; Groh et al. 1989). Studies in which the surface and cytoplasmic expression of TCRγ and TCRδ chains were compared have not identified cells with exclusively cytoplasmic expression of TCRδ chains (Campana et al. 1989). Moreover, cells with exclusively cytoplasmic TCRγ chains were undetectable or extremely rare (<0.1%) in the infant thymic samples examined (D. Campana, unpublished observations).

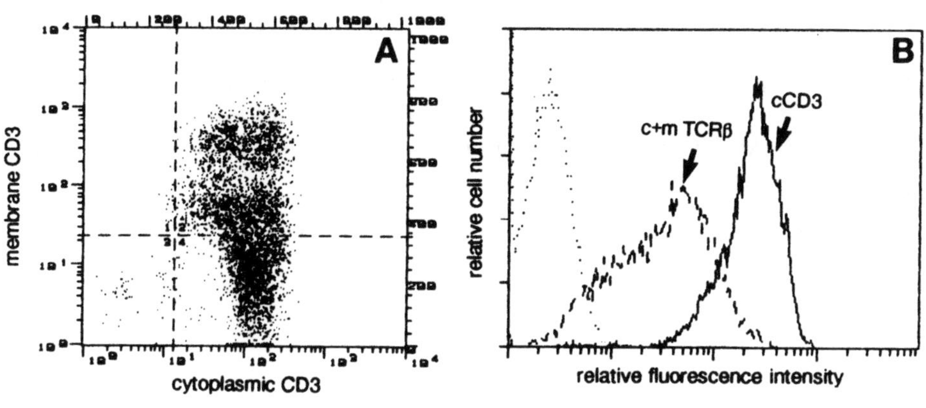

Fig. 1A,B. Membrane and cytoplasmic CD3 and TCRβ expression in infant thymus. **A** Thymocytes were first labeled with UCHT1 (CD3) followed by a goat antiserum to mouse immunoglobilin conjugated to phycocerythrin (Jackson Immunoresearch Labs Inc, West Grove, PA, USA). After adding mouse serum to saturate free combining sites, cells were fixed and permeabilized as described by Schmid et al. (1991). Cytoplasmic CD3 was visualized with Leu4 conjugated to fluorescein isothiocyanate and cells were analyzed with a FACScan (both from Becton Dickinson, San Jose, CA, USA). Membrane $CD3^-$ thymocytes are cytoplasmic $CD3^+$. **B** The intensity of labeling of the same thymocytes with βF1 is illustrated and compared to that of cytoplasmic CD3

Stages of TCR Differentiation in T-Cell Acute Lymphoblastic Leukemia

TCRαβ

Discrete stages of differentiation identical to those observed in the thymus can be defined in T-cell acute lymphoblastic leukemia (T-ALL). In 40 of 68 T-ALL cases studied (58.8%), blasts lacked membrane CD3/TCR expression ($mCD3^-$; Campana et al. 1991; Coustan-Smith et al. manuscript in preparation; Table 1). In 20 of these $mCD3^-$ cases TCRαβ proteins were expressed in the cells' cytoplasm: in 17 samples leukemic blasts were $\beta F1^+$ only, in one case they were $\alpha F1^+$ only, and in two cases blasts expressed both cytoplasmic TCRα and TCRβ chains (Campana et al. 1991; Coustan-Smith et al. manuscript in preparation; Table 1). In the other 20 $mCD3^-$ T-ALLs, blasts did not show membrane or cytoplasmic reactivity with βF1 and αF1 MAbs (Campana et al. 1991; Coustan-Smith et al. manuscript in preparation; Table 1). In only a minority of these latter cases could the lack of TCR protein expression be attributed to the germline configuration of the corresponding genes (Campana et al. 1991). However, when five $\beta F1^+$, $\alpha F1^-$ T-ALL cases were investigated at the DNA level, TCRα genes appeared not to be rearranged, and in four of these five cases cytogenetics studies revealed translocations involving the q11 region of the chromosome 14 (Secker-Walker et al. 1991), where the TCRα locus has been mapped. It is likely that in these cases the lack of TCRα gene rearrangement is the most important limiting factor in the expression of a full TCRαβ receptor.

In the remaining 28 T-ALLs studied (41.2%), blasts expressed membrane CD3/TCR chains: in 23 cases, CD3 molecules were associated with the αβ form of the TCR, as demonstrated by the reactivity with WT31 and/or BMA031 MAbs (Campana et al. 1991; Coustan-Smith et al. manuscript in preparation; Table 1).

Table 1. TCR protein expression in T-ALL: proportion of subtypes

TCR status	Cases (*n*)	(%)
$mCD3^-$		
$\beta F1^-$, $\alpha F1^-$	20	29.4
$\beta F1^+$, $\alpha F1^-$	17	25.0
$\beta F1^-$, $\alpha F1^+$	1	1.5
$\beta F1^+$, $\alpha F1^+$	2	3.0
$mCD3^+$		
$WT31^+$	23	33.8
$TCR\delta 1^+$	5	7.3
Total	68	100

See also Campana et al. (1991) and Coustan-Smith et al. (manuscript in preparation).

In all 68 cases studied, leukemic cells were generally strongly CD7$^+$, with the exception of three mCD3$^+$/TCRαβ$^+$ cases in which blasts expressed CD7 weakly and heterogeneously (Campana et al. 1991; Coustan-Smith et al. manuscript in preparation). Terminal deoxynucleotidyl transferase (TdT) positivity was seen in 63 of 68 cases studied; the TdT$^-$ cases were mCD3$^-$, βF1$^-$, αF1$^-$ (2 cases), mCD3$^+$, WT31$^+$, βF1$^+$, αF1$^+$ (2 cases), and mCD3$^+$/TCRαβ$^-$ (1 case). No clear correlation between stages of TCR differentiation and expression of other surface markers could be found (Campana et al. 1991; Coustan-Smith et al. manuscript in preparation; Table 2).

TCRγδ

The expression of surface TCRγδ proteins was studied with TCRδ1 and δTCS1 MAbs. Five of the 68 cases analyzed had leukemic blasts labeled with both TCRδ1 and δTCS1 MAbs (Campana et al. 1991; Coustan-Smith et al. 1992; Table 1): the reactivity of the latter MAb indicates the usage of the $V_{\delta 1}$-$J_{\delta 1}$ gene regions (Wu et al. 1988; Borst et al. 1989). In these five TCRδ$^+$ cases blasts were also mCD3$^+$ but did not clearly react with WT31. When cytocentrifuge preparations of these samples were labeled with αF1, βF1, and CγM1 MAbs the following observations were made. In all five cases, blasts were positive with CγM1, indicating synthesis of TCRγ chains, and were negative after staining with αF1 MAb (Coustan-Smith et al. manuscript in preparation). Unexpectedly, in one of the five cases blasts were also labeled by βF1 MAb (Coustan-Smith et al. manuscript in preparation). Thus, in this latter case three TCR genes were simultaneously expressed, resembling the observations reported in some leukemic cells lines (Koning et al. 1987; J. Minowada, personal communication). Whether the TCR complex present on these cells' membrane is exclusively formed by TCRγ and TCRδ chains or whether TCRβ chains are included remains to be elucidated.

It has been suggested that mTCRγδ is more frequently seen than mTCRαβ in T-ALL, whereas TCRαβ would be more frequent in T-lymphoblastic lymphoma (Gouttefangeas et al. 1990). In our studies (Campana et al. 1991; Coustan-Smith et al. manuscript in preparation) and in other series (Van Dongen et al. 1991) such a TCRγδ predominance in mCD3$^+$ T-ALL was not found. From these data it appears that blasts expressing mTCRγδ are expected to be found in approximately one fifth of mCD3$^+$ T-ALL cases. Considering that TCRγδ-bearing cells normally represent <1% of fetal and infant thymocytes, the relatively high proportion of TCRγδ T-ALLs may reflect a higher susceptibility to leukemogenesis of the TCRγδ lineage.

We also tested the possibility of an exclusively cytoplasmic expression of TCRγδ chains in cases with no membrane TCRγδ expression. As a control, the five TCRγδ$^+$ cases were labeled by TCRδ1 on cytocentrifuge prep-

Table 2. TCR protein expression in T-ALL: Phenotypic features of subtypes

TCR status	1[b]	2	4	5	6	8	10	21	13	33	Class II	TdT
$mCD3^-$												
$\beta F1^-$, $\alpha F1^-$	9/19[c]	11/20	7/20	16/19	5/16	6/20	7/19	8/19	1/7	0/7	0/9	18/20
$\beta F1^+$, $\alpha F1^-$	11/17	16/17	13/17	16/17	8/9	14/17	9/17	15/17	0/12	1/12	1/12	17/17
$\beta F1^-$, $\alpha F1^+$	1/1	1/1	1/1	1/1	1/1	1/1	0/1	1/1	–	–	–	1/1
$\beta F1^+$, $\alpha F1^+$	2/2	1/2	1/2	2/2	1/1	1/2	0/2	0/1	0/1	0/2	0/2	2/2
$mCD3^+$												
$WT31^+$	15/23	23/23	14/23	23/23	5/6	17/23	6/23	6/22	0/20	0/20	0/21	21/23
$TCR\delta 1^+$	3/5	3/5	2/5	4/5	0/2	2/5	2/5	3/5	0/5	0/4	1/5	4/5

See also Campana et al. (1991) and Coustan-Smith et al. (1992).
[a] All cases studied were $CD7^+$ as well as cytoplasmic and/or membrane $CD3^+$.
[b] CD numbers.
[c] No. of cases with >20% positive cells/no. of cases studied.

arations and blast were brightly stained. By contrast, TCRδ1 invariably failed to react with leukemic blasts from 40 $mCD3^-$ T-ALLs in cytocentrifuge preparation (Campana et al. 1991; Coustan-Smith et al. manuscript in preparation). However, in two of nine $mCD3^-$ cases studied, TdT^+ blasts reacting with CγM1 were seen, suggesting the possibility of cytoplasmic TCRγ chain expression in the absence of TCRδ chains (Coustan-Smith et al. manuscript in preparation; Table 3). Unexpectedly, one of these cases also expressed cytoplasmic TCRβ chains (Coustan-Smith et al. manuscript in preparation; Table 3). Within the $mCD3^+$ leukemias, none of the 23 $TCR\alpha\beta^+$ cases tested expressed cytoplasmic TCRδ chains. The results obtained with CγM1 were again surprising because two of the seven $TCR\alpha\beta^+$ T-ALLs also reacted with CγM1 MAb (Coustan-Smith et al. manuscript in preparation; Table 3).

These observations revealed the occurrence of a promiscuous TCR protein expression in T-ALL which is not seen during normal T-cell development. The occurrence of such deviation from a normal developmental program is also illustrated by the finding that one of the five TCRγδ cases examined had blasts with cytoplasmic TCRβ chains (see above).

Rate of TCR Gene Expression in T-ALL

TCRβ and -γ genes are rearranged in the majority of T-ALLs; in most cases TCRδ genes are either rearranged or, due to the rearrangement of TCRα genes, deleted (reviewed by Van Dongen and Wolvers-Tettero 1991). From our studies a direct estimate of the efficiency of TCR gene expression can be made. The comparative analysis between gene rearrangements and protein expression demonstrates that rearrangements of the TCRα and TCRβ genes have the highest likelihood of resulting in protein expression: 7/8 (87.5%) cases investigated with TCRα rearrangements, indicated by deletions of the

Table 3. Reactivity of CγM1 and TCRα1 with cytospins of T-ALL blasts

TCR status	CγM1	TCRδ1
$mCD3^-$		
$\beta F1^-$, $\alpha F1^-$	1/3[a]	0/20
$\beta F1^+$, $\alpha F1^-$	1/6	0/17
$\beta F1^-$, $\alpha F1^+$	–	0/1
$\beta F1^+$, $\alpha F1^+$	–	0/2
$mCD3^+$		
$WT31^+$	2/7	0/21
$TCR\delta 1^+$	3/3	5/5

See also Coustan-Smith et al. manuscript in preparation.
[a] No. of cases in which TdT^+ blasts labeled by the MAb were seen (range 5%–99%)/no. of cases studied.

TCRδ loci, and 35/48 (72.9%) cases with TCRβ gene rearrangements had leukemic blasts expressing TCRα and TCRβ proteins, respectively (Campana et al. 1991; Coustan-Smith et al. manuscript in preparation; Table 4). By contrast, only 7/19 (36.8%) cases with TCRγ rearrangements and 2/16 (12.5%) cases with TCRδ rearrangements had cells synthesizing the corresponding protein (Campana et al. 1991; Coustan-Smith et al. manuscript in preparation; Table 4). The lower rate of TCRγ and TCRδ expression may be due to a higher incidence of incomplete or out-of-frame rearrangement in these genes and/or to hypothetical control mechanisms for TCR gene expression. The absence of TCRδ chains exclusively expressed in the cytoplasm may also be due to a rapid degradation of these molecules when they are not coupled to the TCRγ chains. It is pertinent that the lack of cytoplasmic TCRδ chains has also been reported in studies on murine (Farr et al. 1990), avian (Bucy et al. 1990), and human thymocytes (Campana et al. 1989).

Conclusions

Over 10 years ago the observation that approximately 25% of B-lineage ALL cases, namely pre-B-ALL, had blasts expressing incomplete antigen recognition structures (μ heavy chains) in the cytoplasm was reported (Vogler et al. 1978). The equivalent developmental stages in T-ALL have now been described (Campana et al. 1991a,b). These appear to be more complex than in the B lineage and cases with a variety of cytoplasmic TCR chains can be found (Fig. 2). TCR receptor protein expression in T-ALL either recapitulates patterns seen during normal development or appears in aberrant combinations. Whether these aberrant patterns reflect the derivation of the neoplastic process from extremely rare cells with such phenotypes or are the consequence of the leukemic process is unknown. The high recombinase activity of immature leukemic cells may justify the second

Table 4. Frequency of TCR gene expression in T-ALL

Gene	No. of cases with rearrangement[a]	No. of cases with protein	%
TCRα[b]	8	7	87.5
TCRβ	48	35	72.9
TCRγ	19	7	36.8
TCRδ	16	2	12.5

See also Campana et al. (1991) and Coustan-Smith et al. (1992).
[a] Cases with at least one allele rearranged.
[b] TCRα gene rearrangement indicated by the deletion of TCRδ genes.

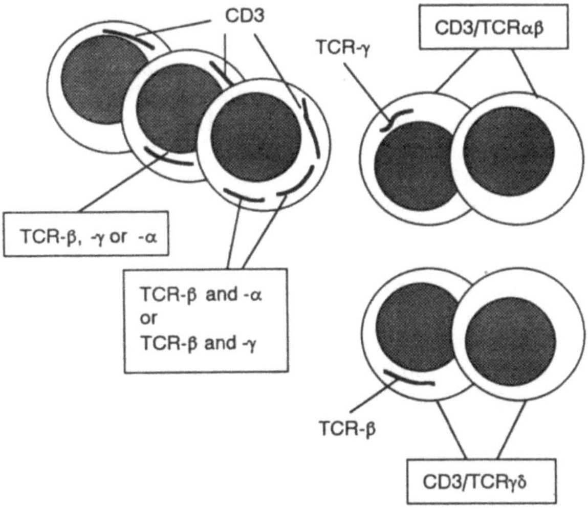

Fig. 2. TCR proteins are heterogeneously expressed in T-ALL. The figure illustrates the different patterns of TCR expression that have been observed (see text and Campana et al. 1991; Coustan-Smith et al. 1992)

possibility, by generating new rearrangements in the TCR loci during the course of the disease.

T-ALL has been previously classified by comparing phenotypic features of leukemic blasts with those seen in the normal thymus (Reinherz et al. 1980; Foon and Todd 1986; First MIC Cooperative Group 1986). The formulation of several stages of development in T-ALL has resulted from such a comparison. The expression of some membrane molecules has been associated with a different clinical outcome. For example, lack of CD2 expression has been interpreted to indicate poor prognosis (Thiel et al. 1989). In other studies, membrane CD3 (Pui et al. 1990) or CD10 (Rivera et al. 1991) has been taken as an indicator of poorer outcome. The investigation of TCR protein expression may provide a more accurate indication of the maturation status of leukemic blasts. It is not yet known whether this information may help to identify patients with different clinical outcomes; studies addressing this question are in progress.

Acknowledgement. This work was supported by the Cancer Center Research Grant No. P30-CA21765 from the National Cancer Institute and by the American Lebanese Syrian Associated Charities (ALSAC).

References

Borst J, Van Dongen JJM, Bolhuis RLH, Peters PJ, Haffler DA, De Vries E, Van de Griend RJ (1988) Distinct molecular forms of human T cell receptor γ/δ detected on viable T cells by a monoclonal antibody. J Exp Med 167:1625

Borst J, Wicherink A, Van Dongen JJM, De Vries E, Comans-Bitter WM, Wassenaar F, Van der Elsen P (1989) Non-random expression of T cell receptor γ and δ variable gene segments in functional T lymphocyte clones from human peripheral blood. Eur J Immunol 19:1559

Brenner MB, McLean J, Scheft H, Warnke RA, Jones N, Strominger JL (1987) Characterization and expression of the human αβ T cell receptor by using a framework monoclonal antibody. J Immunol 138:1502

Brenner MB, Strominger JL, Krangel MS (1988) The γδ T cell receptor. Adv Immunol 43:133

Bucy RP, Chen CLH, Cooper MD (1990) Ontogeny of T cell receptors in the chicken thymus. J Immunol 144:1161

Campana D, Thompson JS, Amlot P, Brown S, Janossy G (1987) The cytoplasmic expression of CD3 antigens in normal and malignant cells of the T lymphoid lineage. J Immunol 138:648

Campana D, Janossy G, Coustan-Smith E, Amlot PL, Tian WT, Ip S, Wong L (1989) The expression of T cell receptor-associated proteins during T cell ontogeny in man. J Immunol 142:57

Campana D, Van Dongen JJM, Mehta A, Coustan-Smith E, Wolvers-Tettero ILM, Ganeshaguru G, Janossy G (1991a) Stages of T-cell receptor protein expression in T-cell acute lymphoblastic leukemia. Blood 77:1546

Coustan-Smith E, Behm FG, Goorha R, Campana D (Manuscript in preparation) Promiscuous T cell receptor protein expression in normal and malignant human T cells.

Clevers H, Alarcon B, Wileman T, Terhorst C (1988) The T cell receptor/CD3 complex: a dynamic protein ensemble. Ann Rev Immunol 6:629

Davis MM, Bjorkman PJ (1988) T cell antigen receptor genes and T cell recognition. Nature 334:395

Farr A, Hosier S, Nelson A, Itohara S, Tonegawa S (1990) Distribution of thymocytes expressing γδ receptors in the murine thymus during development. J Immunol 144:492

First MIC Cooperative Study Group (1986) Morphologic, immunologic, and cytogenetic working classification of acute lymphoblastic leukemias. Cancer Genet Cytogenet 23:189

Foon KA, Todd RF III (1986) Immunological classification of leukemia and lymphoma. Blood 68:1

Furley AJ, Mizutani S, Weilbaecher K, Dhalival HS, Ford AM, Chan LC, Molgaard HV, Toyonaga B, Mak T, Van der Elsen P, Gold D, Terhorst C, Greaves MG (1986) Developmentally regulated rearrangement and expression of genes encoding the T cell receptor-T3 complex. Cell 46:75

Gouttefangeas C, Bensussan A, Boumsell L (1990) Study of the CD3-associated T-cell receptors reveals further differences between T-cell acute lymphoblastic lymphoma and leukemia. Blood 75:931

Groh V, Porcelli S, Fabbi M, Lanier LL, Picker LJ, Anderson T, Warnke RA, Bhan AK, Strominger JL, Brenner MB (1989) Human lymphocytes bearing T cell receptor γ/δ are phenotypically diverse and evenly distributed throughout the lymphoid system. J Exp Med 169:1277

Haynes BF, Denning SM, Singer KH, Kurtzberg J (1989) Ontogeny of T-cell precursors: a model for the initial stages of human T cell development. Immunol Today 10:87

Henry L, Tian WT, Rittershaus C, Ko JL, Marsh HC, Ip SH (1989) Two distinct immunogenic epitopes on the α chain of human T cell antigen receptor. Hybridoma 8:577

Hochstenbach F, Brenner MB (1989) T-cell receptor δ-chain can substitute for α to form a βδ heterodimer. Nature 340:562

Klausner RD, Lippincott-Schwartz J, Bonifacino JS (1990) The T cell antigen receptor: insights into organelle biology. Ann Rev Cell Biol 6:403
Koning F, Maloy WL, Cohen D, Coligan JE (1987) Independent association of T cell receptor β and Vγ chains with CD3 in the same cell. J Exp Med 166:595
Lanier LL, Allison JP, Phillips JH (1986) Correlation of cell surface antigen expression on human thymocytes by multi-color flow cytometric analysis: implications for differentiation. J Immunol 137:2501
Link MP, Stewart SJ, Warnke RA, Levy R (1985) Discordance between surface and cytoplasmic expression of the Leu4 (T3) antigen in thymocytes and in blast cells from childhood T lymphoblastic malignancies. J Clin Invest 76:248
Pardoll DM, Fowlkes BJ, Blueston JA, Krisbeek A, Maloy WL, Coligan JE, Schwartz RH (1987) Differential expression of two distinct T-cell receptors during thymocyte development. Nature 326:79
Pui C-H, Behm FG, Singh B, Schell MJ, Williams DL, Rivera GK, Kalwinsky DK, Sandlund JT, Crist WM, Raimondi SC (1990) Heterogeneity of presenting features and their relation to treatment outcome in 120 children with T-cell acute lymphoblastic leukemia. Blood 75:174
Raulet DH, Garman RD, Saito H, Tonegawa S (1985) Developmental regulation of T cell receptor gene expression. Nature 314:103
Reinherz EL, Kung PC, Goldstein G, Levey RH, Schlossman SF (1980) Discrete stages of human intrathymic differentiation: analysis of normal thymocytes and leukemic lymphoblasts of T cell lineage. Proc Natl Acad Sci USA 77:1588
Rivera GK, Raimondi SC, Hancock ML, Behm FG, Pui C-H, Abromovitch M, Mirro J, Ochs JS, Look AT, Williams DL, Murphy SB, Dahl GV, Kalwinsky DK, Evans WE, Kun LE, Simone JV, Crist WM (1991) Improved outcome in childhood acute lymphoblastic leukaemia with reinforced early treatment and rotational combination chemotherapy. Lancet i:61
Schmid I, Uittenbogaart CH, Giorgi JV (1991) A gentle fixation and permeabilization method for combined cell surface and intracellular staining with improved precision in DNA quantification. Cytometry 12:279
Secker-Walker LM, Campana D, Hawkins JM, Sampson R, Coustan-Smith E (1991) Correlation of karyotype and T-cell receptor expression in T-lineage acute lymphoblastic leukemia. Genes Chromosomes Cancer 4:41
Snodgrass HR, Dembic Z, Steinmetz M, von Boehmer H (1985) Expression of T cell antigen receptor genes during fetal development in the thymus. Nature 315: 232
Spits H, Borst J, Tax W, Capel PJA, Terhorst C, De Vries JE (1985) Characteristics of a monoclonal antibody (WT-31) that recognizes a common epitope on the human T cell receptor for antigen. J Immunol 135:1922
Strominger JL (1989) Developmental biology of T cell receptors. Science 244:943
Thiel E, Kranz BR, Raghavachar A, Bartram CR, Loffler H, Messerer D, Ganser A, Ludwig W-D, Buchner T, Hoelzer D (1989) Prethymic phenotype and genotype of pre-T ($CD7^+/ER^-$)-cell leukemia and its clinical significance within adult acute lymphoblastic leukemia. Blood 73:1247
Transy C, Moingeon PE, Marshall B, Stebbins C, Reinherz EL (1989) Most anti-human CD3 monoclonal antibodies are directed to the CD3 ε subunit. Eur J Immunol 19:947
Van de Griend RJ, Borst J, Tax WJM, Bolhuis RLH (1988) Functional reactivity of WT31 monoclonal antibody with the T cell receptor γ expressing $CD3^+4^-8^-$ T cells. J Immunol 140:1107
Van Dongen JJM, Wolvers-Tettero ILM (1991) Analysis of immunoglobulin and T cell receptor genes: II. Possibilities and limitations in the diagnosis and management of lymphoproliferative diseases and related disorders. Clin Chim Acta 198:93

Van Dongen JJM, Quertermous T, Bartram CR, Gold DP, Wolvers-Tettero ILM, Comans-Bitter WM, Hooijkaas H, Adriaansen HJ, De Klein A, Raghavachar A, Ganser A, Duby AD, Seidman JG, Van der Elsen P, Terhorst C (1987) T cell receptor-CD3 complex during early T cell differentiation. Analysis of immature T cell acute lymphoblastic leukemias at DNA, RNA, and cell membrane level. J Immunol 138:1260

Van Dongen JJM, Krissansen GW, Wolvers-Tettero ILM, Comans-Bitter WM, Adriaansen HJ, Hoijkaas H, Van Vering ER, Terhorst C (1988) Cytoplasmic expression of the CD3 antigen as a diagnostic marker for immature T cell malignancies. Blood 71:603

Van Dongen JJM, Comans-Bitter WM, Wolvers-Tettero ILM, Borst J (1990) Development of human T lymphocytes and their thymus-dependency. Thymus 16:207

Vogler LB, Crist WM, Bockman DE, Pearl ER, Lawton AR, Cooper MD (1978) Pre-B leukaemia: a new phenotype of childhood lymphoblastic leukaemia. N Engl J Med 298:872

Wu YJ, Tian WT, Snider RM, Ritterhaus C, Rogers P, Lamanna L, Ip SH (1988) Signal transduction of γδ T cell antigen receptor with a novel mitogenic anti-δ antibody. J Immunol 141:1476

Flow Cytometric Analysis of Intracellular Myeloperoxidase and Lactoferrin in Leukemia Diagnosis

W. Knapp, O. Majdic, and H. Strobl

Institut für Immunologie der Universität Wien, A-1090 Vienna, Austria

Introduction

The immunological characterization of leukemic blast cells in terms of their lineage commitment and differentiation stage has so far mainly been based on the analysis of surface marker molecules. Mainly for technical reasons, and this is particularly true for flow cytometric analyses, most investigators avoided intracellular markers in their evaluation panel and restricted their studies to easily accessible surface antigens. During the last several years it has become evident, however, that the most reliable lineage markers, already expressed very early in differentiation, are in fact localized within the cytoplasm (reviewed in van Dongen et al. 1988a; Catovsky et al. 1991; Knapp 1991).

The three best studied markers of that kind are cytoplasmic CD3 for the T lineage (Campana et al. 1987; Rani et al. 1988; Van Dongen et al. 1988b; Janossy et al. 1989), cytoplasmic CD22 for the B lineage (Dörken et al. 1986; Mason et al. 1987; Rani et al. 1988; Janossy et al. 1989) and cytoplasmic myeloperoxidase (MPO) for the granulomonocytic lineage (Van der Schoot et al. 1987, 1990; Vainchenker et al. 1988; Catovsky et al. 1991). The standard method for the demonstration of these antigens is immunofluorescence or immunoenzyme staining of dried and fixed cytospin preparations or smears. As shown in this communication, all three markers can also be stained, however, with cells in suspensions and analyzed by flow cytometry. This makes evaluation much easier and allows quantitative analysis. It also facilitates multiparameter analyses, including the simultaneous demonstration of cytoplasmic MPO and lactoferrin (LF) for the distinction between undifferentiated and mature cells of the granulocytic lineage.

Recent Results in Cancer Research, Vol. 131

Materials and Methods

Normal and Leukemic Hemopoietic Cells

Normal blood samples were obtained from healthy individuals. Normal bone marrow was taken from aspirates for allogeneic or autologous bone marrow transplantation. Leukemic cell samples were collected from newly diagnosed patients before therapy.

Mononuclear cells (MNC) were isolated from bone marrow samples using discontinuous Ficoll/Hypaque (Pharmacia, Uppsala) density gradient centrifugation. Interphase cells were removed, washed in phosphate-buffered saline (PBS) with 1% bovine serum albumin and 0.1% sodium azide, and then resuspended at 10^7 cells/ml for further staining. Peripheral blood samples were directly stained without prior isolation of leukocytes.

Antibodies

Fluorescein (FL) or phycoerythrin-R (PE) labeled monoclonal antibody conjugates of the following specificities were used in that study: human myeloperoxidase (clone H-43-5), human lactoferrin (clone 4C5), human CD3 (clone UCHT1), CD22 (clone RFB4), CD13 (clone MY7), CD14 (clone MEM18), CD33 (clone MY9) and CD_w65 (clone VIM2). Apart from MY7 and MY9 (Coulter, Hialeah, FL. USA) all antibody conjugates were obtained from An der Grub (Scandic, Vienna, Austria).

Immunofluorescence Staining Procedures

Membrane Staining. For membrane staining 50 µl isolated MNC (10^7/ml) were incubated for 15 min at 0°–4°C with 20 µl conjugated monoclonal antibody. Afterwards cells were washed and analyzed or submitted to intracellular staining.

Intracellular Staining. For suspension stainings of intracellular antigens we used the commercially available reagent combination Fix & Perm from An der Grub (Scandic, Vienna, Austria) and followed the proposed procedure. In short, cells are first fixed for 15 min at room temperature (50 µl cells plus 100 µl formaldehyde-based fixation medium). After one washing with phosphate-buffered saline (PBS) pH 7.2 cells are resuspended in 50 µl PBS and mixed with 100 µl permeabilization medium plus 20 µl fluorochrome-labeled antibody. After a further incubation for 15 min at room temperature, cells are washed again and analyzed.

Flow Cytometry

Flow cytometric analyses were performed with a FACScan flow cytometer (Becton Dickinson Immunocytometry Systems, Mountain View, CA, USA).

Results and Discussion

Myeloperoxidase in Blood and Bone Marrow Cells

The cytochemical demonstration of myeloperoxidase activity is a classical marker in leukemia diagnosis. In the French-American-British (FAB) classification (Bennett et al. 1985), the presence of more than 3% MPO-containing blasts is, in fact, considered as diagnostic of acute myeloid leukemia (AML). Not infrequently, it is difficult, however, to demonstrate MPO activity in blast cells with conventional light microscopy methods. More sensitive techniques at the ultrastructural level have therefore been proposed (Vainchenker et al. 1988). For routine application, these electron microscopical methods are too work-intensive, however. An attractive alternative has recently been described with the demonstration of MPO and proforms of MPO in the cytoplasm of AML blasts using appropriate monocloncal antibodies directed against MPO. Using conventional fluorescence microscopy on cytospin preparations this method was found by van der Schoot et al. (1987, 1990) to be the most sensitive assay available for the identification of AML blasts. Similar observations have been made by others (Vainchenker et al. 1988; Catovsky et al. 1991), and in our hands too the immunological demonstration of cytoplasmic MPO turned out to be a reliable and highly sensitive marker. Using the monoclonal anti-MPO antibody H-43-5 (Murao et al. 1988) in indirect immunofluorescence combined with conventional fluorescence microscopy we found 48 of 56 AML samples containing more than 90% blasts to be MPO^+ (>20% of blasts MPO^+). On the basis of these observations and the above-mentioned reports in the literature, we decided to go one step further and to establish a suspension staining technique for MPO which would allow flow cytometric single- and multiparameter analyses.

When starting this approach we were able to choose among a variety of published procedures (Slaper-Cortenbach et al. 1988; Halldén et al. 1989; Kastan et al. 1989; Andersson et al. 1989, 1990; Drach et al. 1989, 1991; Gore et al. 1990; Larsen et al. 1991) for the permeabilization of cell membranes to give antibodies access to intracellular antigens. Most of these procedures deal with nuclear antigens often analyzed in lymphoid cells. Only recently were studies reported on the demonstration of cytoplasmic structures such as cytokines (Andersson 1989, 1990; Labalette-Houache et al. 1991). We tried several of these procedures, and it quickly became evident that cells had to be fixed before permeabilization in order to avoid leakage of MPO. We obtained the best results when fixing the cells with a formaldehyde-based fixation medium and then adding fluorescein labeled MPO antibodies together with permeabilization medium (Fig. 1). Details of the procedure are given in "Materials and Methods."

Combined Staining for Myeloperoxidase and Lactoferrin

When evaluating MPO staining of bone marrow cells one has, of course, to consider that the majority of cells in a normal bone marrow sample are myeloid and, therefore, MPO^+. In bone marrow samples of leukemia patients, too, variable proportions of normal bone marrow cells, some of them MPO^+, must be expected. The vast majority of these residual normal MPO^+ cells are differentiated myeloid cells, however, and can, using microscopy, be easily distinguished from MPO^+ leukemic blast cells on the basis of their morphology. In flow cytometry morphological information is much more limited. Other ways must, therefore, be found which allow a distinction between differentiated MPO^+ granulomonocytic cells and undifferentiated MPO^+ cells.

One way to achieve that is combining MPO-staining with lactoferrin-staining. Lactoferrin (LF), an iron-binding protein with bactericidal and bacteriostatic activity, is restricted among hemopoietic cells to the maturation compartment of the granulocytic lineage starting from the myelocyte stage. Normal and malignant myeloblasts and promyelocytes are LF nega-

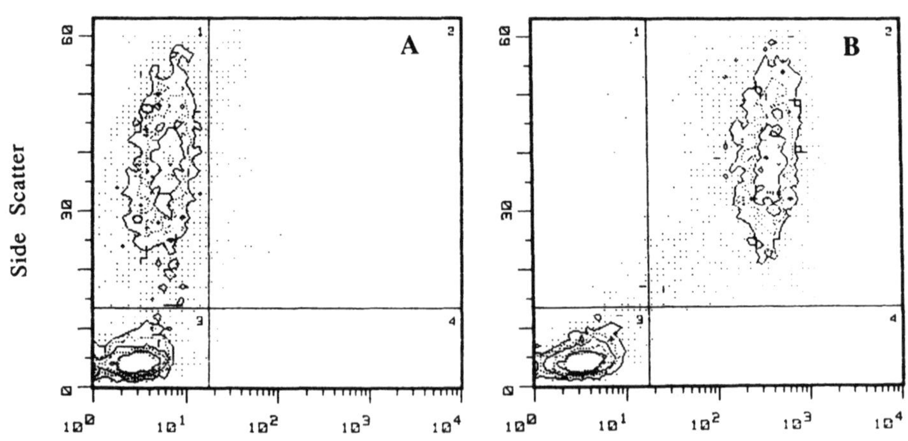

Fig. 1A,B. FACS profile of fixed and permeabilized peripheral blood leukocytes stained with fluorescein-labeled negative control antibody (**A**) or antimyeloperoxidase (MPO) antibody (**B**). Note that side-scatter characteristics of granulocytes and monocytes are maintained and that virtually all cells with scatter characteristics of granulocytes or monocytes are MPO positive

tive (Rado et al. 1984; Cramer et al. 1985; Srivastavar et al. 1991). Typical staining patterns of bone marrow cells obtained with such an anti-MPO/anti-LF conjugate combination can be seen in Fig. 2. As illustrated in Fig. 2A, LF staining clearly divides the MPO^+ population of a normal bone marrow into two subsets. The LF^+MPO^+ subset represents the large granulocytic maturation compartment, while the LF^-MPO^+ subset includes LF^-MPO^+ myeloblasts, promyelocytes and LF^-MPO^+ monocytes. Fig. 2B shows a typical MPO^+ LF^- profile of AML cells.

The same anti-MPO/anti-LF conjugate combination can also be used for the analysis of peripheral blood leukocytes. A typical staining pattern of normal blood leukocytes with MPO^+LF^+ granulocytes, MPO^+LF^- monocytes, and MPO^-LF^- lymphocytes is shown in Fig. 3.

Combined Intracellular Staining for MPO/CD3 and MPO/CD22

In the same way as described above for MPO and LF, staining for MPO can also be combined with cytoplasmic marker molecules of the lymphoid lineage. This allows simultaneous analysis of the most reliable lineage-associated marker molecules of normal and malignant lymphoid progenitor cells. In T cells CD3 can already be detected in the cytoplasm at the earliest

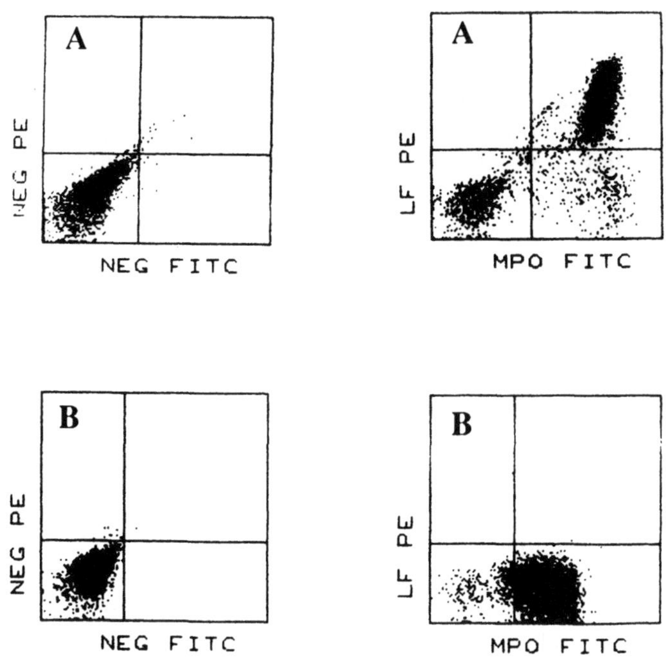

Fig. 2A,B. Myeloperoxidase–lactoferrin double staining of **A** normal bone marrow cell and **B** bone marrow cells from a patient with acute myeloid leukemia

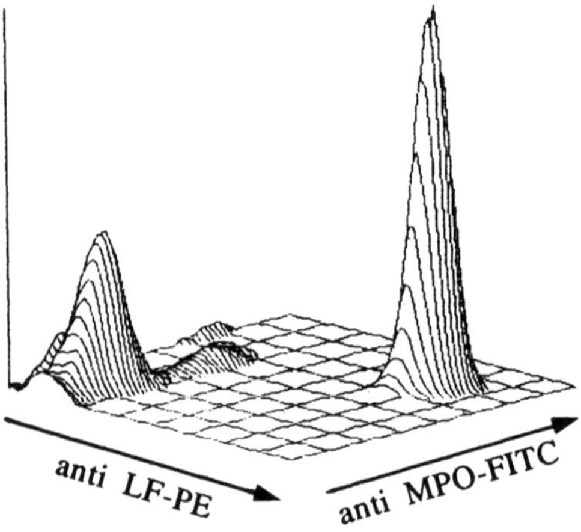

Fig. 3. Contour plot of myeloperoxidase–lactoferrin double-stained peripheral blood leukocytes. As can be seen, neutrophils are $MPO^{+}LF^{+}$, monocytes are $MPO^{+}LF^{-}$, and lymphocytes are $MPO^{-}LF^{-}$

stages of T cell differentiation (Campana et al. 1987; Rani et al. 1988; Van Dongen et al. 1988b; Janossy et al. 1989), while only mature T lymphocytes express CD3 on their surface. In B cells CD22 is first expressed in the cytoplasm, and virtually all acute lymphatic leukemias of B-progenitor cell type are cytoplasmic CD22 positive (Dörken et al. 1986; Mason et al. 1987; Rani et al. 1988; Janossy et al. 1989). Only later in B-cell differentiation at the mature B-lymphocyte stage does CD22 also become surface expressed.

We therefore combined phycoerythrin-conjugated CD3 or CD22 antibodies with fluorescein-conjugated MPO antibodies and stained bone marrow samples essentially as described above for MPO/LF stainings. Typical FACS profiles obtained after such stainings are shown in Fig. 4. As can be seen, even the notoriously weak cytoplasmic CD22 expression in ALL cells can be clearly demonstrated with that procedure.

Combined Surface and Cytoplasmic Stainings of Myeloid Cells

The availability of a staining procedure which labels all myeloid cells containing the classical granulomonocytic marker molecule MPO opens up for the first time the possibility to directly relate the expression of myeloid surface antigens on bone marrow cells to cytoplasmic MPO expression. In such experiments cell samples are first stained for surface antigens in a standard way using PE-labeled antibodies. Cells are then washed, fixed, and permeabilized as described in "Materials and Methods" and counterstained with fluorescein-labeled anti-MPO antibodies. The results of such double-stainings of four normal bone marrow samples using the antibody com-

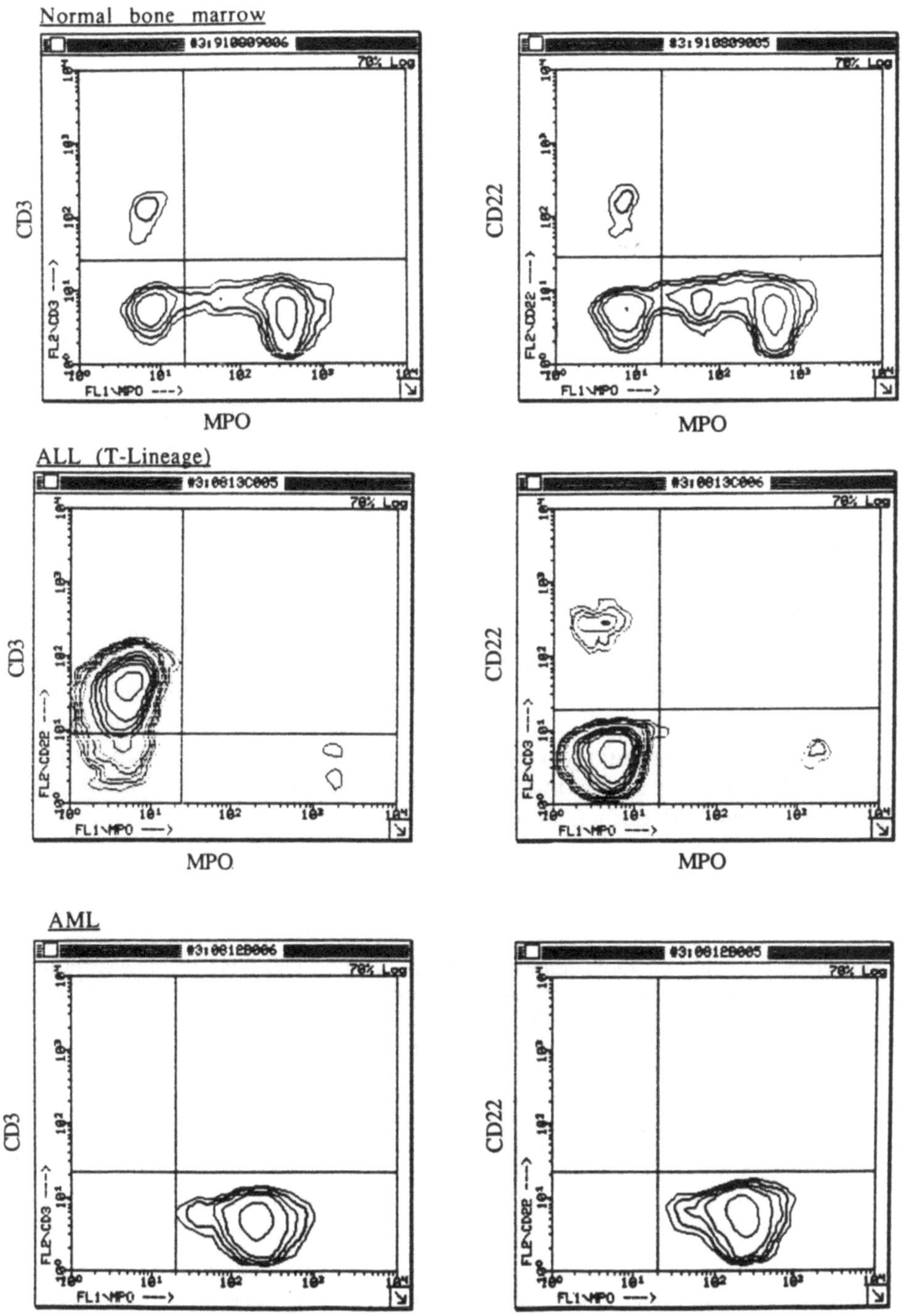

Fig. 4. FACS profiles of bone marrow samples doublestained for intracellular MPO/CD3 or MPO/CD22

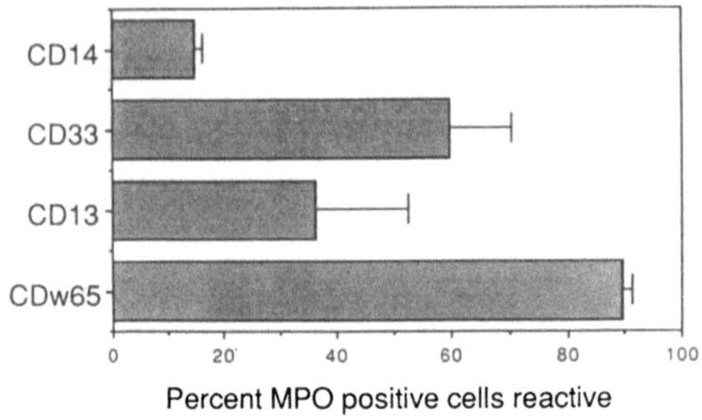

Fig. 5. Coexpression of surface CD14, CD33, CD13, and CD_w65 (VIM2) by myeloperoxidase-positive bone marrow cells

binations MPO/CD14, MPO/CD33, MPO/CD13, MPO/CD_w65 are shown in Fig. 5.

Conclusion

We have showed that suspension staining and flow cytometric analysis of intracellular MPO in bone marrow and blood cells is possible and easy to perform. Both fluorescein-labeled and also larger PE-labeled antibody conjugates can be used. Intracellular MPO staining can be combined with intracellular LF staining, thus allowing distinction of myeloid progenitors from more mature granulocytic cells. Intracellular MPO staining can also be combined with staining for intracellular CD3 or CD22 or with membrane staining for myeloid surface molecules.

References

Andersson U, Adolf G, Dohlsten M, Möller G, Sjögren HO (1989) Characterzation of individual tumor necrosis factor alpha- and β-producing cells after polycloncal T cell activation. J Immunol Methods 123:233

Andersson U, Andersson J, Lindfors A, Wagner K, Möller G, Heusser CH (1990) Simultaneous production of interleukin 2, interleukin 4 and interferon-gamma by activated human blood lymphocytes. Eur J Immunol 20:1591

Bennett JM, Catovsky D, Daniel MT, Flandrin G, Galton DAG, Gralnick HR, Sultan C (1985) Proposed revised criteria for the classification of acute myeloid leukemia. Ann Intern Med 103:620

Campana D, Thompson JS, Amlot P, Brown S, Janossy G (1987) The cytoplasmic expression of CD3 antigens in normal and malignant cells of the T lymphoid lineage. J Immunol 138:648

Catovsky D, Matutes E, Buccheri V, Shetty V, Hanslip J, Yoshida N, Morilla R (1991) A classification of acute leukaemia for the 1990s. Ann Hematol 62:16

Cramer E, Pryzwanski KB, Villeval JL, Testa U, Breton-Gorius J (1985) Ultrastructural localization of lactoferrin and myeloperoxidase in human neutrophils by immunogold. Blood 65:423

Dörken B, Moldenhauer G, Pezzutto A, Schwartz R, Feller A, Kiesel S, Nadler LM (1986) HD39 (B3), a B lineage restricted antigen whose cell surface expression is limited to resting and activated human B lymphocytes. J Immunol 136:4470

Drach J, Gattringer C, Glassl H, Schwarting R, Stein H, Huber H (1989) Simultaneous flow cytometric analysis of surface markers and nuclear Ki-67 antigen in leukemia and lymphoma. Cytometry 10:743

Drach J, Gattringer C, Huber H (1991) Combined flow cytometric assessment of cell surface antigens and nuclear TdT for the detection of minimal residual disease in acute leukaemia. Br J Hematol 77:37

Gore SD, Kastan MB, Goodman SN, Civin CI (1990) Detection of minimal residual T cell acute lymphoblastic leukemia by flow cytometry. J Immunol Methods 132:275

Halldén G, Andersson U, Hed J, Johansson SGO (1989) A new membrane permeabilization method for the detection of intracellular antigens by flow cytometry. J Immunol Methods 124:103

Janossy G, Coustan-Smith E, Campana D (1989) The reliability of cytoplasmic CD3 and CD22 antigen expression in the immunodiagnosis of acute leukemia: a study of 500 cases. Leukemia 3:170

Kastan MB, Stone KD, Civin CI (1989) Nuclear oncoprotein expression as a function of lineage, differentiation stage, and proliferative status of normal human hematopoietic cells. Blood 74:1517

Knapp W (1992) Antibody defined surface molecules of normal and malignant hemopoietic cells. In: Laerum OD, Bjerknes R (eds) Flow cytometry in hematology. Academic, London, p 213

Labalette-Houache M, Torpier G, Capron A, Dessaint JP (1991) Improved permeabilization procedure for flow cytometric detection of internal antigens. J Immunol Methods 138:143

Larsen JK, Christensen IJ, Christiansen J, Mortensen BT (1991) Washless double staining of unfixed nuclei for flow cytometric analysis of DNA and anuclear antigen (Ki-67 or Bromodeoxyuridine). Cytometry 12:429

Mason DY, Stein H, Gerdes J, Pulford KAF, Ralfkiaer E, Falini B, Erber WN, Michaelm K, Gatter KC (1987) Value of monoclonal anti-CD22 (pl35) antibodies for the detection of normal and neoplastic B lymphoid cells. Blood 69:836

Murao SI, Stevens FJ, Ito A, Huberman E (1988) Myeloperoxidase: a myeloid cell nuclear antigen with DNA-binding properties. Proc Natl Acad Sci USA 85:1232

Rado TA, Bollekens J, Laurent GS, Parker L, Benz J Jr (1984) Lactoferrin biosynthesis during granulocytopoiesis. Blood 64:1103

Rani S, de Oliveira MSP, Catopvsky D (1988) Different expression of CD3 and CD22 in leukemic cells according to whether tested in suspension or fixed on slides. Hematol Pathol 2:73

Slaper-Cortenbach ICM, Admiraal LG, Kerr JM, van Leeuwen EF, Von dem Borne AEGK, Tetteroo PAT (1988) Flow cytometric detection of terminal deoxynucleotidyl transferase and other intracellular antigens in combination with membrane antigens in acute lymphatic leukemias. Blood 72:1639

Srivastava CH, Rado TA, Bauerle D, Broxmeyer HE (1991) Regulation of human bone marrow lactoferrin and myeloperoxidase gene expression by tumor necrosis factor-α. J Immunol 146:1014

Vainchenker W, Villeval JL, Tabilio E, Matamis H, Karanakis G, Guichard J, Henri A, Vernant JP, Rochant H, Breton-Gorius J (1988) Immunophenotype of leukemic blasts with small peroxidase-positive granules detected by electron microscopy. Leukemia 2:274

Van der Schoot CE, Von dem Borne AEGK, Tetteroo PAT (1987) Characterization of myeloid leukemias by monoclonal antibodies, with an emphasis on antibodies against myeloperoxidase. Acta Hematol 78:32

Van der Schoot CE, Daams GM, Pinkster J, Vet R, Von dem Borne AE (1990) Monoclonal antibodies against myeloperoxidase are valuable immunological reagents for the diagnosis of acute myeloid leukaemia. Br J Haematol 74:173

Van Dongen JJM, Adriaansen HJ, Hooijkaas H (1988a) Immunophenotyping of leukaemias and non-Hodgkin's lymphomas. Immunological markers and their CD codes. Neth J Med 33:298

Van Dongen JJM, Krissansen GW, Wolvers-Tetteroo ILM et al. (1988b) Cytoplasmic expression of the CD3 antigen as a diagnostic marker for immature T-cell malignancies. Blood 71:603

II. Phenotypic Heterogeneity in Acute Leukemias: Immunological Characterization and Clinical Relevance

Immunological, Ultrastructural and Molecular Features of Unclassifiable Acute Leukaemia

E. Matutes, V. Buccheri, R. Morilla, V. Shetty, M. Dyer, and D. Catovsky

Academic Department of Haematology and Cytogenetics, Royal Marsden Hospital, Fulham Road, London SW3 6JJ, UK

Introduction

The majority of acute leukaemia (AL) cases can be classified as myeloid or lymphoid on the basis of light microscopic morphology, cytochemistry and immunophenotyping by analysing the membrane expression of myeloid and B- and T-lymphoid antigens recognized by lineage-specific monoclonal antibodies (MoAbs) (Chan et al. 1985). Membrane marker analysis was first shown to be essential to characterize acute lymphoblastic leukaemia (ALL) (Greaves et al. 1981), and subsequently this was also possible for acute myeloid leukaemia (AML), particularly in cases with poorly differentiated myeloblasts or those arising from megakaryocytic and erythroid precursors. Despite these advances, the lineage of the leukaemic blasts may still remain uncertain in a minority of AL cases. This is due to the lack of membrane expression of some lymphoid and myeloid antigens or to the expression of a constellation of lymphoid and myeloid antigens on the same cells. Such AL cases are usually of one of two types: (1) undifferentiated AL and (2) biphenotypic or mixed-lineage AL (Campana et al. 1990; Asou et al. 1991; Catovsky et al. 1991).

In the last few years, it has become apparent that at least a proportion of the unclassifiable AL cases can be accurately classified by analysing the cytoplasmic expression of early B, T and myeloid antigens such as CD22, CD3, CD13 and anti-myeloperoxidase (MPO) (Janossy et al. 1989; Van Donghen et al. 1988; Pombo de Oliveira et al. 1988; Buccheri et al. 1992). The problem still exists in the precise classification of AL with biphenotypic features. Furthermore, the lack of a uniform terminology to define such leukaemias has made it difficult to establish whether they have distinct clinical and biological features.

We have analysed the main features of a group of AL unclassifiable by light microscopy examination and standard immunophenotyping by flow cytometry analysis. By investigating the cytoplasmic expression of a

Recent Results in Cancer Research, Vol. 131

number of antigens and applying strict criteria to define biphenotypic cases (Catovsky et al. 1991), we demonstrate that one third of unclassifiable AL are in fact proliferations of poorly differentiated myeloblasts (M0 AML) (Bennett et al. 1991; Matutes et al. 1988) and the remaining ones are biphenotypic AL.

Material and Methods

Samples. Peripheral blood and/or bone marrow samples from 180 patients with AL have been analysed. All the specimens contained over 50% blasts and usually more than 80%. Cases were classified as ALL or AML according to the French–American–British (FAB) criteria (Bennett et al. 1985) by examining May–Grünwald–Giemsa-stained blood and bone marrow films and the cytochemical reactions for myeloperoxidase (MPO), Sudan Black B (SBB) and α-naphthylacetate esterase (ANAE).

Immunophenotyping. This was performed on Lymphoprep (Nycomed, Oslo, Norway) isolated blood and/or bone marrow mononuclear cells by immunofluorescence and/or immunocytochemistry with a panel of anti-lymphoid and myeloid MoAbs, as described elsewhere (Buccheri et al. 1992). The immunofluorescence method was performed on unfixed cells in suspension by an indirect technique using a fluorescein isothiocyanate-conjugated (FITC) goat anti-mouse immunoglobulin (Ig) F $(ab)_2$ fragment as second layer and results were analysed on a FACScan flow cytometer (Becton-Dickinson). In some cases, double labelling with two different MoAbs was performed by a direct immunofluorescence method using FITC and phycoerythrin (PE) directly conjugated to the MoAb. Control preparations were performed in all the cases by replacing the MoAb with a mouse immunoglobulin of the same isotype and/or incubating the cells with the second layer only. Special attention was paid to non-specific binding of MoAb to the Fc receptors. To avoid this, 2% pooled human AB serum was added to the buffer used in all the washes and prior incubation with the antibodies.

The cytoplasmic expression of the antigens recognized by the MoAb (CD3, CD22, CD13 and anti-MPO) was investigated by the immunoalkaline phosphatase anti-alkaline phosphatase (APAAP) technique on cytospin slides or peripheral blood and/or bone marrow smears as previously described (Cordell et al. 1984). Briefly, the slides were fixed for 10 min in acetone, air-dried and incubated with the MoAb at adequate dilution for 30 min at room temperature. Following a 30-min incubation with a rabbit antimouse immunoglobulin (Dakopatts) (1/20) and a 45-min incubation with the APAAP complexes (Dakopatts) (1/60), the reaction was developed with the solution naphthol AS-MX phosphate (Sigma), levamisole, dimethylformamide (Merck) and fast red TR salt (Sigma). The slides were counterstained with haematoloxylin-S and mounted with glycergel (Dakoppatts). The cell reactivity with a MoAb was seen as a red cytoplasmic deposit and allowed us to assess in detail the morphology of the cells. The nuclear enzyme terminal deoxynucleotidyl transferase (TdT) was also investigated by the APAAP technique with a rabbit polyclonal antibody against calf TdT (Sera-Lab); following the incubation with the anti-TdT, an extra-step incubation with a mouse anti-rabbit immunoglobulin was required and, subsequently, the reaction was carried out as described above.

A marker was considered to be positive when over 20% of cells labelled with the MoAb by FACS analysis or over 10% of blasts were positive by immunocytochemistry.

Electron Microscopy. Ultrastructural studies were performed by fixing the cells in 3% glutaraldehyde in 0.1 *M* phosphate buffer (pH 7.6) for 90 min. Post-fixation, dehydration and embedding were performed as described elsewhere (Matutes and Robinson 1991). The MPO activity was investigated on fixed cells following the Graham and Karnovsky method (1966) or on unfixed cells according to the Roels technique (Roels et al. 1975). In some cases, immunoelectronmicroscopy studies were carried out by applying the immunogold method in combination with the cytochemical reaction for peroxidase (Matutes and Robinson 1991).

Molecular Analysis. This was performed by Southern blot on high molecular weight DNA extracted from the leukaemic cells by using standard techniques and digested with the restriction enzymes *Eco*RI, *Hin*dIII and *Bam*HI (Bethesda Research, USA). The DNA probes used were: 2.5-kilobase (kb) *Eco*RI/*Bgl*II fragment for the immunoglobulin heavy chain joining (J_H) region, 0.7-kb *Eco*RI/*Hin*dIII fragment isolated from the constant region of the T-cell receptor (TCR) β chain (TCR-Cβ1), 700-bp *Eco*RI/*Hin*dIII fragment from the clone M13H60 to detect TCR γ rearrangement, the TCR $J_{\delta 1}$ probe (Jδ S16) that detects V-D-$J_{\delta 1}$ rearrangements, and the TCR $C_\delta/J_{\delta 3}$ probe from the clone R21EE which detects rearrangement of the $J_{\delta 3}$ of the TCR δ chain.

Results

Out of 180 AL cases, 20 were unclassifiable by light microscopy morphology and cytochemistry and flow cytometry analysis on cell suspensions. Following cytoplasmic staining with myeloid- and lymphoid-associated antigens and electron microscope cytochemistry to detect MPO, these cases could be divided into two groups: (1) myeloblastic leukaemia with minimal differentiation (AML-M0), and (2) acute leukaemia with biphenotypic features.

Myeloblastic Leukaemia with Minimal Differentiation (AML-M0)

This group included six patients. All but one were adults, with a median age of 59 years (range 36–85); the remaining patient was a 23-month-old infant. Morphologically, the blasts were either undifferentiated or lymphoid looking and were negative with all the cytochemical reactions performed by light microscopy (MPO, SBB and ANAE). As shown in Table 1, blasts from all cases expressed at least one myeloid antigen, shown by the reactivity with CD13 and/or CD33. Membrane expression of CD13 was absent in two of these cases, but in one of them (case 1) a significant proportion of blasts was positive for cytoplasmic CD13. In addition, a minority of blasts from four patients was reactive with anti-MPO despite being negative for MPO by light microscopy cytochemistry. Class II HLA-DR determinants were strongly expressed in all cases, CD34 was positive in three cases, and a proportion of blasts (36% and 86%) in two cases were TdT^+. B- and T-lymphoid associated antigens were negative in all but one case (6) in which 97% of blasts were $CD7^+$. MoAbs against erythroid and megakaryocytic precursors were negative in all cases.

Peroxidase activity could be demonstrated at electron microscopic level in all three cases of AML M0 investigated. The reaction product was often localized to the nuclear membrane, endoplasmic reticulum and small cytoplasmic granules. Samples from three cases were investigated at a molecular level and in all three the immunoglobulin JH and the TCRβ, γ and δ chain genes were shown to be in germline configuration.

Acute Leukaemia with Biphenotypic Features

This corresponded to 14 cases difficult to classify by standard methods because of the coexpression on the same cells of myeloid and lymphoid

Table 1. Findings in six cases of M0 acute myeloid leukaemia

Case no.	CD 13 (%)	CD 33 (%)	Anti-MPO (%)	MPO (EM) (%)
1	40[a]	ND	4	ND
2	95	83	1	ND
3	1[a]	2	6	ND
4	20	55	0	32
5	88	31	3	6
6	97	98	5	7

All cases were negative for MPO by light microscopy and lacked B- and T-lymphoid markers, except TdT, which was positive in cases 3 and 5, and CD7, which was positive in case 6. Immunoglobulin JH and TCR chain genes were in germline configuration in cases 1, 5 and 6.
EM, electron microscopy; ND, not done.
[a] Cytoplasmic expression.

antigens and consistent with the criteria adopted for the definition of biphenotypic AL (Table 2). These patients included nine males and five females, all of whom were adults, with a median age of 33 years (range 13–80), except for an 8-year-old child.

Biphenotypic "ALL". In five of the 14 cases, the blasts were cytochemically negative for MPO, SBB and ANAE and had lymphoid morphology. The phenotype was consistent with common ALL: TdT^+, $CD10^+$, cytoplasmic μ chain negative; cells from four cases were $CD19^+$ and in three out of four tested the cells expressed cytoplasmic CD22 (Table 3). In addition to the lymphoid markers, these leukaemias had a number of myeloid features (Table 3). A high proportion of blasts from these five cases were $CD13^+$; the cells were $CD33^+$ in three cases and the MoAb anti-MPO was positive in a minority of blasts from two of them. Double labelling staining using FITC-CD13 or FITC-CD33 and PE-CD10 or PE-CD19 showed, in all three cases investigated (nos. 8–10), a single cell population (20%–85%) expressing the lymphoid and myeloid antigens.

Electron microscope studies confirmed myeloid features in a minority of blasts by showing peroxidase activity. Analysis of the simultaneous expression of myeloid and lymphoid antigens with peroxidase activity by immunoelectronmicroscopy revealed that in all these four cases the $CD19^+$ and/or $CD10^+$ blasts always lacked peroxidase activity, despite of the coexpression of myeloid and lymphoid antigens by FACS analysis.

Molecular studies carried out in three samples (cases 7,9,10) showed rearrangement of the immunoglobulin JH chain in the three of them; in case 7, the TCRβ chain gene was rearranged and the TCRδ chain gene was deleted, whereas in case 9 rearrangements of the TCR γ and δ chain genes were demonstrated.

Table 2. Scoring system for the diagnosis of biphenotypic acute leukaemia

Scoring points	Lineage		
	B-lymphoid	T-lymphoid	Myeloid
2	cCD22	cCD3	MPO[a]
1	CD19 CD10	CD2 CD5	CD13 CD33
0.5	TdT	TdT CD7	CD14, CD15 CD11b, CD11c

Biphenotypic AL is defined when the score from two separate lineages is greater than 2. Modified (simplified) from our earlier proposal (Catovsky et al. 1991) by not including the information on gene rearrangements as part of the score.
c, cytoplasmic.
[a] MPO demonstrated by cytochemical or immunocytochemical methods.

Table 3. Biphenotypic acute leukaemia with "lymphoid" morphology

Case no.	Lymphoid markers (%)					Myeloid markers (%)				
	CD19	CD10	CD22[a]	TdT	Score	CD13	CD33	Anti-MPO	MPO[b]	Score
7	89	93	37	90	4.5	79	3	8	7	3
8	85	83	ND	0	2[c]	66	3	0	5	3
9	96	82	0	95	2.5	86	86	6	5	4
10	82	26	74	58	4.5	70	34	0	4	4
11	3	32	88	81	3.5	74	40	ND	ND	2[c]

ND, not done.
[a] Cytoplasmic CD22.
[b] By electron microscopy.
[c] The scores were only 2 for the lymphoid and myeloid lineages, respectively, but information was lacking on reliable markers (cytoplasmic CD22 and MPO).

Biphenotypic "AML". Blasts from nine cases were classified as AML according to FAB criteria (M1 or M2 AML), with a varying proportion (4%–85%) of MPO- and/or SBB-positive blasts in eight cases; in case 15, the blasts were MPO negative but showed otherwise marked myeloid differentiation and was classified as AML M2. Immunological markers showed that five cases had a B-lymphoid plus a myeloid phenotype (cases 12–16) and the other four had a T-lymphoid plus myeloid markers (cases 17–20) (Table 4). In addition to the morphological and cytochemical features consistent with AML, all but three cases expressed at least two myeloid antigens recognized by the MoAbs for CD13 and CD33, and anti-MPO was positive in five of six cases tested. Thus, the score points for the myeloid lineage were 3 or more in all these cases. Cells from four cases with B-lymphoid markers were $CD19^+$, three cases were $CD10^+$ and four were also cytoplasmic $CD22^+$. Cells from all four cases with T-lymphoid markers were $CD2^+$ and in three of them a minority of blasts was also cytoplasmic $CD3^+$; the MoAb for CD7 was positive in three and the one for CD10 was positive in two cases. All these "AML" cases scored between 2.5 and 4.5 points for the B- and T-lymphoid lineages. A varying proportion of blasts from nine cases were TdT^+, all were class II $HLA\text{-}DR^+$, and in five out of the nine the cells were $CD34^+$. Double labelling with FITC-CD13 and PE-CD19 and/or PE-CD10 was performed in three cases (12, 13, 15) and with FITC-CD13 or FITC-CD33 and PE-CD2 in case 17; in all four cases, a single population of blasts (14%–85%) coexpressing the myeloid and lymphoid antigens could be identified.

Ultrastructural studies demonstrated MPO activity in all six cases investigated, including case 15 which was MPO negative by light microscopy. The immunogold method showed that in cases 12 and 17 a proportion of blasts that expressed CD19 or CD2, respectively, displayed peroxidase activity, whereas in cases 13 and 15 the MPO^+ blasts did not show reactivity with the anti-lymphoid MoAb; thus these two features were present in different cell populations.

Molecular analysis was carried out in seven cases of biphenotypic AL. In four (nos. 14, 15, 17, 20), the immunoglobulin JH and TCRβ, γ and δ chain genes were in germline configuration. Regarding the remaining three cases, the immunoglobulin JH chain was rearranged in two (nos. 13, 19) and deleted in one (no. 12). Two of these three cases had the TCRδ chain gene deleted (nos. 12, 13) and in the other (no. 19) this gene was rearranged; the TCRβ gene was rearranged in one of these three cases and the TCRγ gene in another.

Discussion

In this study we have examined in detail the cellular features of 20 AL cases which were unclassifiable according to membrane markers and light

Table 4. Biphenotypic acute leukaemia with "myeloid" morphology (percentage of positive blasts)

	Lymphoid markers								Myeloid markers					
Case no.	TdT	CD19	CD10	CD22[a]	CD2	CD7	CD3[a]	Score	CD13	CD33	LM	EM	MoAb	Score
12	61	64	26	0	0	0	0	2.5	61	37	16	30	14	4
13	18	86	0	65	0	0	0	3.5	74	44	4	6	5	4
14	26	19	30	16	0	0	0	4.5	81	2	+	ND	ND	3
15	85	82	26	74	0	0	0	4.5	46	34	0	10	4	4
16	37	0	0	28	0	0	0	2.5	35	0	55	ND	0	3
17	70	0	0	0	79	85	5	2.5	46	60	4	4	42	4
18	11	0	58	0	37	39	12	4.5	68	65	40	35	ND	4
19	50	0	56	0	30	60	26	4.5	8	71	15	28	89	3
20	5	6	9	4	67	8	13	3	59	73	85	ND	ND	4

ND, not done.
[a] Cytoplasmic expression.

microscopy cytochemistry. Most of these patients were adults and they represented 10.5% of a series of 180 AL cases studied over the last 2 years. Our findings demonstrate that within the unclassifiable AL, two scenarios are possible: (1) cases in which the cells display only features characteristic of early myeloid progenitor cells and which may thus be considered as poorly differentiated AML or AML M0 (Bennett et al. 1991; Matutes et al. 1988; Lee et al. 1987); and (2) those cases in which the blasts have features of lymphoid and myeloid cells and for this reason are designated biphenotypic AL.

In the former group, the pure myeloid commitment of the blast cells is demonstrated by: (a) the cytoplasmic and/or membrane expression of myeloid-associated antigens; (b) the presence of MPO activity, shown only by immunocytochemistry with a MoAb that detects the active form of the MPO and the inactive form or properoxidase (Van der Schoot et al. 1987; Buccheri et al. 1992) and/or by ultrastructural cytochemistry using sensitive techniques, e.g. the Roels method on unfixed cells; and (c) the absence of specific lymphoid markers. The enzyme MPO is considered to be highly specific and the hallmark for the myeloid lineage and it is therefore apparent that these cases represent proliferations of early myeloblasts and should be defined as AML M0 with minimal differentiation (Bennett et al. 1991). Further support comes from the lack in these cells of DNA features associated with lymphoid differentiation, as shown in all three cases studied in which the immunoglobulin JH and TCR chain genes were in germline configuration.

The detection of MPO is important as the expression of myeloid antigens recognized by the MoAbs for CD13 and CD33 has been reported in "apparently" bona fide ALL which for this reason is referred to as My$^+$ ALL (Sobol et al. 1987; Davey et al. 1988; Childs et al. 1989; review by Drexler et al. 1991). In most of these studies, application of more sensitive techniques (anti-MPO and ultrastructural cytochemistry) to investigate further myeloid differentiation was not carried out and thus it is possible that some of these cases may well corresponded to AML M0 and/or biphenotypic AL. Indeed, in the series reported by Sobol et al. (1987) seven cases (23%) had a pure myeloid phenotype with no expression of lymphoid antigens; and few cases referred to by Davey et al. (1988) were SBB$^+$, and in one of them Auer rods were present. Furthermore, one of the My$^+$ ALL cases reported by Childs et al. (1989) relapsed as AML with similar cytogenetics and immunoglobulin JH rearrangements at presentation and at relapse, suggesting that it represented a stem-cell or biphenotypic leukaemia rather than an ALL with aberrant expression of one or two myeloid markers.

The recognition of poorly differentiated myeloid leukaemia or M0 AML had been possible in the past by using sensitive methods at the electron microscopic level to demonstrate MPO activity (Lee et al. 1987; Matutes et al. 1988; LeMaistre et al. 1988). In our experience it is now possible to detect most of these cases, which are characteristically negative for lymphoid markers, by a combination of reliable myeloid markers like CD13 and CD33 in addition to the MoAb against the enzyme MPO (Buccheri et al. 1992). To this end, the cytoplasmic detection of myeloid antigens in fixed cells, particularly CD13 and anti-MPO, appears to be highly sensitive and thus this approach should be systematically carried out to clarify the nature of cases with otherwise unclassifiable AL by standard flow cytometry immunophenotyping (Pombo de Oliveira et al. 1988; Buccheri et al. 1992; Campana et al. 1990). In some studies referring to undifferentiated AL (Asou et al. 1991), the cytoplasmic expression of myeloid antigens has not been investigated and therefore the posibility that some such cases are examples of AML M0 cannot be ruled out.

Another issue concerns cases in which the blast cells have a complex composite phenotype which makes them difficult to classify as ALL or AML, and for that reason they have been designated as biphenotypic or mixed-lineage AL. The lack of a uniform terminology to describe such cases is one of the problems for a better understanding of the clinical and biological significance of what we believe corresponds to a distinct entity. Thus, in terms of a definition, the number of myeloid and lymphoid features as well as the degree of specificity for the myeloid and lymphoid lineage of a particular marker should be considered. In an attempt to unify the description of such cases, we have recently proposed a scoring system to define cases of truly biphenotypic AL. This analysis is aimed at distinguishing these cases from those which may be better considered as AML or ALL with unusual or aberrant expression of a marker from the other lineage (Catovsky et al. 1991). This scoring system to qualify biphenotypic AL is illustrated in Table 2 and has been slightly modified. All but two cases examined in this study fulfil the criteria proposed, and thus scored over 2 and usually over 3 points. The information obtained from DNA analysis was initially considered for the definition (Catovsky et al. 1991). However, it has become apparent that high scoring is possible without this information, and for this reason we do not consider this approach essential to define biphenotypic AL. It is of interest that in all four cases classified as biphenotypic AL with "lymphoid" morphology, we could demonstrate MPO activity in a minority of blasts by electron microscopy, thus confirming the myeloid commitment of at least a proportion of the leukaemic cells; however, in none of these cases could we show the coexistence of MPO^+, lymphoid antigen-positive blasts when examined by electron microscopy using the immunogold method. This is in contrast to findings for biphenotypic AL with "myeloid" morphology, where in half (two out of four) of the cases studied such coexpression was documented. At present, we do not know the significance of these findings or whether cases of biphenotypic AL with "lymphoid" and "myeloid" morphology correspond to two different subgroups with different features.

We have examined whether, in our AML cases with high scores for lymphoid antigens designated as biphenotypic AL, there is a correlation with the rearrangement of lymphoid functional genes (immunoglobulin H chain and TCR). This work is still in progress, but preliminary findings suggest that there is a higher incidence of H chain and/or TCR rearrangement in biphenotypic AL (here in three of seven cases). It will be important to extend this work and test our proposed scoring system to see if it may help in disclosing whether these AL cases have distinct biological features (e.g., chromosome translocations) or clinical outcomes and thus in the design of therapeutic strategies.

References

Asou N, Suzushima H, Hattori T, Nishikawa K, Wang J-X, Okubo T, Oura K, Sato M, Kawano F, Shido T, Takatsuki K (1991) Acute unclassified leukemia originating from undifferentiated cells with aberrant rearrangement and expression of immunoglobulin and T-cell receptor genes. Leukemia 5:293–299

Bennett JM, Catovsky D, Daniel MT, Flandrin G, Galton DAG, Gralnick HR, Sultan C (1985) Proposed revised criteria for the classification of acute myeloid leukemia. Ann Intern Med 103:620–625

Bennett JM, Catovsky D, Daniel MT, Flandrin G, Galton DAG, Gralnick HR, Sultan C (1991) Proposal for the recognition of minimally differentiated acute myeloid leukaemia. Br J Haematol 78:325–329

Buccheri V, Shetty V, Yoshida N, Morilla R, Matutes E, Catovsky D (1992) The role of an anti-myeloperoxidase antibody in the diagnosis and classification of acute leukaemia: a comparison with light and electron microscopy cytochemistry. Br J Haematol 80:62–68

Campana D, Hansen-Hagge TE, Matutes E, Coustan-Smith E, Yokota S, Shetty V, Bartram CR, Janossy G (1990) Phenotypic, genotypic, cytochemical and ultrastructural characterization of acute undifferentiated leukemia. Leukemia 9:620–624

Catovsky D, Matutes E, Buccheri V, Shetty V, Hanslip J, Yoshida N, Morilla R (1991) A classification of acute leukaemia for the 1990s. Ann Haematol 62:16–21

Chan LC, Pegram SM, Greaves MF (1985) Contribution of immunophenotype to the classification and differential diagnosis of acute leukaemia. Lancet i:475–479

Childs CC, Hirsch-Ginsberg C, Walters RS, Anderson BS, Reuben J, Trujillo JM, Cork A, Stass SA, Freireich EJ, Zipf TF (1989) Myeloid surface antigen-positive acute lymphoblastic leukemia (My+ ALL). Immunophenotypic, ultrastructural, cytogenetic and molecular characteristics. Leukemia 11:777–783

Cordell JL, Falini B, Erber WN, Ghosh AK, Abdulazaziz Z, MacDonald S, Pulford KAF, Stein H, Mason DY (1984) Immunoenzymatic labelling of monoclonal antibodies using immunocomplexes of alkaline phosphatase and monoclonal alkaline phosphatase (APAAP complexes). J Histochem Cytochem 32:219–229

Davey FR, Mick R, Nelson DA, MacCallum J, Sobol RE, Royston I, Cuttner J, Ellison RR, Bloomfield CD (1988) Morphologic and cytochemical characteristics of adult lymphoid leukemias which express myeloid antigen. Leukemia 2:420–426

Drexler HG, Thiel E, Ludwig WD (1991) Review of the incidence and clinical relevance of myeloid antigen-positive acute lymphoblastic leukemia. Leukemia 5:637–645

Graham RC, Karnovsky MJ (1966) The early stages of absorption of injected horseradish peroxidase in the proximal tubules of mouse kidney: ultrastructural cytochemistry by a new technique. J Histochem Cytochem 14:291–302

Greaves MF, Janossy J, Peto J, Kay H (1981) Immunologically defined subclasses of acute lymphoblastic leukaemia in children: their relationship to presentation features and prognosis. Br J Haematol 48:179–197

Janossy G, Coustan-Smith E, Campana D (1989) The reliability of cytoplasmic CD3 and CD22 antigen expression in the immunodiagnosis of acute leukemia-a study of 500 cases. Leukemia 3:170–181

Lee EJ, Pollak A, Leavitt RD, Testa JR, Schiffer CA (1987) Minimally differentiated acute non-lymphocytic leukemia: a distinct entity. Blood 70:1400–1406

LeMaistre A, Childs C, Hirsch-Ginsberg C, Reuben J, Cork A, Trujillo JMV, Andersson B, McCredie KB, Freireich E, Stass SA (1988) Heterogeneity in acute undifferentiated leukemia. Hematol Pathol 2:79–90

Matutes E, Robinson D (1991) Ultrastructure of lymphoid cells. In: Catovsky D (ed) The leukemic cell. Churchill Livingstone, Edinburgh, pp 127–167

Matutes E, Pombo de Oliveira M, Foroni L, Morilla R, Catovsky D (1988) The role of ultrastructural cytochemistry and monoclonal antibodies in clarifying the nature of undifferentiated cells in acute leukaemia. Br J Haematol 69:205–211

Pombo de Oliveira M, Matutes E, Rani S, Morilla R, Catovsky D (1988) Early expression of MCS2 (CD13) in the cytoplasm of blast cells from acute myeloid leukaemia. Acta Haematol (Basel) 80:61–64

Roels F, Wisse E, De Brest B, van der Meulen J (1975) Cytochemical discrimination between catalases and peroxidases using diaminobenzidine. Histochemistry 41:281–311

Sobol RE, Mick R, Royston I, Davey FR, Ellison RR, Newman R, Cuttner J, Griffin JD, Collins H, Nelson DA, Bloomfield CD (1987) Clinical importance of myeloid antigen expression in adult acute lymphoblastic leukemia. N Engl J Med 316:1111–1117

Van der Schoot CE, von dem Borne AEGK, Tetteroo PAT (1987) Characterization of myeloid leukaemias by monoclonal antibodies with an emphasis on antibodies against myeloperoxidase. Acta Haematol (Basel) 78 [Suppl 1]:32–40

Van Dongen JJM, Krissansen GW, Wolvers-Tettero ILM, Comans-Bitter WM, Adriaansen HJ, Hooijkas H, Van Wering ER, Terhorst C (1988) Cytoplasmic expression of the CD3 antigen as a diagnostic marker for immature T cell malignancies. Blood 71:603–612

Incidence and Clinical Relevance of Myeloid Antigen-Positive Acute Lymphoblastic Leukemia

H.G. Drexler[1] and W.-D. Ludwig[2]

[1] German Collection of Microorganisms and Cell Cultures, Department of Human and Animal Cell Cultures, W-3300 Brunswick, Fed. Red. of Germany
[2] Free University of Berlin, Klinikum Steglitz, Department of Hematology/ Oncology, W-1000 Berlin 45, Fed. Rep. of Germany

Introduction

Acute leukemias are traditionally classified according to their morphological and cytochemical features, being named according to the assumed normal counterparts which they most closely resemble. However, the concordance rate among investigators on the morphological distinction between acute lymphoblastic leukemia (ALL) and acute myeloblastic leukemia (AML) has been found to range from 70%–98% (S.L. Lee et al. 1962; Brincker and Jensen 1972; Viana et al. 1980; Head et al. 1985; Browman et al. 1986). Furthermore, some acute leukemia cases lack features that are currently recognized as diagnostic of ALL or AML within the morphological FAB schema. In several studies, 2%–10% of the cases were defined as morphologically "unclassifiable" (Foon et al. 1979; Mertelsmann et al. 1980; Youness et al. 1980; Bennett et al. 1985; E.L. Lee et al. 1987).

With the availability of heterologous antisera and more recently monoclonal antibodies to differentiation antigens, the diagnostic precision has increased (Drexler and Scott 1989). As early as 1980 the lineage association of acute leukemia cases could be established in 92% of cases (Janossy et al. 1980); the reliable classification with immunodiagnostic methods has then increased to over 99% (Chan et al. 1985; Chen et al. 1986; Drexler et al. 1986; Herrmann et al. 1986; Janossy et al. 1989); even the lineage affiliation of leukemias with unique aberrant features can now be routinely assessed (Janossy et al. 1989; Campana et al. 1990).

Immunophenotyping has also documented the existence of acute leukemia cases in which the blasts express markers supposedly specific for, or predominantly associated with, another cell lineage (Ben-Bassat and Gale 1984; Stass and Mirro 1985, 1986; Greaves et al. 1986; Gale and Ben-Bassat 1987; Mirro et al. 1987; Hoffbrand et al. 1988; Mirro and Kitchingman 1989; Maitreyan and Gale 1989; Altman 1990; Paietta 1990; Schiffer 1990). Descriptively a variety of terms have been used to refer to these acute

Recent Results in Cancer Research, Vol. 131

leukemias, including hybrid, biphenotypic, bilineal, biclonal, simultaneous, metachronous, synchronous, chimeric, and mixed. It appears that the most widely used and relatively well-defined terms are "acute mixed-lineage leukemia" and "hybrid acute leukemia" (Ben-Bassat and Gale 1984; Mirro et al. 1985; Gale and Ben-Bassat 1987).

The best-studied example is positivity of ALL blast cells for cell surface markers regarded as being exclusively associated with the myeloid lineage (mostly referred to as My^+ ALL). However, the expression of myeloid antigens alone is not sufficient to classify these malignancies as hybrid acute leukemia (Gale and Ben-Bassat 1987). While originally ALL cases staining with only one myeloid marker were included into the category acute mixed-lineage leukemia (Mirro et al. 1985), the revised, more stringent criteria excluded these leukemias from the proposed system (Mirro and Kitchingman 1989). Consequently, it was suggested that such cases be described as "lymphoid leukemias with myeloid-associated antigen expression" (Mirro and Kitchingman 1989). The myeloid antigen-associated monoclonal antibodies used for the detection of My^+ ALL are listed in Table 1.

Incidence of My^+ ALL

The frequency with which My-positivity occurs among ALL cases ranges from 5% to nearly 50% as reported in 14 studies (without corrections for obvious misinterpretations), an average of 12% (465 out of 3817; Fig. 1). Fewer reports on My^+ ALL have provided details with regard to children versus adults, T- versus B-lineage ALL, positivity for various CD groups, and prognostic impact.

Table 1. Myeloid lineage-associated CD groups and individual monoclonal antibodies

CD group	Antibodies used
CD13	MY7, MCS-2, WM54
CD14	MY4, Leu-M3, CRIS-6
CD15	MY1, Leu-M1, VIM-D5, 1G10
CD33	MY9, L4F3, WM15
CD_w65	VIM-2

This is not a complete list of all myeloid-associated CD groups but includes only the most commonly used and most strongly lineage-associated CD groups (see also Fig. 4). CD11b (e.g., OKM-1, Mol) does not qualify as a "myeloidassociated cluster" in the context of My^+ ALL (see text).

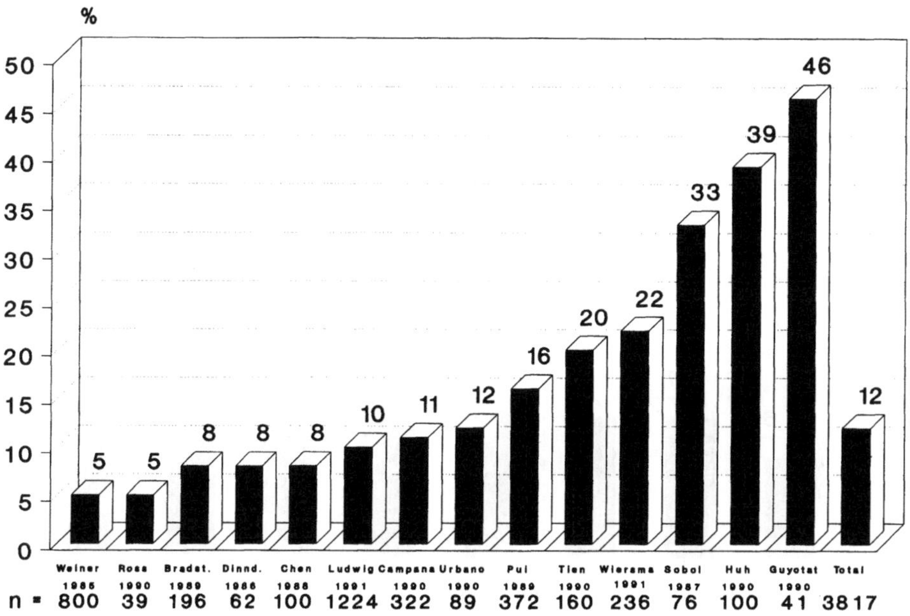

Fig. 1. Incidences of myeloid antigen-positive ALL cases (children and adults). Shown are the percentages of My^+ ALL cases in 14 large series totaling 3817 ALL cases. Figures are not corrected for obvious inconsistencies, e.g., $CD11b^+$ ALL, AML M0 cases, etc. In some studies children and adult ALL cases were not differentiated (for more detailed studies on childhood and adult My^+ ALL, see Fig. 2,3). *References*: Weiner et al. 1985; Ross et al. 1990; Bradstock et al. 1989; Dinndorf et al. 1986; Chen et al. 1988; Ludwig et al. 1989a, 1990, and unpublished results; Campana et al. 1990; Urbano-Ispizua et al. 1990; Pui et al. 1989; Tien et al. 1990; Wiersma et al. 1991; Sobol et al. 1987; Huh et al. 1990; Guyotat et al. 1990

Children. In seven studies of childhood ALL involving 2424 patients, 8% of the cases were labeled by myeloid-associated monoclonal antibodies (range 5%–22%; Fig. 2). However, most series reported incidences in the rather narrow range of 7%–11%. ALL in infants (<1 year of age) was associated with a significantly higher frequency of myeloid antigen coexpression: in the two largest series 19/43 (44%) infant ALL cases were My^+ (Katz et al. 1988; Ludwig et al. 1989b).

Adults. Markedly diverging results were found in adult ALL with regard to positivity for myeloid antigen expression (Fig. 3). While three studies reported an incidence of 13%–15% My^+ ALL cases, three other reports described the significantly higher frequencies of 33%–46%. However, it should be pointed out that in the latter three studies and in the childhood series of Wiersma et al. (1991) (see above) the initial diagnosis of ALL was based strictly on the light microscopic appearance and cytochemical stains of

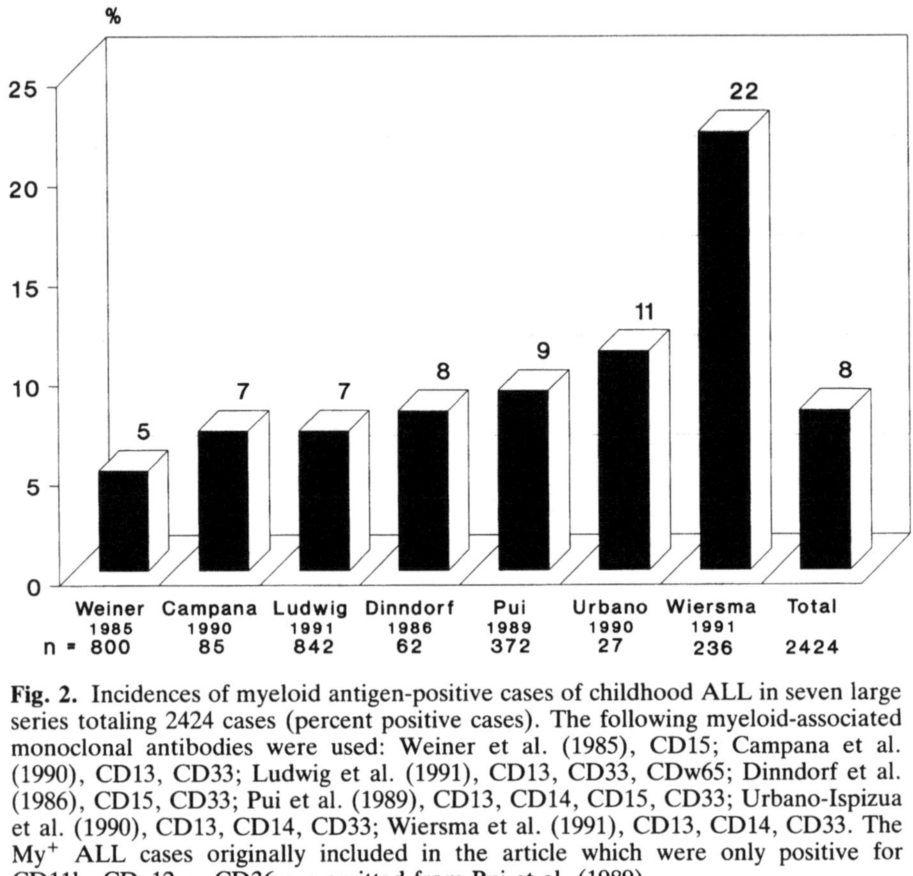

Fig. 2. Incidences of myeloid antigen-positive cases of childhood ALL in seven large series totaling 2424 cases (percent positive cases). The following myeloid-associated monoclonal antibodies were used: Weiner et al. (1985), CD15; Campana et al. (1990), CD13, CD33; Ludwig et al. (1991), CD13, CD33, CDw65; Dinndorf et al. (1986), CD15, CD33; Pui et al. (1989), CD13, CD14, CD15, CD33; Urbano-Ispizua et al. (1990), CD13, CD14, CD33; Wiersma et al. (1991), CD13, CD14, CD33. The My^+ ALL cases originally included in the article which were only positive for CD11b, CD_w12 or CD36 are omitted from Pui et al. (1989)

the blast cells (Sobol et al. 1987; Childs et al. 1989; Guyotat et al. 1990). This led to the curious situation where cases lacking T- and B-cell-associated surface markers and carrying germline configurations for T-cell receptor and immunoglobulin genes were classified as ALL and termed "pure myeloid phenotype ALL" (Sobol et al. 1987; Childs et al. 1989).

Morphological Classification. It appears that morphology of the blast cells cannot be regarded as an independent variable and a reliable indicator for determining leukemic cell lineage and may, in fact, be misleading (Mirro and Kitchingman 1989). In view of the wide acceptance of the need for a multiparameter approach using various diagnostic criteria in addition to morphology, it does not seem advisable to rely on morphology as the sole criterion for leukemia diagnosis (Paietta 1990).

Some "ALL cases" lacking T- or B-cell surface markers but expressing myeloid antigens cannot be identified with the use of conventional FAB

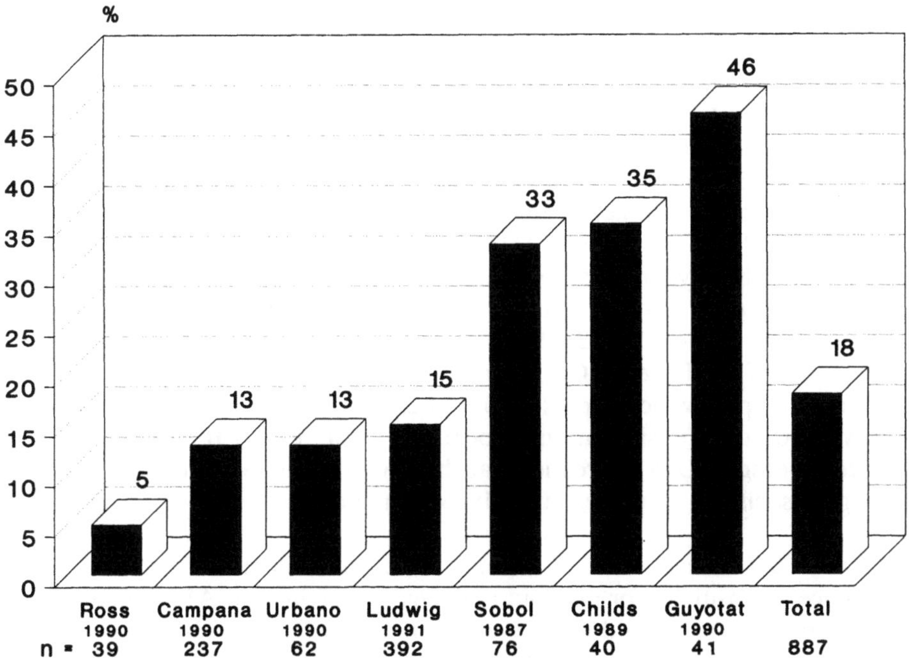

Fig. 3. Incidences of myeloid antigen-positive cases of adult ALL in seven large series totaling 887 cases (percent positive cases). The following myeloid-associated monoclonal antibodies were used: Ross et al. (1990), CD13, CD33; Campana et al. (1990), CD13, CD33; Urbano-Ispizua et al. (1990), CD13, CD14, CD33; Ludwig et al. (1991), CD13, CD33, CD_w65; Sobol et al. (1987), CD13, CD33; Childs et al. (1989), CD13, CD14, CD15; Guyotat et al. (1990), CD13, CD14, CD15, CD33

myeloid scheme parameters. These cases, apparently representing 2%–5% of all morphologically classified ALL cases (Garand et al. 1989), appear to be mostly proliferations of early myeloblasts which can only be recognized by immunological and ultrastructural methods (Kita et al. 1985; Matutes et al. 1988; Vainchenker et al. 1988). To this end the new category AML M0 for this early myeloblastic leukemia with immature morphology (mostly resembling L2) has been introduced into the FAB classification (Catovsky et al. 1991).

Reactivity of Different CD Monoclonal Antibodies. The most commonly studied monoclonal antibodies in the analysis of My^+ ALL cases belong to the CD13, CD14, CD15, CD33, and CD_w65 groups. Figure 4 illustrates the reactivity of individual anti-myeloid monoclonal antibodies combined for each CD group with leukemic cells from patients with ALL. Commonly a case is considered to be positive if 20%–30% or more of the blast cell population were labeled by the respective antibody. No significant differences were found between the CD13, CD14, CD15, CD33, and CD_w65 reactivity percentages (Fig. 4). These results, accumulated from 11 studies from 1987 to 1990, are nearly identical to previously reviewed data on My positivity of ALL cases (Drexler 1987).

Other anti-myeloid monoclonal antibodies assigned to groups CD11b, CD_w12, CD36 and others have been used to characterize the expression of myeloid-associated antigens on ALL cells (Bradstock et al. 1989; Childs et al. 1989; Pui et al. 1989). CD11b expression, though, is not exclusively confined to the myeloid lineage. CD11b is found on a proportion of lymphocytes including natural killer cells (Yamada et al. 1985). Therefore, it is not adequate to include CD11b reagents in the analysis of myeloid antigen expression of ALL cells. CD15 monoclonal antibodies detect the carbohydrate X-hapten which is present on ALL cells in a cryptic form but can be easily exposed by desialylation (Stockinger et al. 1984). It has been questioned whether CD15 expression can be regarded as evidence for myeloid lineage association (Greaves et al. 1986; Mirro et al. 1987).

T-Versus B-Lineage ALL. B-lineage ALL cases demonstrated a higher incidence of positivity for myeloid antigens than T-lineage ALL (on average 12% versus 8%), in children as well as in adults (Fig. 5) (Bradstock et al.

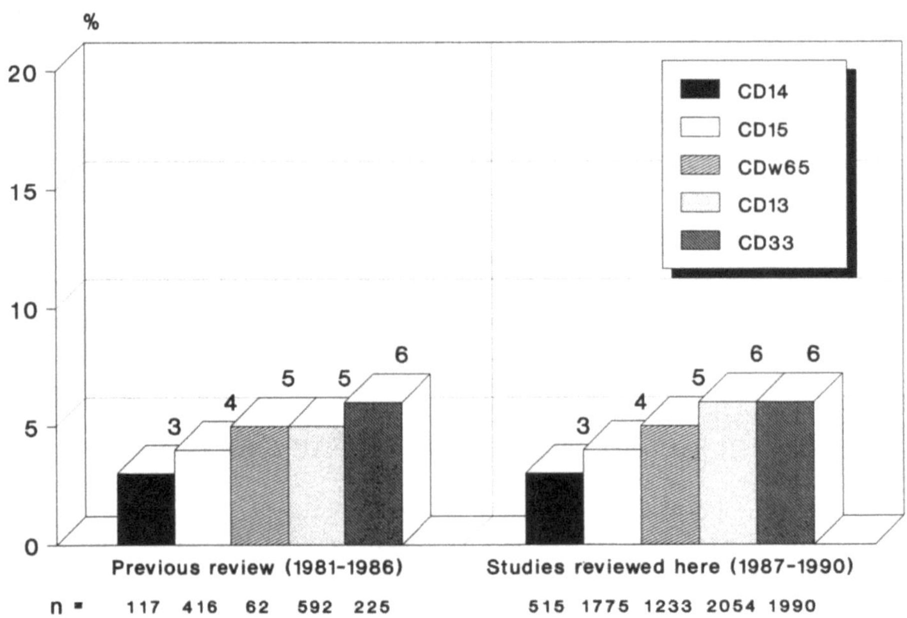

Fig. 4. Expression of myeloid-associated antigens on My^+ ALL detailed for the five different CD groups (percent positive cases). Data from 1987–1990 are compiled from the above studies totaling 3167 ALL cases. Previous data from 1981–1986 were summarized in Drexler (1986)

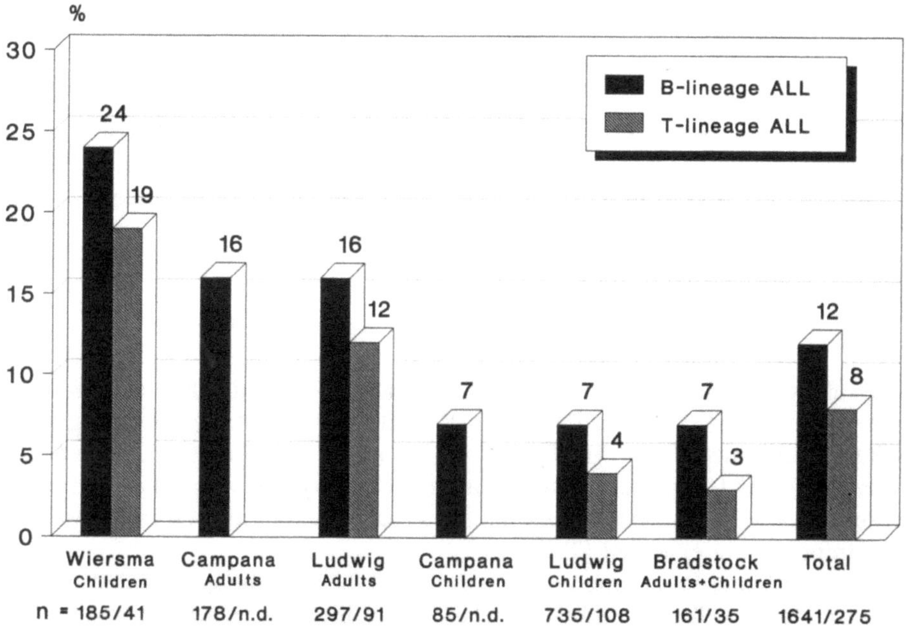

Fig. 5. Incidences of myeloid antigen-positive cases of B- and T-lineage ALL (percent positive cases). The following myeloid-associated monoclonal antibodies were used: Wiersma et al. (1991), CD13, CD14, CD33; Campana et al. (1990), CD13, CD33; Ludwig et al. (1991), CD13, CD33, CD_w65; Bradstock et al. (1989), CD13, CD33. *n.d.*, not described

1989; Campana et al. 1990; W.D. Ludwig et al., unpublished results; Wiersma et al. 1991).

CD34⁺, My⁺ ALL. The surface glycoprotein CD34 (e.g., detected by monoclonal antibody MY10) is expressed in normal human hematopoiesis only on progenitor cells (Strauss et al. 1986). Three studies noted a positive correlation between CD34 and myeloid antigen expression on ALL cells. High percentages of My^+ ALL cases were also $CD34^+$ (66%–93%) and 30% of $CD34^+$ ALL cases were My^+ (Vaughan et al. 1988; Borowitz et al. 1990; Guyotat et al. 1990). These data, which require independent confirmation, were interpreted as follows: ALL involving transformation of a pluripotent stem cell which undergoes limited differentiation after transformation is relatively common (Vaughan et al. 1988).

Chromosomal Aberrations. A nonrandom association of specific chromosomal abnormalities with the development of hybrid acute leukemia, acute mixed-lineage leukemia and My^+ ALL has become apparent (Paietta 1990; Pui et al. 1990). Translocations between chromosomes 4 and 11 were recognized as non-randomly associated with hybrid acute leukemia and acute mixed-lineage leukemia (Mirro et al. 1986; Gale and Ben-Bassat 1987; Mirro et al. 1987; Altman 1990). In particular, a correlation between My^+ ALL and translocations involving 11q23 was reported (Childs et al. 1989; Ludwig et al. 1989b; Guyotat et al. 1990; Hayashi et al. 1990a). Translocations involving 14q32 (Hayashi et al. 1990b; Paietta 1990) and t(9;22) (Chen et al. 1988; Childs et al. 1990; Guyotat et al. 1990) appear to be further non-random chromosome abnormalities in My^+ ALL.

Prognostic Relevance of My^+ ALL

Initially it was thought that cases of hybrid acute leukemia and acute mixed-lineage leukemia comprised a high-risk group with generally poor prognosis (Stass and Mirro 1986; Hoffbrand et al. 1988; Schiffer 1990). However, when My^+ ALL was interpreted as a distinct entity and when the treatment results of My^+ALL cases were analyzed separately for children and adults, a different picture emerged (Table 2).

It is difficult to compare the various studies as these included single institution as well as multicenter trials, used different treatment protocols, and measured different outcome parameters. A further study did not report the data separately for children and adults, and patients were treated with several protocols; however, the treatment outcomes of My^+ ALL cases in that study were not different from those anticipated in My^- ALL patients (Bradstock et al. 1989).

Children. In a series of more than 800 pediatric ALL cases, children with non-T ALL expressing myeloid-associated antigens had an apparently lower complete remission rate when treated with standard induction therapy (Weiner et al. 1985). However, the cells were tested only with CD15 monoclonal antibodies and a longer follow-up was not reported.

The data from three further more detailed studies (Table 2) suggest clearly that, in the context of contemporary intensive multiagent treatment, expression of myeloid-associated antigens on lymphoblasts has no apparent prognostic significance in childhood ALL (Dinndorf et al. 1986; Ludwig et al. 1989a; Pui et al. 1989; W.D. Ludwig et al., unpublished results).

In one of these studies, children with My^+ ALL showed a worse treatment outcome which, however, was confined to ($CD10^-$) pre-pre-B ALL patients and could mainly be attributed to the adverse biological and clinical characteristics (e.g., rearrangements involving band 11q23, age less than 1 year, high white blood cell count) of this subtype (Ludwig et al. 1989a, 1990, and unpublished results).

A recent study identified myeloid antigen expression on ALL cells in children as the most statistically significant predictor of a poor outcome (Wiersma et al. 1991). As noted above, the original diagnosis of ALL was

Table 2. Prognostic relevance of My^+ ALL

Reference	No. of patients	Clinical trial	Prognosis[a]	Parameter[b]
Children				
Dinndorf et al. 1986	62	Multicenter trial (CCSG)	Same	CR, CCR
Pui et al. 1989	372	Single institution (St. Jude)	Same	CR, survival
Ludwig et al. 1989a	570	Multicenter trial (Germany)	Same[c]	CR, EFS
Wiersma et al. 1991	236	Single institution (Los Angeles)	Worse	EFS
Adults				
Sobol et al. 1987	76	Multicenter trial (CALGB)	Worse	CR, survival[d]
Childs et al. 1989	40	Single institution (M.D. Anderson)	Worse	CR[e]
Urbano-Ispizua et al. 1990	62	Single institution (Barcelona)	Worse	CR, CCR, survival
Guyotat et al. 1990	41	Single institution (Lyon)	Worse	CR

[a] Compared with My-negative ALL (statistically significant).
[b] CR, complete remission (rate); CCR, continuous complete remission (duration); EFS, event-free survival.
[c] A worse prognosis was seen for the $CD10^-$ pre-pre-B ALL subtype (see text).
[d] Same prognosis regarding CCR.
[e] Same prognosis regarding survival.

based solely on the morphological appearance of the cells. It is conceivable that a certain number of the My^+ ALL cases in this study might in reality have been examples of AML.

Adults. The situation in adult My^+ ALL is more complicated. Obviously, if some of the cases diagnosed as My^+ ALL do in reality not contain lymphoblastic, but myeloblastic populations (there are ample examples in some studies, see above), then there is reason to believe that the failure of genuine AML cases to respond to ALL therapy will clearly falsify the statistics of treatment outcome of My^+ ALL compared with My^- ALL.

Keeping the above caveat in mind, four out of four studies concluded that adult My^+ ALL patients had a significantly poorer prognosis than those with My^- ALL (Table 2) (Sobol et al. 1987; Childs et al. 1989; Guyotat et al. 1990; Urbano-Ispizua et al. 1990).

Conclusions

While My^+ ALL does not belong to the category hybrid acute leukemia, it represents a subset of acute mixed-lineage leukemia. There are clearly significant differences between childhood and adult My^+ ALL (Table 3). The incidence of My^+ ALL in children is in the range of 5%–10%. There remains controversy regarding the frequency of adult My^+ ALL, but after critical review of technical artifacts, omission of cases labeled only by monoclonal antibodies not entirely specific for the myeloid lineage, and exclusion of obvious cases showing expression of myeloid antigens without immunophenotypic or genotypic evidence of lymphoid commitment, a conservative guess would put the actual incidence in the range of 10%–20%.

Except in one controversial study, no adverse prognostic value of myeloid-associated antigen expression was found in most subtypes of

Table 3. Synopsis of data on My^+ ALL

Incidence of My^+ ALL	
Children:	8% (range 5%–22%)
Adults:	18% (range 5%–46%)
Prognostic Relevance of My^+ ALL versus My^- ALL	
Children: same prognosis in 3 studies (worse prognosis in 1 study)	
Adults: worse prognosis in 1 study	
Biological parameters associated with My^+ ALL	
Higher incidence in B-lineage ALL than in T-lineage ALL	
Nonrandom chromosomal abnormalities: t(9; 22), 11q23, 14q32	
No predominance of individual myeloid-associated antigens	
Possibly positivity for CD34	

childhood ALL. By contrast, a significantly poorer outcome was commonly seen in adults in the myeloid antigen-positive ALL group. My^+ ALL appears to be associated predominantly with B-cell origin, non-random chromosome abnormalities (t(9;22) and translocations involving 11q23 and 14q32), and possibly positivity for the progenitor marker CD34.

In the majority of acute leukemias a diagnosis can be established by standard FAB criteria based on morphology and cytochemistry (Hoffbrand et al. 1988). However, these techniques should be employed in combination with immunophenotypic and cytogenetic analysis. In cases where morpho-cytochemical FAB classification would give an inconclusive result, the application of expanded diagnostic approaches can indicate more clearly the lymphoid or myeloid origin of the neoplastic cells. In particular, with the combined use of a standardized panel of monoclonal antibodies it is possible to safely establish the lineage affiliation and subgrouping of virtually all acute leukemias (Campana and Janossy 1986; Janossy et al. 1989).

Acknowledgements. We are indebted to the participants of the German multicenter trials, ALL/NHL-BFM and ALL/AUL-BMFT, for their cooperation.

References

Altman AJ (1990) Clinical features and biological implications of acute mixed lineage (hybrid) leukemias. Am J Pediatr Hematol Oncol 12:123–133
Ben-Bassat I, Gale RP (1984) Hybrid acute leukemia. Leuk Res 8:929–936
Bennett JM, Catovsky D, Daniel MT, Flandrin G, Galton DAG, Gralnick HR, Sultan C (1985) Proposed revised criteria for the classification of acute myeloid leukemia: a report of the French-American-British Cooperative Group. Ann Intern Med 103:626–629
Borowitz MJ, Shuster JJ, Civin CI, Carroll AJ, Look AT, Behm FG, Land VJ, Pullen DJ, Crist WM (1990) Prognostic significance of CD34 expression in childhood B-precursor acute lymphocytic leukemia: a Pediatric Oncology Group study. J Clin Oncol 8:1389–1398
Bradstock KF, Kirk J, Grimsley PG, Kabral A, Hughes WG (1989) Unusual immunophenotypes in acute leukaemias: incidence and clinical correlations. Br J Haematol 72:512–518
Brincker H, Jensen K (1972) Cytomorphological classification of acute leukemia. Dan Med Bull 19:215–221
Browman GP, Neame PB, Soamboonsrup P (1986) The contributions of cytochemistry and immunophenotyping to the reproducibility of the FAB classification in acute leukemia. Blood 68:900–905
Campana D, Janossy G (1986) Leukemia diagnosis and testing of complement fixing antibodies for bone marrow purging in ALL. Blood 68:1264–1271
Campana D, Coustan-Smith E, Janossy G (1990) The immunologic detection of minimal residual disease in acute leukemia. Blood 76:163–171
Catovsky D, Matutes E, Buccheri V, Shetty V, Hanslip J, Yoshida N, Morilla R (1991) A classification of acute leukaemia for the 1990s. Ann Hematol 62:16–21
Chan LC, Pegram SM, Greaves MF (1985) Contribution of immunophenotype to the classification and differential diagnosis of acute leukaemia. Lancet i:475–479

Chen Z, Sigaux F, Miglierina R, Valensi F, Daniel M, Ochoa-Noguera M, Flandrin G (1986) Immunological typing of acute lymphoblastic leukemia: concurrent analysis by flow cytofluorometry and immunocytology. Leuk Res 10:1411–1417
Chen SJ, Flandrin G, Daniel MT, Valensi F, Baranger L, Grausz D, Bernheim A, Chen Z, Sigaux F, Berger R (1988) Philadelphia-positive acute leukemia: lineage promiscuity and inconsistently rearranged breakpoint cluster region. Leukemia 2:261–273
Childs CC, Hirsch-Ginsberg C, Walters RS, Andersson BS, Reuben J, Trujillo JM, Cork A, Stass SA, Freireich EJ, Zipf TF (1989) Myeloid surface antigen-positive acute lymphoblastic leukemia (My^+ ALL): immunophenotypic, ultrastructural, cytogenetic, and molecular characteristics. Leukemia 3:777–783
Dinndorf PA, Andrews RG, Benjamin D, Ridgway D, Wolff L, Bernstein ID (1986) Expression of normal myeloid-associated antigens by acute leukemia cells. Blood 67:1048–1053
Drexler HG (1987) Classification of acute myeloid leukemias – a comparison of FAB and immunophenotyping. Leukemia 1:697–705
Drexler HG, Scott CS (1989) Morphological and immunological aspects of leukaemia diagnosis. In: Scott CS (ed) Leukaemia cytochemistry – principles and practice. Horwood, Chichester, pp 13–59
Drexler HG, Menon M, Gignac SM, Misra B, Minowada J (1986) Diagnostic value of immunological phenotyping. Acta Haematol 76:1–8
Foon KA, Naiem F, Yale C, Gale RP (1979) Acute myelogenous leukemia: morphologic classification and response to therapy. Leuk Res 3:171–173
Gale RP, Ben-Bassat I (1987) Hybrid acute leukaemia. Br J Haematol 65:261–264
Garand R, Vannier JP, Bene MC, Faure GC, Bernard A (1989) Correlations between acute lymphoid leukemia (ALL) immunophenotype and clinical and laboratory data at presentation. A study of 350 patients. Cancer 64: 1437–1446
Greaves MF, Chan LC, Furley AJW, Watt SM, Molgaard HV (1986) Lineage promiscuity in hemopoietic differentiation and leukemia. Blood 67:1–11
Guyotat D, Campos L, Shi ZH, Charrin C, Treille D, Magaud JP, Fiere D (1990) Myeloid surface antigen expression in adult acute lymphoblastic leukemia. Leukemia 4:664–666
Hayashi Y, Sugita K, Nakazawa S, Abe T, Kojima S, Inaba T, Hanada R, Yamamoto K (1990a) Karyotypic patterns in acute mixed lineage leukemia. Leukemia 4:121–126
Hayashi Y, Pui CH, Behm FG, Fuchs AH, Raimondi SC, Kitchingman GR, Mirro J Jr, Williams DL (1990b) 14q32 Translocations are associated with mixed-lineage expression in childhood acute leukemia. Blood 76:150–156
Head DR, Savage RA, Cerezo L, Graven CM, Bickers JN, Hartsock R, Hosty TA, Saiki JH, Wilson HE, Morrison FS, Coltman CA Jr, Hutton JJ (1985) Reproducibility of the French-American-British classification of acute leukemia: the Southwest Oncology Group experience. Am J Hematol 18:47–57
Herrmann F, Dörken B, Gatzke A, Ludwig WD (1986) Immunological classification of "unclassifiable" acute leukemia. In: Reinherz EL, Haynes BF, Nadler LM, Bernstein ID (eds) Leukocyte typing II: 2. Human B lymphocytes. Springer, Berlin Heidelberg New York, pp 367–375
Hoffbrand AV, Leber BF, Browett PJ, Norton JD (1988) Mixed acute leukaemias. Blood Rev 2:9–15
Huh YO, Kantarjian H, Childs CC, Reuben J, McCredie K (1990) Classification of adult ALL by immunophenotype. Blood 76:282a
Janossy G, Hoffbrand AV, Greaves MF, Ganeshaguru K, Pain C, Bradstock KF, Prentice HG, Kay HEM (1980) Terminal transferase enzyme assay and immunological membrane markers in the diagnosis of leukaemia – a multiparameter analysis of 300 cases. Br J Haematol 44:221–234

Janossy G, Coustan-Smith E, Campana D (1989) The reliability of cytoplasmic CD3 and CD22 antigen expression in the immunodiagnosis of acute leukemia: a study of 500 cases. Leukemia 3:170–181
Katz F, Malcolm S, Gibbons B, Tilly R, Lam G, Robertson ME, Czepulkowski B, Chessells J (1988) Cellular and molecular studies on infant null acute lymphoblastic leukemia. Blood 71:1438–1447
Kita K, Nasu K, Kamesaki H, Doi S, Tezuka H, Tatsumi E, Fukuhara S, Nishikori M, Uchino H, Shirakawa S (1985) Phenotypic analysis of acute lymphoblastic leukemia (ALL) cells which are classified as Non-T Non-B and negative for common ALL antigen. Blood 66:47–52
Lee EJ, Pollak A, Leavitt RD, Testa JR, Schiffer CA (1987) Minimally differentiated acute nonlymphocytic leukemia: a distinct entity. Blood 70:1400–1406
Lee SL, Livings D, James GW, Schroeder L, Selawry O, Stickney JM (1962) Morphological classification of acute leukemias. Cancer Treat Rep 16:151–153
Ludwig WD, Bartram CR, Thiel E, Teichmann JV, Harbott J, Reiter A, Riehm H (1989a) Childhood acute lymphoblastic leukemia with co-expression of myeloid antigens (My$^+$ ALL): incidence, genotype and clinical significance. Blood 74:197a
Ludwig WD, Bartram CR, Harbott J, Köller U, Haas OA, Hansen-Hagge T, Heil G, Seibt-Jung H, Teichmann JV, Ritter J, Knapp W, Gadner H, Thiel E, Riehm HJ (1989b) Phenotypic and genotypic heterogeneity in infant acute leukemia: I. Acute lymphoblastic leukemia. Leukemia 3:431–439
Ludwig WD, Thiel E, Köller U, Bartram CR, Harbott J, Teichmann JV, Seibt-Jung H, Creutzig U, Ritter J, Riehm H (1990) Incidence and clinical implications of acute hybrid leukemia in childhood. Haematol Blood Transfus 33:516–522
Maitreyan V, Gale RP (1989) What is hybrid acute leukemia? Leuk Res 13:725–728
Matutes E, Pombo de Oliveira M, Foroni L, Morilla R, Catovsky D (1988) The role of ultrastructural cytochemistry and monoclonal antibodies in clarifying the nature of undifferentiated cells in acute leukaemia. Br J Haematol 69:205–211
Mertelsmann R, Thaler HT, To L, Gee TS, McKenzie S, Schauer P, Friedman A, Arlin Z, Cirrincione C, Clarkson B (1980) Morphological classification, response to therapy, and survival in 263 adult patients with acute nonlymphoblastic leukemia. Blood 56:773–781
Mirro J Jr, Kitchingman GR (1989) The morphology, cytochemistry, molecular characteristics and clinical significance of acute mixed-lineage leukaemia. In: Scott CS (ed) Leukaemia cytochemistry – principles and practice. Horwood, Chichester, pp 155–179
Mirro J Jr, Zipf TF, Pui CH, Kitchingman G, Williams D, Melvin S, Murphy SB, Stass S (1985) Acute mixed lineage leukemia: clinicopathologic correlations and prognostic significance. Blood 66:1115–1123
Mirro J Jr, Kitchingman G, Williams D, Lauzon GJ, Lin CC, Callihan T, Zipf T (1986) Clinical and laboratory characteristics of acute leukemia with the 4;11 translocation. Blood 67:689–697
Mirro J Jr, Kitchingman GR, Stass SA (1987) Lineage heterogeneity in acute leukemia. Acute mixed lineage leukemia and lineage switch. In: Stass SA (ed) The acute leukemias. Biologic, diagnostic, and therapeutic determinants. Dekker, New York, pp 383–402
Paietta E (1990) Ambiguous phenotypes in acute leukemia. Leuk Lymph 2:17–33
Pui CH, Behm FG, Singh B, Rivera GK, Schell MJ, Roberts WM, Crist WM, Mirro J Jr (1989) Myeloid-associated antigen expression lacks prognostic value in childhood acute lymphoblastic leukemia treated with intensive multiagent chemotherapy. Blood 75:198–202
Pui CH, Crist WM, Look AT (1990) Biology and clinical significance of cytogenetic abnormalities in childhood acute lymphoblastic leukemia. Blood 76:1449–1463

Ross CW, Stoolman LM, Schnitzer B, Schlegelmilch JA, Hanson CA (1990) Immunophenotypic aberrancy in adult acute lymphoblastic leukemia. Am J Clin Pathol 94:590–599

Schiffer CA (1990) Hybrid leukemias. In: Gale RP, Hoelzer D (eds) Acute lymphoblastic leukemia. Wiley-Liss, New York, pp 129–142 (UCLA symposia on molecular and cellular biology, vol 108)

Sobol RE, Mick R, Royston I, Davey FR, Ellison RR, Newman R, Cuttner J, Griffin JD, Collins H, Nelson DA, Bloomfield CD (1987) Clinical importance of myeloid antigen expression in adult acute lymphoblastic leukemia. N Engl J Med 316:1111–1117

Stass SA, Mirro J Jr (1985) Unexpected heterogeneity in acute leukemia: mixed lineages and lineage switch. Hum Pathol 16:864–866

Stass SA, Mirro J Jr (1986) Lineage heterogeneity in acute leukaemia: acute mixed-lineage leukaemia and lineage switch. Clin Haematol 15:811–827

Stockinger H, Majdic O, Liszka K, Aberer W, Bettelheim P, Lutz D, Knapp W (1984) Exposure by desialylation of myeloid antigens on acute lymphoblastic leukemia cells. J Natl Cancer Inst 73:7–11

Strauss LC, Rosely SD, LaRussa VF, Sharkis SJ, Stuart RK, Civin CI (1986) Antigenic analysis of hematopoiesis: V. Characterization of My10 antigen expression by normal lymphohematopoietic progenitor cells. Exp Hematol 14:878–886

Tien HF, Wang CH, Wu HS, Su IJ, Chien SH, Chen YC, Lin DT, Lin KH, Shen MC (1990) Immunoglobulin and T-cell receptor gene rearrangements in acute lymphoblastic leukemia – A higher incidence of dual genotype in patients with myeloid antigen expression. Blood 76:327a

Urbano-Ispizua A, Matutes E, Villamor N, Ribera JM, Feliu E, Montserrat E, Granena A, Vives-Corrons JL, Rozman C (1990) Clinical significance of the presence of myeloid associated antigens in acute lymphoblastic leukaemia. Br J Haematol 75:202–207

Vainchenker W, Villeval JL, Tabilio A, Matamis H, Karianakis G, Guichard J, Henri A, Vernant JP, Rochant H, Breton-Gorius J (1988) Immunophenotype of leukemic blasts with small peroxidase-positive granules detected by electron microscopy. Leukemia 2:274–281

Vaughan WP, Civin CI, Weisenburger DD, Karp JE, Graham ML, Sanger WG, Grierson HL, Joshi SS, Burke PJ (1988) Acute leukemia expressing the normal human hematopoietic stem cell membrane glycoprotein CD34 (MY10). Leukemia 2:661–666

Viana MB, Maurer HS, Ferenc C (1980) Subclassification of acute lymphoblastic leukaemia in children: analysis of the reproducibility of morphological criteria and prognostic implications. Br J Haematol 44:383–388

Weiner M, Borowitz M, Boyett J, Civin K, Metzger R, McKolnis J, Crist W, Dowell B, Pullen J (1985) Clinical pathologic aspects of myeloid antigen positivity in pediatric patients with acute lymphoblastic leukemia (ALL). Proc Am Soc Clin Oncol 4:172

Wiersma S, Ortega J, Sobel E, Weinberg K (1991) Clinical importance of myeloid-antigen expression in acute lymphoblastic leukemia of childhood. N Engl J Med 324:800–808

Yamada H, Martin PJ, Bean MA, Braun MP, Beatty PG, Sadamoto K, Hansen J (1985) Monoclonal antibody 9.3 and anti-CD11 antibodies define reciprocal subsets of lymphocytes. Eur J Immunol 15:1164–1168

Youness E, Trujillo JM, Ahearn MJ, McCredie KB, Cork A (1980) Acute unclassified leukemia. A clinicopathologic study with diagnostic implications of electron microscopy. Am J Hematol 9:79–88

Myeloid-Associated Antigen Expression in Childhood Acute Lymphoblastic Leukemia

F.M. Fink[1,4], U. Köller[2], H. Mayer[1], O.A. Haas[1], E.R. Grümayer[1], C. Urban[3], K. Dengg[4], I. Mutz[5], H. Tüchler[1], I. Gatterer-Menz[1], W. Knapp[2], and H. Gadner[1], for the Austrian Pediatric Oncology Group

[1] St. Anna Children's Hospital, Vienna, Austria
[2] Institute of Immunology, University of Vienna, Austria
[3] Department of Pediatrics, University of Graz, Austria
[4] Department of Pediatrics, University of Innsbruck, Anichstraße 35, Innsbruck, Austria
[5] Department of Pediatrics, Regional Hospital Leoben, Austria

Introduction

Coexpression of myeloid-associated antigens has been demonstrated in several studies on acute lymphoblastic leukemia (ALL). The proportion of cases with this aberrant antigen expression (myA$^+$ ALL) ranged from 5% to over 20% in pediatric series (Weiner et al. 1985; Ludwig et al. 1990; Pui et al. 1990; Wiersma et al. 1991) and was even higher in adult ALL (Sobol et al. 1987; Childs et al. 1989). The prognostic relevance of myeloid-associated antigen expression in childhood ALL remains controversial (Ludwig et al. 1990; Pui et al. 1990; Wiersma et al. 1991). In adults, however, myA$^+$ ALL represents a high-risk group as demonstrated by fewer complete remissions and shorter survival time (Sobol et al. 1987; Childs et al. 1989). This prospective study of childhood ALL reports clinical features and treatment outcome in relation to myeloid-associated antigen expression.

Patients and Methods

Two hundred and fifty one consecutive children up to 18 years of age with immunologically verified B-cell precursor ALL (surface immunoglobulin, sIg, negative) or T-cell ALL (T-ALL) were enrolled in two consecutive protocols (ALL-A-84 and ALL-BFM-86). From 1984 to 1990 they were diagnosed and treated in 11 pediatric centers in Austria. Complete immunophenotyping including adequate evaluation of myeloid-associated antigen expression was performed in 206 patients (82%). Patients with 3% or more myeloperoxidase-positive blast cells and children with mature B-cell ALL (B-ALL) (surface immunoglobulin positive) were excluded.

Recent Results in Cancer Research, Vol. 131

Diagnosis

All specific diagnostic procedures were performed in a reference laboratory. May–Grünwald–Giemsa-stained bone marrow smears were morphologically classified according to the FAB classification (Bennett et al. 1976). Standard techniques were applied for cytochemical staining (periodic acid-Schiff reagent, acid phosphatase, myeloperoxidase, and α-naphthylesterase staining). For immunophenotyping peripheral blood (PB) and bone marrow (BM) specimens were collected at diagnosis prior to any therapy. Following isolation (Ficoll-Hypaque density gradient) mononuclear cells (MNC) were exposed to a panel of monoclonal antibodies (MAbs) with the following specificities: (1) precursor cells, anti-HLA-D (VID1); (2) lymphoid lineage, CD1 (VIT6), CD2 (9.6), CD3 (VIT3b), CD5 (MT61), CD7 (CD7-6B7, WT1), CD10 (VIL-A1), CD19 (HD37), CD24 (VIB-C5), sIgM; granulocyte/monocyte lineage, CD11b (VIM12), CD13 (My7), CD33 (My9), CD_w65 (VIM2); granulocyte lineage, CD15 (VIM-D5); monocyte lineage, CD14 (VIM13, 63D3); erythroid lineage, anti-glycophorin A (VIE-G4); erythroid/megakaryocyte lineage, anti-blood-group H (CLB-ERY3); megakaryocytic lineage, anti-platelet glycoprotein IIb/IIIa–CD41 (VIPL1, C17–27), anti-platelet glycoprotein IIIa (VIPL2). Acetone- fixed cytospin preparations of leukemic blasts were analyzed for cytoplasmic IgM and terminal deoxyribonucleotidyl transferase (TdT) (Supertech Inc., Bethesda, MD, USA) reactivity. The specificity and reaction pattern of the MAbs has been reported elsewhere (Majdic et al. 1984; Knapp et al. 1989; Köller et al. 1989; Ludwig et al. 1989). Nonspecific Fc receptor binding was blocked by adding human IgG (Serogam, Sero, Vienna, Austria) to the cell suspension. The binding of MAb was assessed by indirect immunofluorescence staining with fluorescein (FITC) conjugated $F(ab)_2$ fragments of sheep anti-mouse IgG and IgM antibodies. Membrane and cytoplasmic or nuclear fluorescence were analyzed using an epiilluminated fluorescence microscope (Leitz Ortholux, Wetzlar, FRG). Mature myeloid cells were excluded from the count.

Results were considered positive if at least 20% of blast cells expressed a particular surface antigen, or if more than 10% expressed a cytoplasmic antigen, respectively. Based on the results of immunophenotyping leukemias were classified as pre-pre-B-ALL (CD10-negative B-cell precursor ALL), common ALL (CD10-positive B-cell precursor ALL), pre-B-ALL (cytoplasmic Ig-positive common ALL), B-ALL (surface Ig-positive, TdT-negative, B-lineage ALL) and T-ALL (Foon et al. 1982).

Definitions and Statistical Analysis

Complete remission (CR) was defined as less than 5% blast cells in the bone marrow together with regeneration of peripheral blood cell counts without evidence of leukemia. Relapse was diagnosed with unequivocal reappearance of >5% blast cells in the bone marrow or any extramedullary, histologically documented appearance of leukemic blasts after CR had been achieved.

Event-free survival was defined as the time from diagnosis until relapse or death in CR. Failure to achieve CR (nonresponse or early death) was considered an event at zero time. Life table analyses were performed by the Kaplan–Meier product-limit method (Kaplan and Meier 1958). Differences in event-free survival among groups were compared by the log-rank test (Mantel 1966). Univariate and multivariate Cox proportional-hazards methods were used to evaluate the prognostic impact of covariates (Cox 1972). Differences of variables at diagnosis were analyzed by the continuity adjusted χ^2 test for categorical variables, by the Wilcoxon two-sample test for continuous variables. Differences with $p < 0.05$ were considered significant.

Treatment Protocol

All patients were intensively treated according to a modified (ALL-A-84; Gruemayer et al. 1990) or the original (ALL-BFM-86, a modified successor of the ALL-BFM-83 protocol; Riehm et al. 1987) protocol of the BFM group. Treatment was risk-adapted in both protocols, and apart from minor differences the treatment schedules were similar in both studies. All patients received protocol I (an induction therapy with prednisone, vincristine, daunorubicin, and *l*-asparaginase for 4–5 weeks and an intensive early consolidation with cyclophosphamide, 6-mercaptopurine, cytosine arabinoside, and methotrexate intrathecally for 4 weeks). Following an 8-week period with oral 6-mercaptopurine and four intravenous doses of intermediate- (ALL-A-84) or high-dose (ALL-BFM-86) methotrexate (protocol M), an early reinduction with dexamethasone, vincristine, doxorubicin, *l*-asparaginase, cyclophosphamide, 6-thioguanine, cytosine arabinoside, and methotrexate intrathecally for 4 (protocol III) to 6 weeks (protocol II) was applied. Maintenance treatment consisted of daily oral 6-mercaptopurine and weekly methotrexate until 2 years from diagnosis. High-risk patients of study ALL-A-84 received an intensification protocol including teniposide and cytosine arabinoside for 2 weeks before protocol II. High-risk patients of the ALL-BFM-86 study were treated with high-dose methotrexate, high-dose cytosine arabinoside, ifosfamide, mitoxantrone, and prednisone (protocol E) instead of protocol M. In study ALL-A-84 age-adapted cranial irradiation was given to all children at a dose of 12–18 Gy. In study ALL-BFM-86 standard-risk patients and children younger than 1 year were not irradiated. All other children received, age- and risk-adapted, 12–18 Gy radiation.

Results

One hundred and thirteen children suffered from common ALL (including eight cases not tested for cytoplasmic immunoglobulin), 50 from pre-B-ALL, 12 from pre-pre-B, and 31 from T-ALL. Atypical myeloid marker expression was found in 23 out of 175 patients (13.1%) with B-cell precursor ALL, and in one out of 31 patients (3.2%) with T-ALL (Table 1).

Among 18 cases with expression of one myeloid marker only, CD_w65 (9 patients) was the most common one, followed by CD13 (4 patients), CD15 (2 patients), CD33, and blood group H (2 patients each). Expression of two myeloid-associated antigens was found in five patients (3 cases with CD15/CD_w65, 1 case with CD13/CD33, 1 case with CD_w65/blood group H) (Table 2).

Atypical myeloid antigen expression was found in any subtype of B-cell precursor ALL. However, there was a significant association with CD10-negative cases (pre-pre-B-ALL) ($p < 0.0001$, Table 1).

Compared to myA^- cases, children with myA^+ ALL presented with higher initial leukocyte counts (median 8.45 vs 21.8×10^{12}/l, $p = 0.056$) and higher hemoglobin values (median 7.45 vs 8.7 g/dl, $p = 0.054$). Other parameters (age at diagnosis, sex distribution, hepatosplenomegaly, platelet count, FAB-L1/L2 ratio, frequency of CNS and thymus involvement) were similar in both groups.

Myeloid-associated antigen expression did not influence remission induction rates: 95.7% and 98.7% of children with myA^+ ALL and myA^- ALL, respectively, achieved CR. However, the probability of event-free survival (p_{EFS}) after 5 years (median observation time in remission 44 months) was significantly lower for myA^+ ALL (37.8% vs 74.6%, $p = 0.0001$, Fig. 1). This was not explained by differences in leukocyte counts as demonstrated by life table analysis stratified for leukocyte count (cut-off

Table 1. Immunological subtypes of childhood ALL and corresponding cases with myeloid antigen expression

	Cases		myA^+	
	(*n*)	(%)	(*n*)	(%)
Common ALL[a]	113	54.9	9	8.0
Pre-B-ALL	50	24.3	4	8.0
Pre-pre-B-ALL	12	5.8	10	83.3
B-cell precursor ALL	175	85.0	23	13.1
T-ALL	31	15.0	1	3.2
Total	206	100.0	24	11.7

[a] Eight patients not tested for cytoplasmic immunoglobulin.

Table 2. Results of immunophenotyping in 23 cases of B-cell precursor ALL with myeloid-associated antigen expression (% positive bone marrow blast cells)

Patient	Diagnosis	CD13	CD15	CD33	CD_w65	CLB-ERY3
1	c-ALL	30	0	0	0	0
2rd	c-ALL	0	40	ND	5	ND
3[r]	c-ALL	0	0	90	0	0
4	c-ALL	0	ND	50	10	ND
5[r]	c-ALL	0	0	0	20	0
6rd	c-ALL	0	0	0	30	0
7	c-ALL	0	ND	0	50	ND
8	c-ALL[a]	0	0	0	60	0
9	c-ALL	70	0	70	0	10
10[r]	pb-ALL	35	0	0	0	15
11	pb-ALL	50	0	0	0	0
12	pb-ALL	0	80	0	10	0
13	pb-ALL	0	5	0	0	20
14[r]	ppb-ALL	20	0	0	0	0
15	ppb-ALL	0	15	5	20	0
16[r]	ppb-ALL	0	0	0	20	0
17	ppb-ALL	0	10	0	20	0
18	ppb-ALL	ND	ND	ND	80	ND
19nd	ppb-ALL	0	0	0	0	40
20[cd]	ppb-ALL	0	30	0	40	0
21rd	ppb-ALL	0	60	0	60	0
22rd	ppb-ALL	0	20	0	50	0
23	ppb-ALL	0	0	50	2	30

All blast cells tested for CD11b ($n = 19$) and CD14 ($n = 21$) were negative. ND, not done; CD, cluster of differentiation designation; c-ALL, common-ALL; pb-ALL, pre-B-ALL; ppb-ALL, pre-pre-B-ALL. [nd] Died after nonresponse; [r] relapsed but alive; [rd] died after relapse; [cd] died in remission. [a] Differentiation between c- and pb-ALL not possible (cIgM not tested).

point 50×10^{12}/l, data not shown). Even after exclusion of patients with CD10-negative disease (pre-pre-B-ALL) as well as of infants below the age of 1 year at diagnosis, the negative prognostic influence of myeloid antigen expression was still evident from the analysis: p_{EFS} was 76.1% (SE 4.0%) for 148 children older than 1 year with myA^- common/pre-B-ALL and 35.9% (SE 18.8%) for 13 corresponding cases with myA^+ disease (p = 0.005, log-rank test).

As demonstrated by multivariate analysis, the expression of myeloid-associated antigens was the most important covariate for prognosis (p_{EFS}) of children with B-cell precursor ALL (Table 3). Of all the other variables tested (initial leukocyte count, age, sex, CNS involvement) the initial leukocyte count was the only one of independent prognostic significance.

Among 31 children with T-ALL only one case with myeloid coex-pression was found (CD_w65). Remission was achieved in this patient and he is still alive in remission 16 months after diagnosis.

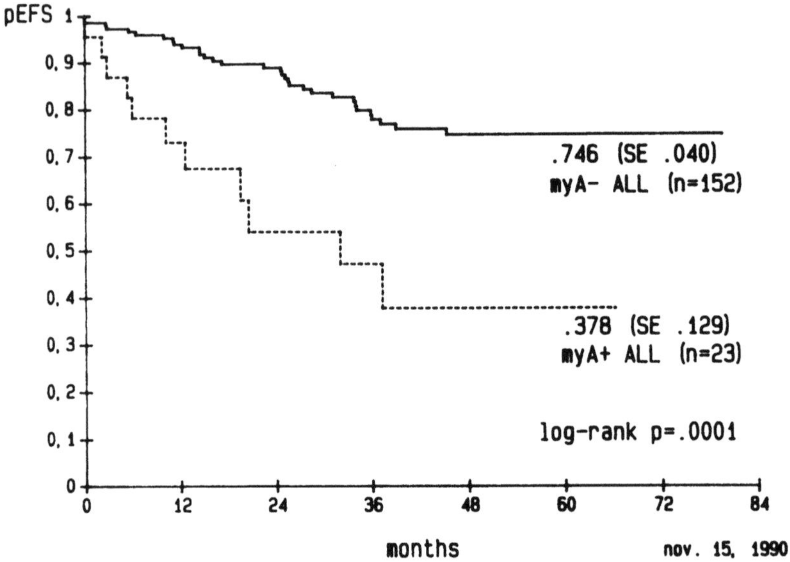

Fig. 1. B-cell precursor ALL (n = 175), probability of event-free survival (p_{EFS}). myA$^+$, cases with myeloid antigen expression; *my*A$^-$, cases without myeloid antigen expression

Table 3. Prognostic significance of presenting variables for probability of event-free survival in children with B-cell precursor ALL (n = 175)

Variable	Univariate *p* value	Multivariate *p* value	Relative risk
Myeloid-associated antigen expression	0.0001	0.0007	3.9039
WBC $\geqslant 50 \times 10^{12}/1$	0.0011	0.0075	2.7393
CNS involvement	0.0168	0.0840	3.4800
Age <1 or >10 years	0.0897	0.7176	–
Male sex	0.8373	0.5500	–

Discussion

Lymphoblasts from 13.1% of children with B-cell precursor ALL expressed myeloid-associated antigens. This frequency is comparable with that reported by Pui et al. (1990), who also applied a broad panel of MAbs (CD11b, CD_w12, CD13, CD14, CD15, CD33, CD36). Ludwig et al. (1990), testing for CD13, CD15, CD33 and CD_w65, and Weiner et al. (1985), testing for CD13 and CD15, found a lower frequency, which is probably explained by the restricted number of myeloid-associated antigens analyzed.

However, Wiersma et al. (1991) found a higher percentage of myA$^+$ ALL, although they tested for three myeloid-associated antigens only (CD13, CD14, CD33).

In our series, atypical expression of myeloid markers was associated with pre-pre-B-ALL. Whereas 83.3% of this undifferentiated subgroup of B-cell precursor ALL were positive for at least one myeloid-associated antigen, only 8% of common or pre-B-ALL showed a similar pattern. In T-ALL expression of myeloid markers was only sporadically seen. Pui et al. (1990) and Wiersma et al. (1991) did not observe any differences within the immunologically defined subgroups. However, results similar to our own series where found by Weiner et al. (1985) and Ludwig et al. (1990).

CD_w65 – in our series the most frequently identified myeloid-associated antigen – has only been reported by Ludwig et al. (1990) on ALL blast cells. In both series it was predominantly associated with pre-pre-B-ALL. Three cases showed reactivity with anti-blood-group H. While this antigen is restricted to erythroid and megakaryocytic cell lines within normal hematopoiesis it had been detected on blasts from de novo as well as secondary leukemias, irrespective of lineage involvement, and in chronic myelocytic leukemia blast crisis (Dunstan et al. 1985; Köller et al. 1987).

In contrast to previous reports, we did not find a single case with CD11b (Pui et al. 1990) or CD14 (Wiersma et al. 1991) expression. Since CD11b is not an antigen exclusively found on normal myeloid cells but also on monocytes and lymphoid cells (NK cells), it may not be a marker of lineage infidelity of lymphoblasts. Despite the assignment of MAbs to specific CD antigens by the International Workshops on Human Leukocyte Differentiation Antigens (Knapp et al. 1989), the conflicting results on the antigens CD11b and CD14 may point to problems arising with the usage of different MAbs and/or techniques.

Children with myA$^+$ ALL had a significantly shorter event-free survival time than those with myA$^-$ ALL. Initial leukocyte count was an additional independent prognostic factor. However, by multivariate analysis as well as univariate analysis stratified for leukocyte counts, myeloid-associated antigen expression was identified as the most important prognostic variable for p_{EFS}. More than 40% of cases with myA$^+$ ALL belonged to the most immature CD10-negative pre-pre-B-ALL, a phenotype often seen in infants below 1 year of age. However, a separate analysis restricted to CD10-positive B-cell precursor ALL (common and pre-B-ALL) in children older than 1 year of age showed the same independent prognostic significance of myeloid-associated antigen expression.

At the present time the discussion about the prognostic relevance of myeloid-associated antigen expression in childhood ALL is controversial. While our group, together with other authors (Wiersma et al. 1991), identified myeloid antigen expression as a significant prognostic factor for event-free survival, others (Ludwig et al. 1990; Pui et al. 1990) did not find an impact on prognosis. Further studies with adequate phenotyping, sufficiently large patient numbers, and long-term follow-up are necessary to clarify the issue.

References

Bennett JM, Catovsky D, Daniel MT, Flandrin G, Galton DAG, Gralnick HR, Sultan C (1976) Proposals for the classification of acute leukaemias. Br J Haematol 33:451–458

Childs CC, Hirsch-Ginsberg C, Walters RS et al. (1989) Myeloid surface antigen-positive acute lymphoblastic leukemia (myA$^+$ ALL): immunophenotypic, ultrastructural, cytogenetic, and molecular characteristics. Leukemia 3:777–783

Cox DR (1972) Regression models and life-tables. J R Stat Soc (B) 34:187–220

Dunstan RA, Simpson MB, Knowles RW et al. (1985) The origin of ABH antigens on human platelets. Blood 65:615–619

Foon KA, Schroff RW, Gale RP (1982) Surface markers on leukemia and lymphoma cells: recent advances. Blood 60:1–19

Gruemayer ER, Gadner H, Mutz I et al. (1990) Childhood acute lymphoblastic leukemia: results of the Austrian cooperative study group with the ALL-A-84 protocol. Med Pediatr Oncol 18:6–14

Kaplan EL, Meier P (1958) Nonparametric estimation from incomplete observations. J Am Stat Assoc 53:457–481

Knapp W, Dörken B, Rieber P, Schmidt RE, Stein H, von dem Borne AEGK (1989) CD antigens 1989. Blood 74:1448–1450

Köller U, Bettelheim P, Majdic O et al. (1987) Expression of bloodgroup H antigen on blast cells in leukemias and CML blast crises. In: Grignani F, Martelli MF, Mason DY (eds) Genotypic, phenotypic and functional aspects of haematopoiesis, vol 41. Raven, New York, pp 109–115 (Serono symposia publications)

Köller U, Haas OA, Ludwig W-D et al. (1989) Phenotypic and genotypic heterogeneity in infant acute leukemia: II. Acute nonlymphoblastic leukemia. Leukemia 3:708–714

Ludwig W-D, Bartram CR, Harbott J et al. (1989) Phenotypic and genotypic heterogeneity in infant acute leukemia: I. Acute lymphoblastic leukemia. Leukemia 3:431–439

Ludwig WD, Thiel E, Köller U et al. (1990) Incidence and clinical implications of acute hybrid leukemia in childhood. In: Büchner T, Schellong G, Hiddemann W, Urbanitz D, Ritter J (eds) Acute leukemias II. Springer, Berlin Heidelberg New York, pp 516–522 (Haematology and blood transfusion, vol 33)

Majdic O, Bettelheim P, Stockinger H et al. (1984) M2, a novel myelomonocytic cell surface antigen and its distribution on leukemic cells. Int J Cancer 33:617–623

Mantel N (1966) Evaluation of survival data and two new rank order statistics arising in its consideration. Cancer Chemother Rep 50:163–170

Pui C-H, Behm FG, Singh B et al. (1990) Myeloid-associated antigen expression lacks prognostic value in childhood acute lymphoblastic leukemia treated with intensive multiagent chemotherapy. Blood 75:198–202

Riehm H, Feickert HJ, Schrappe M et al. (1987) Therapy results in five ALL-BFM studies since 1970: implications of risk factors for prognosis. In: Büchner T, Schellong G, Hiddemann W, Urbanitz D, Ritter J (eds) Acute leukemias. Springer, Berlin Heidelberg New York, pp 161–166 (Haematology and blood transfusion, vol 30)

Sobol RE, Mich R, Royston I et al. (1987) Clinical importance of myeloid antigen expression in adult acute lymphoblastic leukemia. N Engl J Med 316:1111

Weiner M, Borowitz M, Boyett J et al. (1985) Clinical pathological aspects of myeloid antigen positivity in pediatric patients with acute lymphoblastic leukemia (ALL). Proc Am Soc Clin Oncol 4:172 (abstr)
Wiersma S, Ortega J, Sobel E, Weinberg KI (1991) Clinical importance of myeloid antigen expression in acute lymphoblastic leukemia of childhood. N Engl J Med 324:800–808

Contribution of Electron Microscopy to the Classification of Minimally Differentiated Acute Leukemias in Children

E.R. van Wering[1], P. Brederoo[2], G.J. van Staalduinen[1], J. van der Meulen[2], B.E.M. van der Linden-Schrever[1], and J.J.M. van Dongen[3]

[1] Dutch Childhood Leukemia Study Group, P.O. Box 60604, 2506 LP The Hague, The Netherlands
[2] Laboratory for Electron Microscopy, University of Leiden, Leiden, The Netherlands
[3] Department of Immunology, University Hospital Dijkzigt/Erasmus University, Rotterdam, The Netherlands

Introduction

In recent multiparameter studies, ultrastructural morphology and cytochemistry of undifferentiated or minimally differentiated acute leukemias have been investigated (Lee et al. 1987; Matutes et al. 1988; Campana et al. 1990; Van Wering et al. 1990; Heil et al. 1991). Detection of myeloperoxidase (MPO) and platelet peroxidase (PPO) at the ultrastructural level appeared to be useful for myeloid leukemias (Bennett et al. 1991) and supportive for the diagnosis of megakaryocytic leukemias (Breton-Gorius et al. 1978; Bennett et al. 1985). We investigated 12 light-microscopically unclassifiable acute childhood leukemias by immunological marker analysis and by electron microscopy (EM), including peroxidase cytochemistry. The combined results appeared to provide information to diagnose conclusively cases of minimally differentiated acute myeloid leukemias (AML M0; Bennett et al. 1991) and acute megakaryoblastic leukemia (AML M7; Bennett et al. 1985).

Patients

In the Netherlands air-dried blood and bone marrow smears of children below 16 years of age with acute leukemia or suspected of having leukemia are sent to the laboratory of the Dutch Childhood Leukemia Study Group. A response of more than 95% of such patients has been achieved (van Steensel-Moll et al. 1983).

From 1986 and until 1991 (55 months), a diagnosis of acute leukemia was made in 483 consecutive cases. In this period 22 patients were unclassifiable by light microscopy alone. Twenty one of these patients were immunophenotyped. Criteria for ultrastructural investigation were:

Recent Results in Cancer Research, Vol. 131

- Inconclusive cytomorphology, possibly myeloid, or suspected to be an acute megakaryoblastic leukemia or
- Low peroxidase positivity (1%–10%)
- Availability of sufficient cells

Following these criteria, 12 patients were studied by EM including peroxidase cytochemistry. Included is one patient (no. 1) with 7% peroxidase positivity, which should be considered as a myeloid leukemia according to the FAB criteria. Three patients had Down's syndrome. Clinical data are summarized in Table 1. Patients 1, 2, 3, and 7 were published before as patients 4, 2, 6, and 8 respectively (van Wering et al. 1990).

Material and Methods

Light Microscopy

Bone marrow and blood slides were stained with May–Grünwald–Giemsa, periodic acid–Schiff, peroxidase, Sudan Black B, α-naphthylacetate esterase, and acid phosphatase. The diagnosis of acute lymphoblastic leukemia (ALL) or acute myeloid leukemia (AML) was made on the basis of the criteria of the FAB classification (Bennett et al. 1976, 1985).

Immunophenotyping

A standard panel of monoclonal antibodies was assessed on cytocentrifuge preparations by an indirect immunoperoxidase (IPOX) staining technique. In cases of doubt as well as in cases of suspected myeloid leukemia, antibody reactivity was also evaluated by indirect immunofluorescence stainings of cells in suspension, or if necessary by double immunofluorescence stainings. The following antibodies were used: anti-terminal deoxynucleotidyl transferase (TdT) from Supertechs (Bethesda, MD, USA); anti-HLA-DR, CD22 (Leu-14), and CD3 (Leu-4) from Becton-Dickinson (Sunnyvale, CA, USA); CD34 (BI-3C5) from Sanbio (Uden, The Netherlands); CD10 (VIL-A1) and CD_w65 (VIM-2), a gift from Dr. W. Knapp (Vienna, Austria); CD19 (B4), CD20 (B1), CD13 (My-7), CD33 (My-9) from Coulter Clone (Hialeah, FL, USA); CD61 (CLB-thrombo/1) and anti-glycophorin A (anti-GpA, CLB-ery-1) from the Central Laboratory of the Blood Transfusion Service (Amsterdam, The Netherlands); anti-human immunoglobulin M (IgM) from De Beer Medicals (Hilvarenbeek, The Netherlands); and CD7 (3A1) from American Type Culture Collection (Rockville, MD, USA).

Cell samples were obtained from patients at initial diagnosis. Mononuclear cells were isolated from bone marrow (BM) and peripheral blood

Table 1. Clinical data concerning the 12 leukemia patients

Patient	Age (years)	Sex	WBC ($\times 10^9$/l)	Thrombocytes ($\times 10^9$/l)	FAB LM	Remarks
1	12	F	65.0	346	Ml[a]	Down's syndrome
2	2	M	10.7	8	AUL	
3	1	M	4.4	2	AUL	
4	0	F	12.2	299	AUL	
5	2	F	7.3	10	AUL	
6	2	F	15.8	24	AUL	Down's syndrome
7	0	M	45.4	14	AUL	Down's syndrome
8	1	M	39.3	13	AUL	
9	1	M	14.5	11	AUL	
10	3	M	75.3	55	AUL	
11	8	M	43.0	265	AUL	
12	0	M	14.0	202	AUL	

AUL, acute undifferentiated leukemia; F, female; LM, light microscopy; M, male; WBC, white blood cells.
[a] 7% peroxidase positive cells were detected by light microscopy, which is sufficient for the diagnosis AML Ml according to the FAB criteria.

(PB) by Ficoll density centrifugation (Ficoll Paque; density 1.077 g/ml) for 15 min (room temperature, 1000*g*). All standard washings of cells in suspension were performed with phosphate-buffered saline (PBS, pH 7.8), supplemented with 1% bovine serum albumin (BSA). Washing centrifugations were performed for 5 min at 4°C with 400*g*. Cells incubated in suspension were adjusted to a concentration of 10^7 cells/ml. Blasts were counted in cytocentrifuge preparations made with 50 µl of a cell suspension containing 10^6 cells/ml PBS-BSA and dried over silica gel.

IPOX. Cytocentrifuge preparations were fixed in buffered formaldehyde acetone (pH 7.4, 4°C, 30 s), rinsed in water, washed in PBS (pH 7.4) and incubated with 50 µl of the relevant monoclonal antibody (room temperature, 60 min). After this incubation, preparations were washed twice and incubated with 50 µl peroxidase-conjugated rabbit anti-mouse antiserum with 2% pooled AB human serum added, again washed with PBS (2×) and stained with diaminobenzidine 0.5 mg/ml with 0.05 *M* imidazole in 0.05 *M* Tris HCl buffer (pH 7.6) and 0.02% H_2O_2 (10 min, room temperature). Cells were counterstained with hematoxylin.

TdT Detection. Cytocentrifuge preparations were fixed in methanol (30 min, 4°C), washed in PBS, and incubated with 15 µl rabbit anti-TdT antiserum in a moist chamber (30 min, room temperature). After the incubation, cells were washed in PBS and subsequently incubated with 15 µl fluorescein isothiocyanate- (FITC-)conjugated goat anti-rabbit immunoglobulin antiserum, washed, and mounted in glycerol with 1 mg *p*-phenylenediamine/ml (van Dongen et al. 1987).

Immunofluorescence. 50 µl of a cell suspension was incubated (30 min, 4°C) with 50 µl of the relevant monoclonal antibody, washed in PBS, and incubated with 50 µl FITC-conjugated goat anti-mouse-immunoglobulin antiserum (30 min, 4°C), washed in PBS, and mounted in glycerol with 1 mg *p*-phenylenediamine/ml (van Dongen et al. 1987).

Double Immunofluorescence. 50 µl of a cell suspension was incubated as for immunofluorescence, but with rhodamine-conjugated goat anti-mouse-immunoglobulin antiserum as the second step. After the washings, cytocentrifuge preparations were made and incubated for TdT staining (van Dongen et al. 1987).

Electron Microscopy

Leukocytes from PB or BM samples of untreated patients were processed either directly from a buffy coat or after separation on a Ficoll-Isopaque gradient (1.077 g/ml), followed by cryopreservation. For morphology, cells were prefixed for 30 min with 0.1% glutaraldehyde in a 0.1 *M* cacodylate buffer (pH 7.4) and postfixed with 1% osmium tetroxide in a phosphate buffer. For peroxidase cytochemistry, cells were prefixed for 30 min with 0.1% glutaraldehyde in 0.1 *M* cacodylate buffer and incubated for 60 min in a medium containing 20 mg diaminobenzidine 4HCl and 0.003% H_2O_2 per 10 ml Ringer solution in the dark at room temperature (Roels et al. 1975). After incubation cells were washed and postfixed with 1% osmium tetroxide in phosphate buffer. Ultrathin sections were stained with uranyl acetate followed by lead hydroxide (in case of peroxidase studies with lead hydroxide alone) and examined with a Philips EM 410 LS electron microscope (Philips, Eindhoven, The Netherlands) at 80 kV.

Results

Clinical data are shown in Table 1, immunophenotyping data in Table 2, EM data in Table 3, and a summary of the observations leading to the final diagnosis in Table 4.

Patients 1 and 2. Both leukemias were unclassifiable by marker analysis, although case 1 is possibly myeloid, with some CD33 positivity in addition to HLA-DR positivity. EM studies showed immature cells with some chromatin condensation in the nuclei, a small Golgi area, and some granules dispersed through the cytoplasm. Peroxidase activity was found in the rough

Table 2. Immunophenotype of the 12 leukemias

Patient	Blasts (%)	TdT	HLA-DR	CD34	CD19	CD10	CD22	CD3	CyCD3	CD7	CD2	CD13	CD33	CD_w65	CD61	anti-GpA	
1	59	0	72	0	0	0	–	–	22[a]	79	1	2	26	1	3	2	AUL
2	68	3	8	–	4	0	–	13	–	50	8	1	3	–	3	3	AUL
3	57	0	18	–	0	0	–	–	–	–	–	9	–	–	0	0	AUL?
4	60	0	70	–	14	0	–	–	–	75	17	11	14	2	35	2	MKB
5	52	0	20	0	0	1	–	–	29[a]	38	–	0	2	1	20	1	MKB
6	77	0	9	0	7	2	4	–	21[a]	46	–	50	65	16	46	0	MKB
7	80	0	51	–	0	6	1	2	2	41	–	0	0	0	4	0	AUL
8	60	0	6	83	7	0	5	0	–	8	–	69	85	3	5	–	AML
9	78	3	26	41	15	14 (95)	12	13	8	86 (1)	–	32	69 (0)	9	37	0	MKB
10	73	52	88 (84)	33 (100)	47 (50)	0	15	4	6	8	–	0	6	51 (44)	–	1	null-ALL
11	60	49	12 (7)	1	4 (0)	30 (36)	–	1	63	68 (51)	–	38 (0)	39 (30)	8	0	0	T-ALL
12	81	77	90	67	95	64	–	–	0	14	3	1	7	–	–	–	common ALL

–, not tested; AUL, acute unclassifiable leukemia; MKB, megakaryoblastic leukemia.
Immunophenotypic data are given as percentages per mononuclear cells after Ficoll density centrifugation. Figures in parentheses represent percentage positivity of TdT^+ cells as determined by double-immunofluorescence stainings.
[a] Although membrane CD3 was not tested on cells in suspension in patients 1, 5, and 6, CyCD3 expression was interpreted as membrane CD3 expression of mature T lymphocytes. These cells probably represent remaining mature T lymphocytes.

Table 3. Electron microscopic analysis of the 12 leukemias

Patient	Cell sample	Peroxidase positivity				Conclusion
		%	RER	NE	Granules	
1	BM	48	+	+	+	AML
2	BM	74	+	+	+	AML
3	BM	22	+	+	–	AML (M7?)
4	BM	30	+	+	–	AML (M7?)
5	PB	38	+	+	–	AML (M7?)
6	BM	–	+	+	–	AML (M7?)
7	BM	96	+	+	– (Θ/f⁻)	AML MΘ (M7?)
8	BM	90	+	+	– (Θ/f⁻)	AML MΘ (M7?)
9	PB	0	–	–	– (Θ/f⁻)	AML MΘ
10	PB	0	–	–	–	ALL
11	BM	0	–	–	–	ALL
12	PB	0	–	–	–	ALL

Θ, presence of theta granules (see text); f⁻, no ferritin molecules found in the theta granules.

Table 4. Summary of observations and final diagnosis

Patient	FAM LM	Immuno-phenotype	EM	Diagnosis
1	MI[a]	AUL	AML	AML M1
2	AUL	AUL	AML	AML M0
3	AUL	AUL?	AML (M7?)	AML M0
4	AUL	MKB	AML (M7?)	AML M7
5	AUL	MKB	AML (M7?)	AML M7
6	AUL	MKB	AML (M7?)	AML M7
7	AUL	AUL	AML MΘ (M7?)	AML M0/MΘ
8	AUL	AML	AML MΘ (M7?)	AML M0/MΘ
9	AUL	MKB	AML MΘ	AML M7/MΘ
10	AUL	null ALL⁺	ALL	ALL
11	AUL	T-ALL⁺	ALL	ALL
12	AUL	common ALL	ALL	ALL

AUL, acute undifferentiated leukemia; MKB, megakaryoblastic leukemia; Θ, presence of theta granules (see text); ALL⁺, myeloid marker expression was found (see Table 2).
[a] Patient 1: 7% peroxidase-positive cells were found by light microscopy.

endoplasmic reticulum (RER), nuclear envelope (NE), and granules, which pattern is specific for MPO. Therefore, ultrastructurally these leukemias were of the myeloid lineage. A final diagnosis of AML M1 was made in patient 1, because peroxidase positivity was also found, at low frequency, by light microscopy. The final diagnosis of patient 2 was AML M0.

Patients 3–6. The leukemic cells of patient 3 could not be immunophenotyped sufficiently and were therefore unclassifiable. In cases 4 and 5 without positivity for TdT or B-cell markers, but with CD7 positivity combined with CD61 positivity, a megakaryoblastic population seemed to be present. In case 6 myeloid marker expression (CD13, CD33) was found in addition to CD61 expression.

These four cases showed on EM a population of immature cells with short cisternae of RER and occasionally small granules or blebs; bull's eye granules were not observed. Peroxidase activity was found in NE and RER but not in the granules, which pattern has been suggested to represent PPO (Breton-Gorius et al. 1978) and therefore supportive for a diagnosis of acute megakaryoblastic leukemia (Fig. 1). Based on immunological marker analysis, especially CD61 expression, a final diagnosis of AML M7 was made in patients 4–6, which was supported by the EM data. In patient 3 a number of myeloid markers could not be tested but no CD61 expression was found, which was in contrast to the ultrastructurally "PPO-like" peroxidase

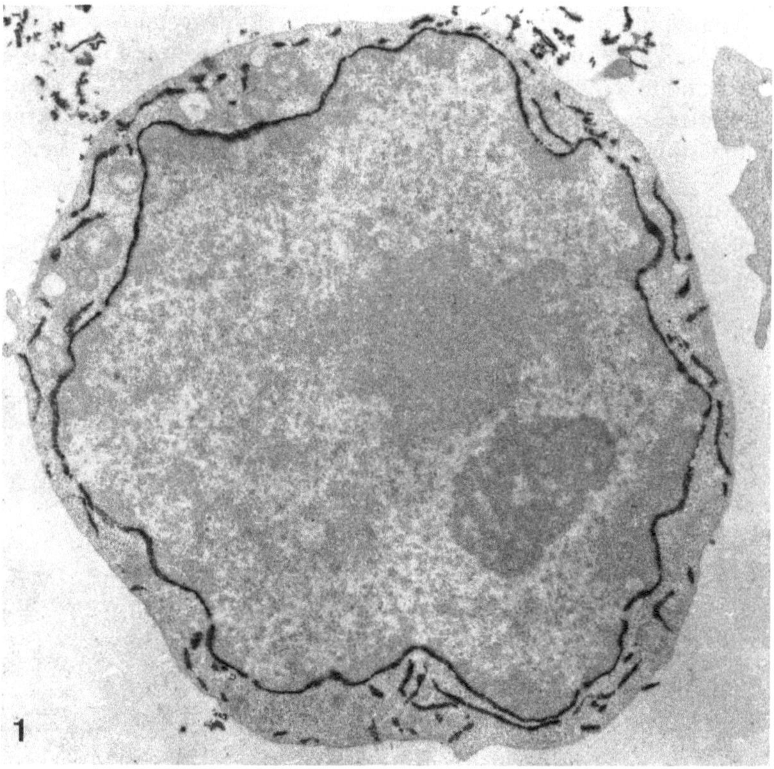

Fig. 1. Peroxidase positivity present in the nuclear envelope and the rough endoplasmic reticulum (patient 5; M7). ×13 800

pattern. Therefore the leukemia of patient 3 was diagnosed as AML M0 and not as AML M7.

Patients 7–9. The leukemia of patient 7 was unclassifiable by immunological marker analysis. No markers were expressed except for CD7. Case 8 was a myeloid leukemia ($CD34^+$, $CD13^+$, and $CD33^+$) and case 9 expressed myeloid markers as well as the CD61 antigen. In the latter case low percentages positivity for TdT, CD19, and CD10 were also found. Double-marker analysis demonstrated that the great majority of the TdT-positive cells (3% of the mononuclear cells) expressed CD10 but not CD7 or CD33. Therefore these TdT^+ cells most probably represented remaining normal precursor B-cells. EM studies in patients 7–9 showed immature cells, some of which contained small round granules at the concave side of the kidney-shaped nucleus. The granules contained a kind of nucleoid or barr in a light flocculent matrix (Figs. 2, 3). These granules, called theta (Θ) granules, did not contain ferritin at high magnifications. Peroxidase activity was found in cases 7 and 8, in the RER and NE, but not in the theta granules. This pattern of peroxidase positivity suggested a minimally differentiated myeloid leukemia with theta granules or a megakaryoblastic leukemia, but immunophenotyping did not reveal positivity for the thrombocytic lineage marker CD61. Therefore patients 7 and 8 were diagnosed as AML M0/MΘ. In patient 9 approximately 16% of the leukemic blasts contained theta granules, but no peroxidase positivity was found at the ultrastructural level, suggesting that it concerned a minimally differentiated acute leukemia.

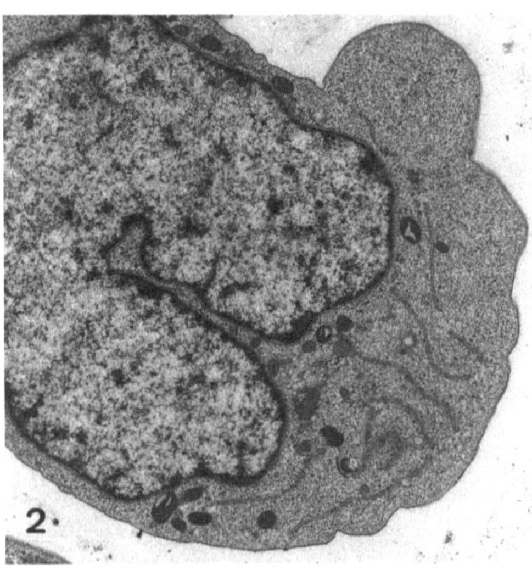

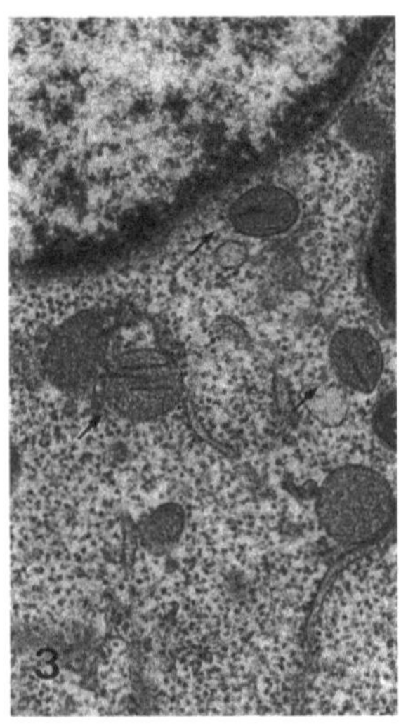

Fig. 2. Immature cell with theta granules (patient 7; AML M0/MΘ). ×6700
Fig. 3. Enlargement of the theta granules (*arrows*) of Fig. 2. ×24600

However, positivity for the myeloid markers CD13 and CD33 as well as for the thrombocytic lineage marker CD61 allowed us to make the final diagnosis of AML M7/MΘ.

Patients 10–12. The leukemias of patients 10–12 were immunophenotyped as ALL, i.e., as null ALL, T-cell ALL, and common ALL, respectively. The leukemic cells of patients 10 and 11 exhibited myeloid marker expression (CD_w65 and CD33, respectively), which was confirmed by double-marker analysis (Table 2). On EM, peroxidase activity was not found in any of these cases, confirming the ALL origin of the blasts.

Discussion

Generally, the diagnosis of ALL or AML can be made by light microscopy supported by standard immunological marker analysis (Bennett et al. 1976, 1991). In a few leukemias, like in patient 1, a very low peroxidase positivity by light microscopy (3%–10%) is sufficient for a diagnosis of AML by FAB criteria, although immunological markers are inconclusive. In such cases, EM studies, especially peroxidase cytochemistry, are an additional aid in diagnosis. Peroxidase activity in these leukemias is found in RER, NE and granules, which pattern is regarded as representing MPO (Breton-Gorius et al. 1978; Bennett et al. 1985). EM can also support the immunophenotypic diagnosis of acute megakaryoblastic leukemia, with peroxidase activity only in RER and NE and not in granules (patients 4–6; Breton Gorius et al. 1978; Bennett et al. 1985). In ALL with cross-lineage expression of myeloid markers (patients 10 and 11), the absence of peroxidase activity confirms the diagnosis of ALL.

In a number of cases, however, light microscopy and immunological marker analysis are inadequate and their results inconclusive. Such leukemias are therefore unclassifiable, but by EM they can sometimes be diagnosed conclusively. From the 12 patients described here, patients 2 and 7 had such an unclassifiable leukemia. Case 2 without lineage-specific markers by immunophenotyping did show peroxidase activity in RER, NE, and granules, which defined the leukemia ultrastructurally as a minimally differentiated myeloid leukemia (AML M0), as recently, proposed by the FAB group (Bennett et al. 1991). In patient 7, the leukemic cells had a comparable immunophenotype, whereas peroxidase activity was only found in RER and NE, but not in the granules. Such a pattern of peroxidase activity has been described as PPO and diagnoses a megakaryocytic leukemia by FAB criteria (Bennett et al. 1985). However, a similar "PPO-like" pattern of peroxidase positivity has been found in erythroblastic leukemias (Breton-Gorius et al. 1987). In addition, the first (so-called nucleated) granules appearing in early promyelocytes are also devoid of peroxidase activity (Brederoo et al. 1986), which implies that peroxidase positivity in RER and NE but not in the granules can fit with a diagnosis of AML M0. Therefore, patient 7 as well as patients 3 and 8 were diagnosed as AML M0, because the "PPO-like" peroxidase pattern was not supported by the expression of the CD61 antigen in these cases.

Interestingly, the granules in patient 7 as well as in patients 8 and 9 were not morphologically identical to the granules in early neutrophilic promyelocytes or in megakaryocytes. They had a homogeneously flocculent matrix with an inclusion. Such so-called theta granules were first described in a Ph-negative chronic myeloid leukemia (CML) and were reported to be related to basophil granulopoiesis (Parkin et al. 1980). A similar type of granule has been described by Breton-Gorius et al. (1987) in patients with Down's syndrome and CML. At high magnification they found the granules to contain ferritin molecules and considered this a marker for erythroid blasts. In our three cases with theta granules (patients 7–9), ferritin molecules were not found, which is in agreement with observations of Eguchi et al. (1989), who detected these granules in blasts of acute megakaryoblastic leukemias in children with Down's syndrome. Based on these data we conclude that the presence of theta granules in cases 7–9 may be associated with minimally differentiated AML. In patients 7 and 8 this was supported by the results of immunological marker analysis, but in patient 9 a final diagnosis of AML M7 was made because of positivity for the CD61 antigen. Since we have no ultrastructural evidence for specific association of theta granules with a particular differentiation lineage, we propose to add the code "MΘ" in cases of AML with theta granules.

In conclusion, EM proved to be an additional aid for further classification of acute unclassifiable childhood leukemias. It allowed us to diagnose conclusively cases of minimally differentiated AML (AML M0). The immunological diagnosis of acute megakaryocytic leukemia was supported by the presence of ultrastructural "PPO-like" peroxidase positivity in most cases, although exceptions were found in which immunophenotyping results and the "PPO-like" peroxidase pattern did not correlate. In our material theta granules did not contain ferritin and, at least in this series of patients, these granules were not associated with acute erythroblastic leukemia.

Acknowledgements. We gratefully acknowledge Dr. J.P.M. Bokkerink, M.V.A. Bruin, Dr. P.J. van Dijken, Dr. K. Hählen, Dr. W.A. Kamps, Dr. E.F. van Leeuwen, F.A.E. Nabben, A. Postma, J.A. Rammeloo, I.M. Risseeuw-Appel, Dr. G.A.M. de Vaan, E.T. van't Veer-Korthof, Prof. Dr. A.J.P. Veerman, Dr. F.C. de Waal, M. van Weel-Sipman and Dr. R.S. Weening, board members of the DCLSG, for providing cell samples.

References

Bennett JM, Catovsky D, Daniel MR, Flandrin G, Galton DAG, Granick HR, Sultan C (1976) Proposals for the classification of the acute leukemias: French-American-British Cooperative Group. Br J Haematol 33:451–458

Bennett JM, Catovsky D, Daniel MT, Flandrin G, Galton DAG, Gralnick HR, Sultan C (1985) Criteria for the diagnosis of acute leukaemia of megakaryocyte lineage (M7). Ann Intern Med 103:460–462

Bennett JM, Catovsky D, Daniel MT, Flandrin G, Galton DAG, Gralnick HR, Sultan C (1991) Proposal for the recognition of minimally differentiated acute myeloid leukaemia (AML-M0). Br J Haematol 78:325–329

Brederoo P, Van der Meulen J, Daems WTH (1986) Ultrastructural localization of peroxidase activity in developing neutrophil granulocytes from human bone marrow. Histochemistry 84:445–453

Breton-Gorius J, Reyes F, Duhamel G, Najman A, Gorin NC (1978) Megakaryoblastic acute leukemia: Identification by the ultrastructural demonstration of platelet peroxidase. Blood 51:45–60

Breton-Gorius J, Villeval JL, Mitjavilla MT, Guichard J, Rochant H, Flandrin G, Vainchenker W (1987) Ultrastructural and cytochemical characterization of blasts form early erythroblastic leukemias. Leukemia 1:173–181

Campana D, Hansen-Hagge TE, Matutes E, Coustan-Smith E, Yokota S, Shetty V, Bartram CR, Janossy G (1990) Phenotypic, genotypic, cytochemical, and ultrastructural characterization of acute undifferentiated leukemia. Leukemia 4: 620–624

Eguchi M, Sakakibara H, Suda J, Ozawa T, Hayashi Y, Sato T, Kojima S, Furukawa T (1989) Ultrastructural and ultracytochemical differences between transient myeloproliferative disorder and megakaryoblastic leukaemia in Down's syndrome. Br J Haematol 73:315–322

Heil G, Gunsilius E, Raghavachar A, Bartram CR, Ganser A, Kurrle E, Aydemir U, Loffler H, Hoelzer D, Thiel E, Heimpel H (1991) Ultrastructural demonstration of peroxidase expression in acute unclassified leukemias correlation to immunophenotype and treatment outcome. Blood 77:1305–1312

Lee EJ, Pollak A, Leavitt RD, Testa JR, Schiffer CA (1987) Minimally differentiated acute nonlymphocytic leukemia: a distinct entity. Blood 70:1400–1406

Matutes E, Pombo de oliveira M, Foroni L, Morilla R, Catovsky D (1988) The role of ultrastructural cytochemistry and monoclonal antibodies in clarifying the nature of undifferentiated cells in acute leukaemia. Br J Haematol 69:205–211

Parkin JL, McKenna RW, Brunning RD (1980) Ultrastructural features of basophil and mast cell granulopoiesis in blastic phase philadelphia chromosome-positive leukemia. J Natl Cancer Inst 65:535–546

Roels F, Wisse E, De Prest B, Van der Meulen J (1975) Cytochemical discrimination between catalases and peroxidases using diaminobenzidine. Histochemistry 41: 281–311

Van Dongen JJM, Adriaansen HJ, Hooijkaas H (1987) Immunological marker analysis of cells in the various hematopoietic differentiation stages and their malignant counterparts. Application of monoclonal antibodies in tumor pathology. Nijhoff, Dordrecht, pp 87–116

Van Steensel-Moll HA, Valkenburg HA, Van Zanen GE (1983) Incidence of childhood leukaemia in the Netherlands (1973–1980). Br J Cancer 47:471–475

Van Wering ER, Brederoo P, Van Dijk-de Leeuw JHS, Van Der Meulen J, Van't Veer MB (1990) Electron microscopy: a contribution to further classification of acute unclassifiable childhood leukemia. Blut 60:291–296

III. Biological and Clinical Significance of Cytogenetic Abnormalities in Acute Leukemias

Molecular Cytogenetic Applications in Leukemias

S. Knuutila

Department of Medical Genetics, University of Helsinki, Haartmaninkatu 3, 00290 Helsinki, Finland

Introduction

Slow proliferation and low mitotic index, indistinct chromosome morphology, and inadequate chromosome banding often hamper the cytogenetic study of hematologic neoplasms. The fact that leukemias and lymphomas are heterogeneous regarding involvement of various bone marrow cell lineages renders standard cytogenetic analysis less than ideal, as it does not allow the study of cell lineage. The recently developed chromosome-specific probes and their use in situ hybridization (Rappold et al. 1984; Pinkel et al. 1986, 1988; Willard and Waye 1987; Hopman et al. 1988a,b; Cremer et al. 1986, 1988; Lichter et al. 1988a,b) as well as the MAC (morphology antibody chromosomes) methodology (Teerenhovi et al. 1984; Wessman and Knuutila 1988; Knuutila and Teerenhovi 1989; Tiainen et al. 1992), allowing the simultaneous analysis of chromosomes, cell morphology, and immunophenotype, have done much to remove the aforementioned problems. In the following, in situ hybridization and its adaptation to MAC preparations will be briefly described, the use of these methods in leukemia research will be discussed, and a few clinical examples presented.

Methodological Considerations

Preparations for In Situ Hybridization

The cell material for in situ hybridization is usually in the form of slide preparations. The target chromosomes and a labeled DNA probe are first denatured. Complementary sequences of the probe and target are then allowed to hybridize (reanneal). After washing and incubation in affinity reagents the reporting signal is visible at the sites of hybridization.

Recent Results in Cancer Research, Vol. 131

Many types of preparations can be used, including standard acetic acid/ methanol-fixed chromosome preparations, blood or bone marrow smears stained by cytochemical techniques (Wessman et al. 1993), cytocentrifuge preparations stained by immunocytochemical techniques (MAC preparations; Knuutila and Teerenhovi 1989), and paraffin-embedded sections (Emmerich et al. 1989; Hopman et al. 1988a,b, 1989).

In Situ Hybridization Procedures

Details of in situ hybridization procedures have been described elsewhere for standard chromosome preparations (e.g., Eastmont and Pinkel 1989; Perez Losada et al. 1991), for morphologically and immunologically classified MAC preparations (Wessman and Knuutila 1988; Knuutila and Teerenhovi 1989; Tiainen et al. 1991), and for section material (Emmerich et al. 1989; Hopman et al. 1988a,b, 1989).

Repetitive alphoid probes, chromosome library probes, oligonucleotide probes, and cosmid clones containing DNA inserts (Lichter et al. 1990; Kievits et al. 1990) can be used for metaphase cells (metaphase molecular cytogenetics), whereas repetitive alphoid and oligonucleotide probes are the most reliable for interphase cytogenetics. Also, single-copy probes have been employed in interphase cells, not only for detecting structural chromosome abnormalities, but also for spotting numerical abnormalities (e.g., Arnoldus et al. 1990; Tkachuk et al. 1990).

Both enzymatic reactions (Burns et al. 1985; Wessman et al. 1989) and fluorochromes (e.g., Pinkel et al. 1986; Eastmond and Pinkel 1989; Nederlof et al. 1990) can be used in detecting hybridization of probes. The simultaneous use of two or more probes is also possible by two-color or polycolor fluorescence staining (e.g., Nederlof et al. 1990; Tiainen et al. 1992; Trask et al. 1991). The polycolor detection systems enhance the success rate of scoring structural abnormalities on poor-quality metaphases (Tiainen et al. 1992). We have in collaboration with T. Cremer's group in Heidelberg, for instance, demonstrated the Philadelphia chromosome in very poor MAC preparations by using biotinylated and digoxigenin-labeled chromosome 9 and 22 library probes and fluorescein isothiocyanate (FITC), tetramethylrhodamine isothiocyanate (TRITC), and/or 7-amino-4-methylcoumarin-3-acetic acid (AMCA) fluorescence detection (Tiainen et al. 1992).

The double-color system also enables the detection of translocations in interphase cells. For example, Arnoldus et al. (1990) have demonstrated the Philadelphia translocation in interphase cells by using cosmid clones of *bcr* and *abl* genes and two-color detection. Two-color in situ hybridization also helps to detect the specific but hard-to-spot inversion encountered in acute myeloid leukemia (AML) M4 (Dauwerse et al. 1990).

Molecular Cytogenetic Applications

Complementation of Chromosome Banding (Metaphase Molecular Cytogenetics)

It is a regrettable fact still today that the quality of chromosome banding of leukemic cells is not always sufficient for accurate interpretation of an abnormality. Molecular cytogenetics is clearly alleviating this problem, as evidenced by some earlier reports (Cremer et al. 1990; Jauch et al. 1990; Smit et al. 1990; Kibbelaar et al. 1991) and also by the following examples.

G-banding analysis in one of our patients with AML yielded an abnormal chromosome 8 resembling isochromosome 8q in a small proportion of metaphase cells (Fig. 1). The presence of a translocation between 8 and some other chromosome could not, however, be ruled out. The use of a 8-specific library probe confirmed that the abnormality really was an isochromosome (Fig. 1). The second example concerns a patient with AML, in whom two different abnormal clones were detected in G-banded metaphases of fairly poor quality (Fig. 2). In the first one of these clones, chromosomes 17, 18, and 21 were replaced with an abnormal chromosome 4 and two marker chromosomes; in the second one, chromosomes 17, 18, and 21 were replaced with an abnormal 15 and two marker chromosomes. The interpretation of the karyotype was 45,XX,−17,−18,−21,+2mar,?4q+/45,XX,−17,−18,−21,+2mar,?15q+ (Fig. 2). Molecular cytogenetics using 15- and 17-specific library probes demonstrated a translocation between the long arms of chromosomes 4 and 17 (first clone) and a translocation between the long arms of chromosomes 15 and 17 (second clone) (Fig. 2). Thus, use of molecular cytogenetics yielded information about these translocations, which can be considered to have general significance from the viewpoint of elucidation of the biological and clinical aspects of cancer.

In some leukemias the frequency of abnormal cells may be very low. Especially in acute promyelocytic leukemia (APL) we have seen cases in which the frequency of metaphase cells with the 15;17 translocation is less than 5%. The extreme was a patient in whom only 2% of bone marrow metaphases exhibited the translocation and in whom the abnormality was not detected until the 52nd metaphase analyzed. Furthermore, the poor quality of metaphases containing the translocation (often seen in APL and other leukemias) may cause preferential selection of normal cells for analysis. In such cases, chromosome painting can be used to ensure accurate cytogenetic interpretation.

We have started using molecular cytogenetics to demonstrate abnormalities in cases where cell morphology and/or immunophenotype point to a specific chromosome abnormality but where the karyotype appears normal. The possibility of screening large numbers of cells rapidly and reliably has won this methodology important applications also in disease follow-up and in the detection of minimal residual disease, as will be discussed below.

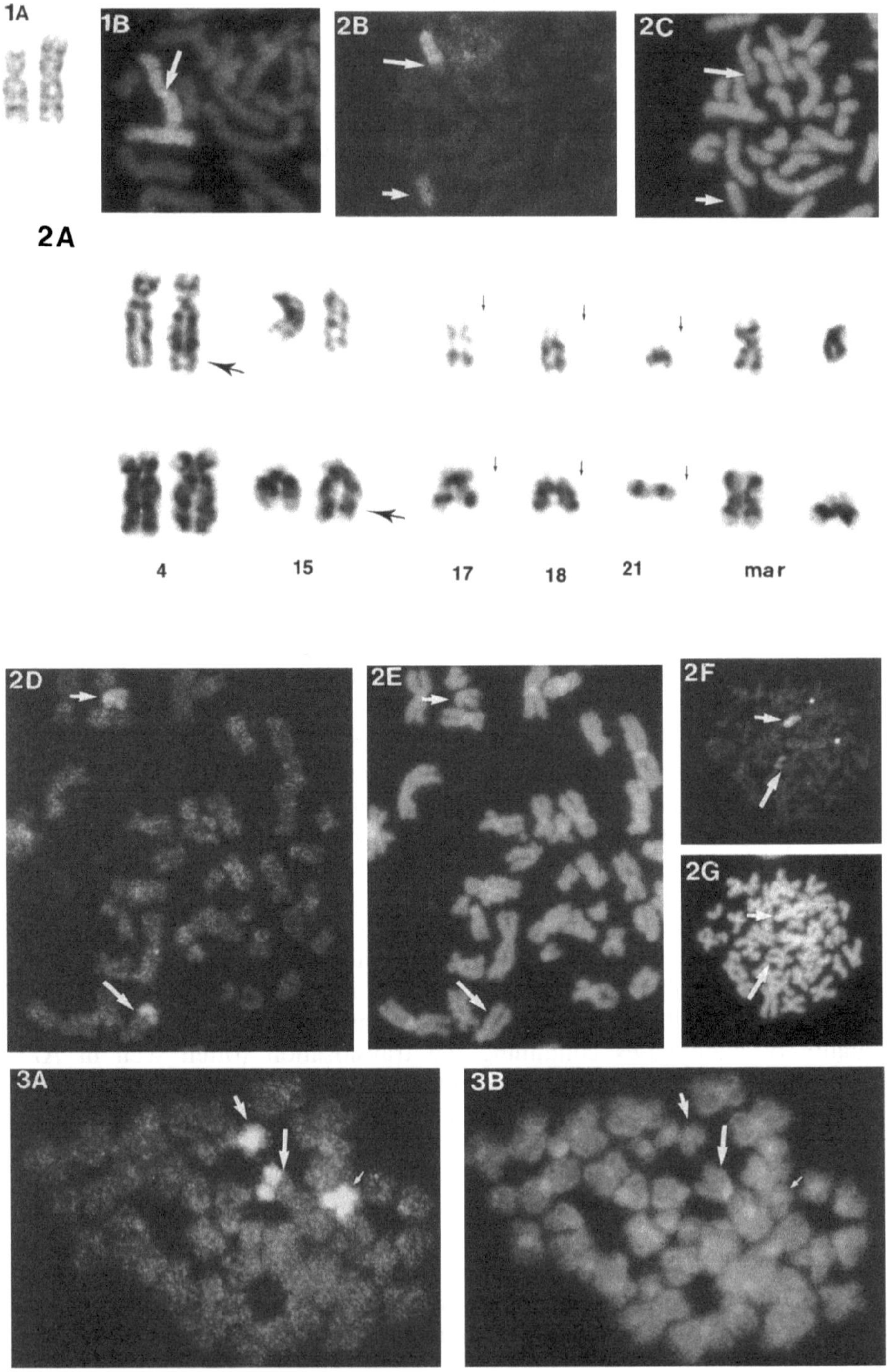
1A
1B
2B
2C
2A
4
15
17
18
21
mar
2D
2E
2F
2G
3A
3B

Slow Proliferation or Total Absence of Mitotic Cells (Interphase Molecular Cytogenetics)

In some leukemias proliferation activity in vitro is very low. The karyotypes encountered, for example, in chronic lymphocytic leukemia (CLL), multiple myeloma, and Hodgkin's disease are often normal (10%–60% of cases), or no mitosis is seen because the neoplastic cells do not enter mitosis whereas normal cells do (Knuutila et al. 1986; Autio et al. 1987; Teerenhovi et al. 1988). Our series of patients with CLL demonstrated that the frequency of trisomy 12, the most common abnormality in CLL, is higher when analyzed by interphase cytogenetics than when the result is based on karyotype analysis of metaphase cells. Two out of 13 patients with a normal karyotype had the trisomy by interphase cytogenetics (Perez Losada et al. 1991).

Disease Follow-up (Metaphase and Interphase Molecular Cytogenetics)

Chromosome abnormalities provide highly cancer-specific markers for the follow-up of the disease. We have started using metaphase and interphase molecular cytogenetics along with karyotype analysis for follow-up of cases exhibiting a suitable chromosome abnormality on G-banding analysis at

---

Fig. 1. A Cut-out normal chromosome 8 and isochromosome 8q (on the right) from a G-banded metaphase of a patient with AML. **B** A metaphase from the same patient after hybridization with chromosome 8-specific library probe (obtained from the American Type Culture Collection (ATCC, LL08NSO2). The biotinylated probe was detected with avidin conjugated with fluorescein isothiocyanate (FITC). The cells were counterstained with propidium iodide. Isochromosome 8q is indicated by the *arrow*

Fig. 2. A Cut-out G-banded chromosomes 4, 15, 17, 18, and 21 and marker chromosomes from two metaphases demonstrating two different abnormal clones seen in a patient with AML. *Large arrows* indicate abnormal chromosomes 4 and 15 and *small arrows* indicate missing chromosomes. **B–G** Chromosome 15 painted (**B**) plus DAPI stained (**C**) and 17 painted (**D, F**) plus DAPI stained (**E, G**): metaphases demonstrate a translocation between the long arms of chromosomes 15 and 17 (**B, D**, compare to the *lower line* in **A**) and a translocation between the long arms of chromosomes 4 and 17 (**F**, compare to the *upper line* in **A**). *Small arrows* indicate normal chromosomes 15 (**B, C**) and 17 (**D–G**) and *large arrows* indicate translocated chromosomes 15, i.e., der(15)t(15;17) (**B–E**) and translocated chromosome 4, i.e., der(4)t(4;17) (**F, G**). The biotinylated probes were detected with avidin conjugated with FITC. Counterstaining was done with propidium iodide

Fig. 3. A A patient with acute promyelocytic leukemia, exhibiting the 15;17 translocation, was followed up by in situ hybridization with a chromosome 17-specific probe (from ATCC, LL17NSO2), using FITC fluorescence plus propidium iodide counterstaining. **B** Same metaphase after DAPI staining. The translocation can be readily distinguished: *small arrows* indicate normal chromosome 17, *medium-sized arrows* translocated 17 [der(17)t(15;17)], and *large arrows* translocated 15 [der(15)t(15;17)] diagnosis. MAC preparations have been used in those cases in which a single immunophenotype of clonal cells is known to be present. Such cases mainly consist of B-cell leukemias and lymphomas and infiltration of bone marrow by neuroblastoma cells.

The number of cases is so far too small and the follow-up period too short to allow evaluation of the clinical importance of our results (Table 1). Nevertheless, it seems that molecular cytogenetics in combination with MAC methodology provides a reliable and sensitive technique for the detection of minimal residual cells and of bone marrow infiltration by solid tumor cells. Below, some of the cases in Table 1 are described in detail for discussion of the usefulness of our approach.

Leukemia-Specific Translocations. Many of the translocations seen in leukemias are very specific and are not seen in nonleukemic bone marrow. Such translocations offer very reliable cancer-specific markers for follow-up. In patients 1 and 2 (Table 1), who had the 15;17 translocation, we used 17- and 15-specific library probes (Fig. 3). Long colcemid treatment (ca. 12 h) enabled us to collect high numbers of metaphases. Up to 1000 metaphases could be analyzed within 2–3 h. The fact that a distinct chromosome morphology was retained made the analysis very reliable (Fig. 3). With standard karyotype analysis one is not able to screen 1000 cells in order to detect a translocation: even 50–100 metaphases is too great a number for accurate analysis of a translocation.

Numerical Abnormalities Studied by Metaphase Molecular Cytogenetics. In patients 3–11 a trisomy, mostly trisomy 8, was used as the marker of a leukemic cell. Trisomy 8 is the most common abnormality in hematological malignancies, but it is not strictly limited to any leukemia subgroup. Metaphase molecular cytogenetics allows very reliable and rapid diagnosis of this and other trisomies. The question can be raised, however, whether a single trisomic cell among about 500–5000 cells analyzed is a sign of minimal residual disease. There are no controlled studies on the frequency of trisomy 8 in nonneoplastic cells. In patient 4, who was in remission after chemotherapy, there was one metaphase with trisomy 8 among 596 metaphases analyzed. Still in remission after bone marrow transplantation, the patient had two trisomic metaphases among 500 analyzed. Interestingly, one of the two was donor in origin, as it contained the Y chromosome (the donor was the female patient's brother) detected with 4′,6-diamidino-2-phenylindole-dihydrochloride (DAPI) counterstaining. That normal bone marrow cells may have trisomy 8 was confirmed in the interphase cytogenetic study by Kibbelaar et al. (1991). There are also reports of trisomy 9 and monosomy 7 in normal and leukemic cells (Anastasi et al. 1990; Kolluri et al. 1990).

The reliability of metaphase molecular cytogenetics in detecting minimal residual diseases is improved if there are trisomies of two or more separate chromosomes available, firstly because trisomy of several chromosomes is

Table 1. Leukemia/lymphoma patients followed up by molecular cytogenetics

Patient no.	Patient code	Date of birth/sex	Date of sampling	Diagnosis/date	Karyotype at diagnosis[a]	Clinical stage	Karyotype during the study	Molecular metaphase (M) or interphase (I) cytogenetics			
								Probe	M/I	Normal	Abnormal
1	910139	02.09.55/M	08.02.91	AML M3/08.02.91	46,XY,t(15;17)[20]**	Dg	Same	17 library	M	1	78
	910225		06.03.91	08.02.91	See above	Rm	46,XY[20]	17 library	M	262	6
2	910361	07.11.65/F	01.04.91	AML M3/01.08.87	46,XX[8]/46,XX, t(15;17)[12]	Rm	46,XX[20]	17 library	M	500	0
3	900885	30.06.67/M	05.09.90	AML/05.12.89	46,XY[15]/47,XY, +8[6]	Rm	46,XY[20]	8 library	M	195	1
4	910216	29.06.39/F	04.03.91	AML 10.10.90	46,XX[5]/47,XX,+8, t(16;21)(q24;22)[15]	Rm	46,XX[20]	8 library	M	596	1
	910441		24.04.91			Rm after BMT	46,XY[20]	8 library	M	500	2
5	910078	11.08.77/F	24.01.91	AML M4/02.04.90	46,XX[9]/48,XX,+8, +14[8]	Rm	46,XX[20]	8 library	M	400	0
6	901232	30.05.75/M	04.12.90	AML M4/04.12.90	47,XY,+8,t(9;11)	Dg	Same	8 library	M	3	155
7	910003	19.11.26/F	14.01.91	AML 04.07.89	45,XX,−7	Rm	46,XX[1]/47,XX, +8[5]	8 library	M	32	123
	910844		05.08.91			Rl	46,XX[3]/47,XX, +8[20]	8 library	M	8	80
8	910207	31.07.56/M	28.02.91	AML M4/01.10.90	Not done	Active disease	46,XY[7]/49,XY, +6,+8,+14[10]	8 library	M	89	200
								8 and 14 library	M	0	6
	910464		29.04.91			Rm	46,XY[20]	8 library	M	210	0
9	901266	27.10.65/F	31.12.90	Anaplastic large cell lymphoma ($CD30^+$)/ 31.12.90	LN:47,XX,+7,t(2;5) (p23;q35)	Dg	Same	Under study			
	910415		17.04.91		See above	Rm	BM:46,XX[15]/ 47,XX,+7, t(2;5)[3]	7 rep.	I	123 ($CD30^-$)	5 ($CD30^+$)
	910783		15.07.91		See above	Rm	BM:46,XX[20]	7 rep.	I	667	2

Table 1. *Continued*

Patient no.	Patient code	Date of birth/sex	Date of sampling	Diagnosis/date	Karyotype at diagnosis[a]	Clinical stage	Karyotype during the study	Molecular metaphase (M) or interphase (I) cytogenetics			
								Probe	M/I	Normal	Abnormal
10	910569	13.07.52/M	27.05.91	AML/27.05.91	46,XY[5]/51,XY, +8+19,+3mar, 22q-[15]	Dg	Same	8 library	M	18	68
11	910047	09.02.85/M	15.01.91	ALL/15.01.91	46,XY[13]/56,XY,+X, +8,+8,+10,+10, +18,+19,+20,+21, +22[9]	Dg	Same	8 library	M	429	40

ALL, acute lymphocytic leukemia; AML, acute myeloid leukemia; BMT, bone marrow transplantation; Dg, diagnosis; rep., repetitive; Rl, relapse; Rm, remission. Dates are given as day, month, year.

[a] Numbers in brackets indicate numbers of cells studied.

unlikely in normal bone marrow cells and secondly because simultaneous hybridization artifacts with two different probes are unlikely. Such cases can be investigated by simultaneous detection of the two or more chromosomes by means of polycolor techniques. For instance, in patient 5, who had trisomy 14 in addition to trisomy 8, chromosome 8 can be painted red and chromosome 16 green. In this special case, even a monocolor system demonstrated the trisomies reliably, as the trisomic chromosomes belonged to different chromosome groups.

Interphase cytogenetics is a highly sensitive technique in the detection of trisomic cells (Knuutila et al. 1992). When studying minimal residual cells with a single trisomy the following pitfalls must, however, be taken into consideration: (1) unspecific banding of the probe, (2) cross-hybridization of the probe with other chromosomes, and (3) two adjacent signals (representing either a double signal from a single chromosome, which is a normal enough situation, or two signals from two adjacent chromosomes). Reliability can be improved by using two different probes for the same chromosome in a two-color detection system.

The reliability of detecting neoplastic cells is also improved if immunophenotyped cells can be used. For example, one of our patients (no. 9) with large cell anaplastic (Ki-1) lymphoma exhibits the specific 2;5 translocation in association with trisomy 7. In this disease, neoplastic cells are positive for anti-CD30. CD30 is what is known as a proliferation antigen which may be encountered also in normal bone marrow. Thus the finding of cells positive for anti-CD30 in the bone marrow does not necessarily indicate the presence of neoplastic cells. In our patient, we found that a small proportion (ca. 4%) of interphase cells presented three hybridization signals with a chromosome 7-specific repetitive probe. Most of these cells were CD30-positive. This association of CD30-positivity and trisomy 7 allowed us to conclude with a fair amount of certainty that we were dealing with infiltration of the bone marrow by lymphoma cells. According to other parameters, the patient was considered to be in remission. The patient's future follow-up will be based on a combination of MAC and molecular cytogenetic methods.

Involvement of Various Cell Lineages in Clonal Chromosome Abnormalities

We have studied lineage involvement since 1984 using G-banded chromosomes of morphologically and immunologically classified cells (Teerenhovi et al. 1984; Knuutila and Teerenhovi 1989). Adaptation of molecular cytogenetics to the MAC technique (Wessman and Knuutila 1988; Tiainen et al. 1992) has enhanced the analysis of lineage involvement dramatically by allowing the detection of chromosome abnormalities, not only in immunologically classified metaphase cells, but also in interphase cells (Perez Losada et al. 1991; Parlier et al. 1992).

The case of large cell anaplastic (Ki-1) lymphoma with trisomy 7, discussed above, is an example of the determination of the cell lineage of abnormal (neoplastic) cells. In this patient, the determination of lineage involvement facilitated the demonstration of neoplastic cells during follow-up. Regarding therapy, the demonstration of neoplastic lineages will assume added importance in the future when target-specific treatment of leukemias is introduced, but until then, it is still important to know whether the leukemia to be treated is restricted to a single lineage or whether it is a multilineage, stem-cell disease. We are currently conducting studies to determine lineage involvement in some of the most common chromosomal abnormalities in leukemias.

Concluding Remarks

Molecular cytogenetics removes many of the problems inherent in the conventional karyotype analysis of metaphase chromosomes in leukemias. It can be justifiably argued that molecular cytogenetics should be actively employed in every cancer cytogenetic laboratory. It should be borne in mind, however, that molecular cytogenetics is complementary to, rather than a substitute for, the standard karyotype analysis of metaphase chromosomes.

Acknowledgments. The in situ hybridization team at the Department of Medical Genetics consists of the following persons: Mervi Heiskanen, M.Sc., Paula Kvick, laboratory technician, Marianne Tiainen, M.Sc., Tiina Wirtanen, laboratory technician, Maija Wessman, Ph.L., Tapani Ruutu, M.D., Erkki Elonen, M.D., Kaarle Franssila, M.D., Lasse Teerenhovi, M.D. I would also like to acknowledge the help of Thomas Cremer, M.D., Ph.D., and his group in Heidelberg, and Anton Hopman, Ph.D., in setting up our laboratory. Studies conducted by the in situ hybridization team are supported by grants from the Sigrid Juselius Foundation, Finnish Cancer Society, Finnish Academy of Science, and University of Helsinki.

References

Anastasi J, Le Beau MM, Vardiman JW, Westbrook CA (1990) Detection of numerical chromosomal abnormalities in neoplastic hematopoietic cells by in situ hybridization with a chromosome-specific probe. Am J Pathol 136:131–139

Arnoldus EPJ, Wiegant J, Noordermeer IA, Wessels JW, Beverstock GC, Grosveld GC, van der Ploeg M, Raap AK (1990) Detection of the Philadelphia chromosome in interphase nuclei. Cytogenet Cell Genet 54:108–111

Autio K, Elonen E, Teerenhovi L, Knuutila S (1987) Cytogenetic and immunologic characterization of mitotic cells in chronic lymphocytic leukemia. Eur J Haematol 39:289–298

Burns J, Chan VTW, Jonasson JA, Fleming KA, Taylor S, McGee JO'D (1985) Sensitive system for visualising biotinylated DNA probes hyridised in situ: rapid sex determination of intact cells. J Clin Pathol 38:1085–1092

Cremer T, Landegent J, Brückner A, Scholl HP, Schardin M, Hager HD, Devilee P, Pearson P, van der Ploeg M (1986) Detection of chromosome aberrations in the human interphase nucleus by visualization of specific target DNAs with radioactive and nonradioactive in situ hybridization techniques: diagnosis of trisomy 18 with probe L1.84. Hum Genet 74:346–352

Cremer T, Lichter P, Borden J, Ward DC, Manuelidis L (1988) Detection of chromosome aberrations in metaphase and interphase tumor cells by in situ hybridization using chromosome-specific library probes. Hum Genet 80:235–246

Cremer T, Popp S, Emmerich P, Lichter P, Cremer C (1990) Rapid metaphase detection of radiation-induced chromosome aberrations in human lymphocytes by chromosomal suppression in situ hybridization. Cytometry 11:110–118

Dauwerse JG, Kievits T, Beverstock GC, van der Keur D, Smit E, Wessels HW, Hagemeijer A, Pearson PL, Ommen G-JB, Breuning MH (1990) Rapid detection of chromosome 16 inversion in acute nonlymphocytic leukemia, subtype M4: regional localization of the breakpoint in 16p. Cytogenet Cell Genet 53:126–128

Eastmond DA, Pinkel D (1989) Aneuploidy detection by analysis of interphase nuclei using fluorescence in situ hybridization with chromosome-specific probes. In: Resnick MA, Vig BK (eds) Mechanisms of chromosome distribution and aneuploidy. Progress in clinical and biological research. Liss, New York, pp 277–286

Emmerich P, Jauch A, Hofmann M-C, Cremer T, Walt H (1989) Interphase cytogenetics in paraffin embedded sections from human testicular germ cell tumor xenografts and in corresponding cultured cells. Lab Invest 61:235–242

Hopman AHN, Raap AK, Landegent JE, Wiegant J, Boerman RH, van der Ploeg (1988a) Non-radioactive in situ hybridization. In: Van Leeuwen FM, Buijis RM, Pool CW, Pach O (eds) Molecular neuroanatomy. Elsevier, Amsterdam, pp 43–53

Hopman AHN, Ramaekers FCS, Raap AK, Beck JLM, Devilee P, van der Ploeg M, Vooijs GP (1988b) In situ hybridization as a tool to study numerical chromosome aberrations in solid bladder tumors. Histochemistry 89:307–316

Hopman AHN, Poddighe, PJ, Smeets AWGB, Moesker, O, Beck JLM, Voojis GP, Ramaekers FCS (1989) Detection of numerical chromosome aberrations in bladder cancer by in situ hybridization. Am J Pathol 135:1105–1117

Jauch A, Daumer C, Lichter P, Murken J, Schroeder-Kurth T, Cremer T (1990) Chromosomal in situ suppression hybridization of human gonosomes and autosomes and its use in clinical cytogenetics. Hum Genet 85:145–150

Kibbelaar RE, van Kamp H, Dreef EJ, Wessels JW, Beverstock GC, Raap AK, Fibbe WE, Ottolander GJ, Kluin PM (1991) Detection of trisomy 8 in hematological disorders by in situ hybridization. Cytogenet Cell Genet 56: 132–136

Kievits T, Dauwerse JG, Wiegant J, Devilee P, Breuning MH, Cornelisse CJ, van Ommen G-JB, Pearson PL (1990) Rapid subchromosomal localization of cosmids by nonradioactive in situ hybridization. Cytogenet Cell Genet 53:134–136

Knuutila S, Teerenhovi L (1989) Immunophenotyping of aneuploid cells. Cancer Genet Cytogenet 41:1–17

Knuutila S, Elonen E, Teerenhovi L, Rossi L, Leskinen R, Bloomfield CD, de la Chapelle A (1986) Trisomy 12 in B cells of patients with B-cell chronic lymphocytic leukemia. N Engl J Med 314:865–870

Knuutila S, Wessman M, Tiainen M (1992) Combination of in situ hybridization cytogenetics and immunologic cell identification in diagnosing minimal residual disease. In: Hiddeman W, Büchner T, Plunkett W et al. (eds) Acute leukemias III. Springer, Berlin Heidelberg New York, (Hämatologie und Bluttransfusion, vol 34), pp 190–195

Kolluri RV, Manuelidis L, Cremer T, Sait S, Cezer S, Raza A (1990) Detection of monosomy 7 in interphase cells of patients with myeloid disorders. Am J Hematol 33:117–124

Lichter P, Cremer T, Borden J, Manuelidis L, Ward DC (1988a) Delineation of individual human chromosomes in metaphase and interphase cells by in situ suppression hybridization using recombinant DNA libraries. Hum Genet 80: 224–234

Lichter P, Cremer T, Chang Tang CJ, Watkins PC, Manuelidis L, Ward DC (1988b) Rapid detection of chromosome 21 aberrations by in situ hybridization. Proc Natl Acad Sci USA 85:9664–9668

Lichter P, Tang C-JC, Call K, Hermanson G, Evans GA, Housman D, Ward DC (1990) High-resolution mapping of human chromosome 11 by in situ hybridization with cosmid clones. Science 247:64–69

Nederlof PM, Van der Flier S, Wiegant J, Raap AK, Tanke HJ, Ploem JS, Van der Ploeg M (1990) Multiple fluorescence in situ hybridization. Cytometry 11:126–131

Parlier V, Tiainen M, Beris Ph, Mischer PA, Knuutila S, Jotterand Bellomo M (1992) Trisomy 8 detection in granulo-monocytic, erythrocytic and megakaryocytic lineages by chromosomal in situ suppression hybridization in a case of refractory anemia with ringed sideroblasts complicating the course of paroxysmal nocturnal hemoglobinuria. Br J Haematol 81:296–304

Perez Losada A, Wessman M, Tiainen M, Hopman AHN, Willard HF, Sole F, Caballin MR, Woessner S, Knuutila S (1991) Trisomy 12 in chronic lymphocytic leukemia - an intenphase cytogenetic study. Blood 78:775–779

Pinkel D, Straume T, Gray JW (1986) Cytogenetic analysis using quantitative, high sensitivity, fluorescence hybridization. Proc Natl Acad Sci USA 83:2934–2938

Pinkel D, Landegent J, Collins C, Fusco J, Segraves R, Lucas J, Gray JW (1988) Fluorescence in situ hybridization with human chromosome specific libraries: detection of trisomy 21 and translocations of chromosome 4. Proc Natl Acad Sci USA 85:9138–9142

Rappold GA, Cremer T, Hager HD, Davies KE, Müller CR, Yang T (1984) Sex chromosome positions in human interphase nuclei as studied by in situ hybridization with chromosome specific DNA probes. Hum Genet 67:317–325

Smit VTHBM, Wessels JW, Mollevanger P, Schrier PI, Raap AK, Beverstock GC, Cornelissa CJ (1990) Combined GTG-banding and nonradioactive in situ hybridization improves characterization of complex karyotypes. Cytogenet Cell Genet 54:20–23

Teerenhovi L, Knuutila S, Ekblom M, Borgström GH, Tallman JK, Andersson L, de la Chapelle A (1984) A method for simultaneous study of the karyotype, morphology, and immunologic phenotype of mitotic cells in hematologic malignancies. Blood 64:1116–1122

Teerenhovi L, Lindholm C, Pakkala A, Franssila K, Stein H, Knuutila S (1988) Unique display of a pathologic karyotype in Hodgkin's disease by Reed-Sternberg cells. Cancer Genet Cytogenet 34:305–311

Tiainen M, Popp S, Parlier V, Emmerich P, Jotterand Bellomo M, Ruutu T, Cremer T, Knuutila S (1992) Chromosomal in situ suppression hybridization of immunologically classified mitotic cells in hematological malignancies. Genes Chromosomes Cancer 4:135–140

Tkachuk DC, Westbrook CA, Andreeff M, Donlon TA, Cleary ML, Suryanarayan K, Homge M, Redner A, Gray J, Pinkel D (1990) Detection of bcr-abl fusion in chronic myelogeneous leukemia by in situ hybridization. Science 250:559–562

Trask BJ, Massa H, Kenwrick S, Gitschier J (1991) Mapping of human chromosome Xq28 by two-color fluorescence in situ hybridization of DNA sequences to interphase cell nuclei. Am J Hum Genet 48:1–15

Wessman M, Knuutila S (1988) A method for the determination of cell morphology, immunologic phenotype and numerical chromosomal abnormalities on the same mitotic or interphase cancer cell. Genet (Life Sci Adv) 7:127–130

Wessman M, Ruutu T, Volin L, Knuutila S (1989) In situ hybridization using a Y-specific probe – a sensitive method for distinguishing residual male recipient cells from female donor cells in bone marrow transplantation. Bone Marrow Transpl 4:283–286

Willard HF, Waye JS (1987) Hierarchial order in chromosome-specific human alpha satellite DNA. Trends Genet 3:192–198

Wessman M, Popp S, Ruutu T, Volin L, Cremer T, Knuutila S (1993) Detection of residual host cells after bone marrow transplantation using non-isotopic in situ hybridization and karyotype analysis. Bone Marrow Transpl (in press)

Cytogenetic Abnormalities Associated with Childhood Acute Myeloblastic Leukemia

O.A. Haas, M. Kronberger, and L. Mayerhofer

Children's Cancer Research Institute (CCRI), St. Anna Children's Hospital, Kinderspitalgasse 6, A-1090 Vienna, Austria

Introduction

Within the last two decades several nonrandom acquired karyotype abnormalities have been identified in acute myeloblastic leukemia (AML). These abnormalities are specifically associated with morphologically and/or immunologically defined subgroups and define subentities with distinct biological and clinical features (Fig. 1). Consequently, they provide objective disease markers and suggest a specific diagnosis. Furthermore, they reveal the location of genes relevant to disease etiology or progression and have been shown to indicate a patient's prognosis. Since the various types of abnormalities result from causative leukemogenic factors and the genetic background of the patient, their incidence varies within different geographic areas and ethnic subgroups. Although practically all of the specific changes have been observed both in adult as well as in childhood AML, the incidence of individual abnormalities also varies considerably within different age groups. In the following we present a comprehensive overview of published cytogenetic studies in childhood AML and discuss some of the recent cytogenetic findings together with their clinical and biological implications.

General Considerations

AML comprises approximately 10% of all childhood leukemias. It is therefore understandable that, in contrast to adult AML, only few and comparatively small cytogenetic studies of childhood AML have been published within the last decade. A short review of our patients has recently been reported by Kronberger (1991). For comparison of these studies, it is particularly important to analyze the cytogenetic data in context with the age distribution of the respective patients and the morphological classification of their leukemias (Tables 1, 2). The age distribution is unfortunately only

Recent Results in Cancer Research, Vol. 131

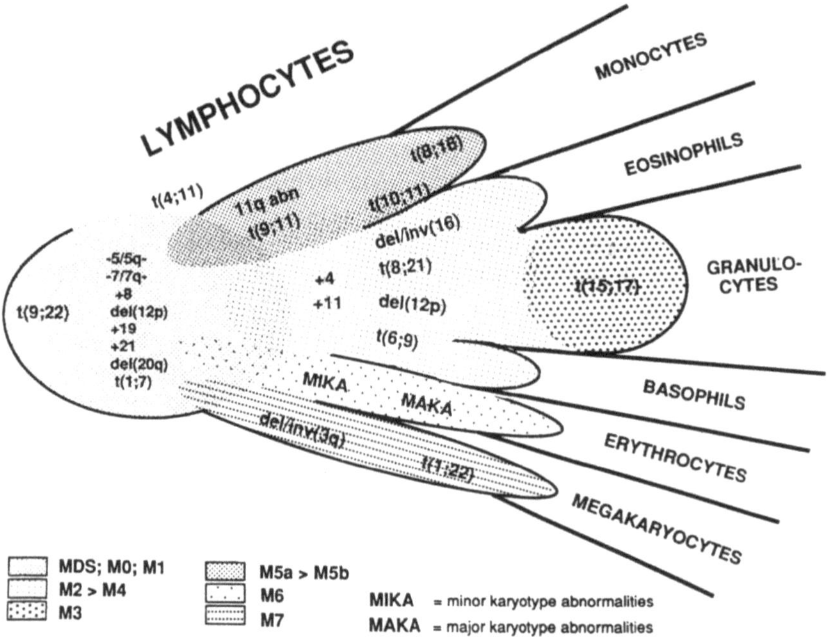

Fig. 1. Schematic representation of specific and typical acquired karyotype abnormalities seen in particular subgroups of acute myeloid leukemia with regard to their association with different maturation stages and cell type involvement

available for the earlier studies with only small numbers of patients. The differences in the distribution of morphological subentities is reflected to a certain extent in the distribution of the various cytogenetic abnormalities. The overall incidence of cytogenetic abnormalities lies between 67% and 79%. The incidence of specific, FAB-associated abnormalities is, with one exception (Olah et al. 1988), between 40% and 50%. Since nearly half of the cases reported by Slater et al. (1983) were of M2 morphology, it is not surprising that, compared to larger studies, approximately twice as many cases had a t(8;21). Interestingly, this abnormality as well as the t(15;17) which is highly specific for AML M3 was rather uncommon in our patients. Inv(16), which was decribed for the first time in 1983, has been reported only in the later and larger studies, with an incidence ranging from 3% to 16%. Although we observed approximately the same incidence of M5 leukemias as others, we had nearly twice as many leukemias with 11(q23) abnormalities. This finding may be explained by our relative large number of infant leukemias, a group which is considered difficult to treat, and by the fact that some of the leukemias with 11(q23) abnormalities were morphologically classified as either M1 or M4 or, in some instances, even resembled acute lymphoblastic leukemia (ALL) AML. M6 seems to be overrepresented in smaller studies

Table 1. Age distribution and morphological subtypes in cytogenetic studies of childhood AML

	Kaneko et al. (1982)		Slater et al. (1983)		Bernstein et al. (1984)		Olah et al. (1988)		Leverger et al. (1988)		Raimondi et al. (1989)		Ritterbach et al. (1990)		Vienna (1978–1989)	
Patients (*n*)	26		16		26		30		130		121		169		71	
Male/female	13/13		8/8		20/6		?		68/62		?		?		37/34	
	(*n*)	(%)	(*n*)	(%)	(*n*)	(%)	(*n*)	(%)	(*n*)	(%)	(*n*)	(%)	(*n*)	(%)	(*n*)	(%)
Age																
0–1 year	3	11	2	12	2	8	?	?	?	?	?	?	?	?	16	23
1–5 years	8	31	5	31	3	11	?	?	?	?	?	?	?	?	21	29
5–10 years	7	27	3	19	13	50	?	?	?	?	?	?	?	?	17	24
over 10 years	8	31	6	38	8	31	?	?	?	?	?	?	?	?	17	24
FAB																
M n.o.s.	–	–	–	–	–	–	–	–	11	9	1	1	?	?	–	–
M1	4	15	–	–	3	11	9	30	21	16	28	23	?	?	14	20
M2	8	31	7	44	8	31	6	20	29	22	30	24	?	?	17	24
M3	3	12	1	6	5	20	–	–	11	8	9	7	?	?	1	1
M4	4	15	4	25	4	16	11	37	25	19	26	22	?	?	15	21
M5	6	23	1	6	3	11	1	3	23	18	25	21	?	?	14	20
M6	1	4	3	19	3	11	3	10	5	4	–	–	?	?	2	3
M7	–	–	–	–	–	–	–	–	5	4	2	2	?	?	3	4
L or L + M	–	–	–	–	–	–	–	–	?	?	–	–	?	?	5	7

n.o.s., not otherwise specified; L, with lymphoblastic morphology, but pure myeloid immunophenotype; L + M, lympho- and myeloblastic cell populations

Table 2. Cytogenetic findings in childhood AML

	Kaneko et al. 1982		Slater et al. 1983		Bernstein et al. 1984		Olah et al. 1988		Leverger et al. 1988		Raimondi et al. 1989		Ritterbach et al. 1990		Vienna 1978–89	
No. of patients	26		16		26		30		130		121		169		71	
	(*n*)	(%)	(*n*)	(%)	(*n*)	(%)	(*n*)	(%)	(*n*)	(%)	(*n*)	(%)	(*n*)	(%)	(*n*)	(%)
Normal	5	19	3	19	7	27	10	33	41	32	25	21	54	32	24	25
Abnormal	21	81	13	81	19	73	20	67	89	68	96	79	115	68	47	75
Specific abnormalities[a]	8	38	5	39	9	47	4	20	46	52	52	56	46	40	25	53
t(9;22)	–	–	–	–	2	10	–	–		–	–	–	–	–	1	2
t(8;21)	3	14	4	31	4	21	2	10	17	19	14	15	16	14	3	6
t(15;17)	3	14	1	8	2	10	–	–	10	11	9	9	5	4	1	2
inv/del (16)	–	–	–	–	1	5	–	–	5	5	15	16	4	3	4	9
t/del(11)(q23)	2	10	–	–	–	–	2	10	14	17	16	17	21	18	16	34
Typical abnormalities[b]	6	29	3	22	3	16	4	20	14	16	6	6	20	17	8	17
+8	–	–	1	8	–	–	4	20	2	2	–	–	?	?	6	13
−7/del(7q)	–	–	–	–	3	16	–	–	5	4	6	6	?	?	2	4
−5/del(5q)	–	–	–	–	–	–	–	–	–	–	–	–	?	?	–	–
complex[c]	6	29	2	14	–	–	–	–	9	10	–	–	?	?	–	–
Other abnormalities	7	33	5	39	7	38	12	60	29	33	36	38	49	43	14	30
Single	1	4	–	–	6	33	10	50	12	14	36	38	?	?	10	21
Multiple	6	29	5	39	1	5	2	10	17	19	–	–	?	?	4	9

[a] FAB-associated.
[b] Not FAB-associated.
[c] Combinations of +8, −7/del(7q) and/or −5/del(5q).

and, for reasons pointed out later, acute megakaryocytic leukemia (AML M7) are not seen in earlier studies. The cases summarized in the group "other abnormalities" make up between 30% and 40% and comprise single and multiple abnormalities which, due to their rare incidence, have not been assigned to a specific biological and/or clinical subentity. They include recurrent abormalities such as +4, +11, t(1;7), inv/del(3q), t(8;16), and t(1;22), which will discussed in more detail later on.

The brief analysis of these data suggests that the differing incidences of cytogenetic abnormalities observed in these studies correlate with the distribution of morphological subgroups for which these abnormalities are characteristic. It should be noted, however, that they also depend on the age distribution of the patients. In order to obtain a representative overview about the incidence and distribution of these cytogenetic abnormalities in childhood AML, a large number of cases must be collected and analyzed. These facts need to be taken into consideration when different studies are compared.

AML in Patients with Down's Syndrome

Individuals with Down's syndrome have an increased risk of developing either a transient myeloproliferative disorder (TMD) or progressive acute leukemia. Despite extensive studies and the detection of a characteristic phenotypic pattern associated with these abnormal myeloproliferations, it is generally impossible to distinguish these two conditions by means of blast cell morphology, clinical signs, or even immunophenotype (Haas et al. 1990; Ravindranath et al. 1990). Moreover, it has been shown that TMD results from a monoclonal expansion of immature cells (Kurahashi et al. 1991), which otherwise is a criterion for a neoplastic process. Comparing patients with TMD and AML M7, which is the most common form of AML in Down's syndrome, Hayashi et al. (1988) found that individuals with TMD are significantly younger and generally have higher leukocyte and platelet counts as well as hemoglobin levels. Most strikingly, however, they found acquired complex karyotype abnormalities in all leukemia patients, whereas individuals with TMD had no chromosome changes in addition to their constitutional abnormalities. Provided these findings are confirmed, cytogenetic analysis may be a useful contribution for delineating TMD from overt leukemia in Down's syndrome with abnormal myelopoiesis.

t(1;22) in Infant Megakaryocytic Leukemia (AML M7)

Owing to the difficulties formerly encountered in distinguishing de novo (AML M7) from other forms of leukemias and, in particular, myelodysplastic syndromes, cytogenetic data on this form of leukemia are scarce.

However, with the help of immunological phenotyping it has been shown that AML M7 seems to constitute at least 5% of all childhood leukemias and as much as 20% of infant AML (Köller et al. 1989; Lion et al. 1992). Lion et al. recently described a new nonrandom karyotype abnormality – a balanced translocation t(1;22)(p13;q13) (Fig. 2) – which was found in 5 of 445 children with AML who were cytogenetically investigated in four European centers. This unique chromosome abnormality constituted 17% (5 of 30 cases) of children with AML M7, and 45% (5 of 11 cases) of infants with megakaryocytic leukemia. Since this abnormality has only previously been reported once, also in a girl with congenital megakaryocytic leukemia, this finding suggests that Lion et al. have identified a novel cytogenetic marker specific for AML M7 in infants.

Chromosome 11q23 Abnormalities

In infant leukemia both lympho- as well as myeloblastic subtypes occur. They are characterized by rather heterogeneous immunophenotypic and genotypic features (Ludwig et al. 1989; Köller et al. 1989). Cytogenetic results from more than 150 cases of infant leukemias have been published so far. Chromosome 11 abnormalities, in particular of region q23–q24, are very common and are observed in both forms. They constitute approximately half of the abnormal karyotypes seen in infant ALL cases. The most frequently encountered specific anomaly is a t(4;11)(q21;q23) which, furthermore, is strongly associated with a mixed pre-pre-B/myeloid phenotype (Ludwig et al. 1989). In infant AML the most common form is monocytic

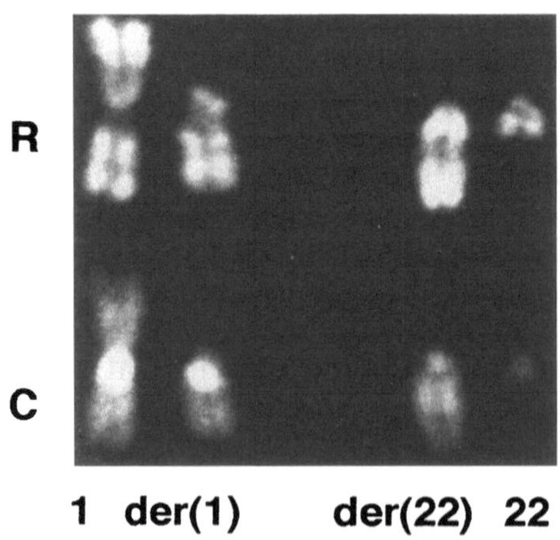

Fig. 2. Partial karyotype of normal and translocated chromosomes 1 and 22 from an infant with megakaryocytic leukemia and a t(1;22)(p13;q13). The chromosomes were R- (*top*) and C-banded (*bottom*) with chromomycin A3 and distamycin A/DAPI and the karyotype generated with a Genevision 121 chromosome analysis system

leukemia. Its characteristic specific karyotype change is a t(9;11)(p21;q23). Interestingly, translocations t(4;11) are exceptionally rare in pure myeloid leukemias, whereas translocations t(9;11) have also been described in ALL and mixed leukemias. Bearing in mind, however, that such particular forms of lympho- and myeloblastic leukemia may be very difficult to distinguish by morphological means, a reliable delineation is only possible by immunological phenotyping. Thus, the combination of immunological phenotyping and cytogenetic analysis allows a more precise delineation and classification of such leukemias, which may have important bearings on treatment decisions.

Another intriguing finding in 11q23 abnormalities is that they have been reported in secondary leukemias, following successful treatment of childhood ALL, particularly T-cell ALL (Pui et al. 1989). One explanation proposed was a certain undefined biological predisposition in such patients. Another, more plausible reason for this complication may be the preceding treatment of all the affected patients with epipodophyllotoxin, a relatively new anti-leukemic and most likely carcinogenic drug. Indeed, such secondary AMLs with t(9;11) have also been observed in children and adults with solid tumors following treatment with epipodophyllotoxin (Weh et al. 1986; Ratain et al. 1987; Pui et al. 1990).

New Clues to Leukemia Pathogenesis and Therapeutic Implications

Tumor-associated, acquired karyotype abnormalities reveal the locations of genes involved in the pathogenesis of the respective neoplasms. However, there are so far only few examples in which the genes involved in specific translocations have been identified, the first and best known being the t(9;22) of chronic myeloid leukemia. The important genetic event in this translocation occurs on chromosome 22. The importance of this region is further underlined by the facts that duplication of the derivative chromosome 22 can be part of the clonal evolution, and that variant or masked translocations always affect chromosome 22. It is therefore interesting to note that in two of the patients with a t(1;22) reported by Lion et al. (1991) duplication of the chromosome 1 translocation product was observed, which accordingly suggests that in these leukemias the critical genetic event occurs on the chromosome 1 breakpoint.

Similar conclusions can be drawn from observations made with leukemias bearing a t(9;11). In our patients we not only observed a high incidence of typical, but also of complex and unusual translocations t(9;11). Only few such variants have been reported thus far (Kaneko et al. 1982; Harris et al. 1988). In all instances the secondary changes exclusively affected the region 9p21, which may indicate the critical role of a gene residing in this chromosomal region.

The identification of genes affected and disturbed by such specific translocations may have important implications for the development of new treatment modalities. It has recently been shown that the translocation t(15;17), the specific cytogenetic marker for acute promyelocytic leukemia, fuses the retinoic acid receptor α on chromosome 17 to a novel transcribed gene on chromosome 15 (de The et al. 1990). At the same time, all-*trans*-retinoic acid has been successfully applied as differentiation therapy for this type of leukemia (Castaigne et al. 1990). Although the relationship between the underlying genetic defect and the efficacy of treatment is still unclear, this finding nevertheless provides the first direct evidence that an acquired genetic alteration can be specifically influenced by a specific growth and/or differentiation factor.

Cytogenetic abnormalities have been found to have independent prognostic significance in adult AML (Berger et al. 1987; Arthur et al. 1989; Fenaux et al. 1989; Schiffer et al. 1989). This is probably also true for childhood AML. Owing to the small numbers of cases and the continuously improving treatment, the prognostic significance of individual abnormalities will be difficult to establish unequivocally. Undoubtedly, however, chromosome abnormalities are closely related to the pathogenesis and progression of leukemias and will therefore, as the t(15;17) elegantly exemplifies, help to individualize therapy and to design more sophisticated and less harmful treatment approaches.

Acknowledgements. Supported by the Jubiläumsfonds der Österreichischen Nationalbank, grant no. 3838, and the Fonds zur Förderung der wissenschaftlichen Forschung, grant no. P-7777.

References

Arthur DC, Berger R, Golomb HM, Swansbury GJ, Reeves BR, Alimena G, Van Den Berghe H, Bloomfield CD, de la Chapelle A, Dewald GW et al. (1989) The clinical significance of karyotype in acute myelogenous leukemia. Cancer Genet Cytogenet 40:203–216

Berger R, Flandrin G, Bernheim A, Le Coniat M, Vecchione D, Pacot A, Derre J, Daniel MT, Valensi F, Sigaux F, Ochoa-Nogueira ME (1987) Cytogenetic studies on 519 consecutive de novo acute nonlymphocytic leukemias. Cancer Genet Cytogenet 29:9–21.

Bernstein R, Macdougall LG, Pinto MR (1984) Chromosome patterns in 26 South African children with acute nonlymphocytic leukemia (ANLL). Cancer Genet Cyogenet 11:199–214.

Castaigne S, Chomienne C, Daniel MT, Ballerini P, Berger R, Fenaux P, Degos L (1990) All-trans retinoic acid as differentiation therapy for acute promyelocytic leukemia: I. Clinical results. Blood 76:1704–1709

Cuneo A, Mecucci C, Kerim S, Vandenberghe E, Dal Cin P, Van Orshoven A, Rodhain J, Bosly A, Michaux JL, Martiat P, Carli MG, Castoldi G, Van den Berghe H (1989) Multipotent stem cell involvement in megakaryoblastic leukemia: cytologic and cytogenetic evidence in 15 patients. Blood 74:1781–1790

de The H, Chomienne C, Lanotte M, Degos L, Dejean A (1990) The t(15;17) translocation of acute promyelocytic leukaemia fuses the retinoic acid receptor a gene to a novel transcribed locus. Nature 347:558–561

Fenaux P, Preudhomme C, Lai JL, Morel P, Beuscart R, Bauters F (1989) Cytogenetics and their prognostic value in de novo acute myeloid leukaemia: a report on 283 cases. Br J Haematol 73:61–67

Haas OA, Köller U, Fink FM, Zoubek A, Knapp W, Gadner H (1990) Transient myeloproliferative disorder in Down's syndrome is characterised by an unique immunological phenotype. Klin Pädiatr 202:291 (abstr)

Harris BN, Davis EM, Le Beau MM, Bitter MA, Kaminer LS, Morgan E, Rowley JD (1988) Variant translocations (9;11): identification of the critical genetic rearrangement. Cancer Genet Cytogenet 30:171–175

Hayashi Y, Eguchi M, Sugita K, Nakazawa S, Sato T, Kojima S, Bessho F, Konishi S, Inaba T, Hanada R, Yamamoto K (1988) Cytogenetic findings and clinical features in acute leukemia and transient myeloproliferative disorder in Down's syndrome. Blood 72:15–23

Kaneko Y, Rowley JD, Maurer HS, Variakojis D, Moohr JW (1982) Chromosomal pattern in childhood acute nonlymphocytic leukemia. Blood 60:389–99

Köller U, Haas OA, Ludwig WD, Bartram CR, Harbott J, Panzer-Grümayer R, Hansen-Hagge T, Ritter J, Creutzig U, Knapp W, Gadner H (1989) Phenotypic and genotypic heterogeneity in infant acute leukemia: II. Acute nonlymphoblastic leukemia. Leukemia 3:708–714

Kronberger M (1991) Cytogenetic aspects of acute non-lymphatic leukemia (ANLL) in childhood. Wien Klin Wochenschr 103:95–97

Kurahashi H, Hara J, Yumura-Yagi K, Murayama N, Inoue M, Ishihara S, Tawa A, Okada S, Kawa-Ha K (1991) Monoclonal nature of transient abnormal myelopoiesis in Down's syndrome. Blood 77:1161–1163

Leverger G, Bernheim A, Daniel MT, Flandrin G, Schaison G, Berger R (1988) Cytogenetic study of 130 childhood acute nonlymphocytic leukemias. Med Pediatr Oncol 16:227–232

Lion T, Haas OA, Harbott J, Bannier E, Ritterbach J, Jankovic M, Fink M, Stojimirovic A, Herrmann J, Riehm H, Lampert F, Ritter J, Koch H, Gadner H (1992) The translocation t(1;22)(p13;q13) is a nonrandom marker specifically associated with acute megakaryocytic leukemia in infants. Blood 79:3325–3330

Ludwig WD, Bartram CR, Harbott J, Köller U, Haas OA, Hansen-Hagge T, Heil G, Seibt-Jung H, Teichmann JV, Ritter J, Knapp W, Gadner H, Thiel E, Riehm H (1989) Phenotypic and genotypic heterogeneity in infant acute leukemia: I. Acute lymphoblastic leukemia. Leukemia 3:431–439

Olah E, Balogh E, Szollar J, Szakmary E, Kovacs I, Schuler D, Karmazsin L (1988) Cytogenetic investigations on children with acute non-lymphocytic leukemia. Blut 56:249–255

Pui CH, Behm FG, Raimondi SC, Dodge RK, George SL, Rivera GK, Mirro J Jr, Kalwinsky DK, Dahl GV, Murphy SB (1989) Secondary acute myeloid leukemia in children treated for acute lymphoid leukemia. N Engl J Med 321:136–142

Pui CH, Hancock ML, Raimondi SC, Head DR, Thompson E, Williams J, Kun LE, Bowman LC, Crist WM, Pratt CB (1990) Myeloid neoplasia in children treated for solid tumours. Lancet 336:417–421

Raimondi SC, Kalwinsky DK, Hayashi Y, Behm FG, Mirro J, Williams DL (1989) Cytogenetics of childhood acute nonlymphocytic leukemia. Cancer Genet Cytogenet 40:13–27

Ratain MJ, Kaminer LS, Bitran JD, Larson AR, LeBeau MM, Skosey C, Purl S, Hoffmann PC, Wade J, Vardiman JW, Daly K, Rowley JD, Golomb HM (1987) Acute nonlymphocytic leukemia following etoposide and cisplatin combination therapy for advanced non-small-cell carcinoma of the lung. Blood 70:1412–1417

Ravindranath Y, Abella E, Kirschner J, Civin CI, Harris M, Chauvenet A, Alvarado C, Dubowy R, Ritchey AK, Land V, Steuber CP (1990) Acute myeloid leukemia (AML) in Down's syndrome (DS): a highly curable disease? Blood Suppl 76:311a (Abstract 1235)

Ritterbach J, Harbott J, Ritter J, Lampert F (1990) Chromosomal aberrations in childhood acute nonlymphoblastic leukemia. Haematol Bluttransfus 33:153–156

Schiffer CA, Lee EJ, Tomiyasu T, Wiernik PH, Testa JR (1989) Prognostic impact of cytogenetic abnormalities in patients with de novo acute nonlymphocytic leukemia. Blood 73:263–270

Slater RM, Behrendt H, de Waal FC (1983) Chromosome studies on acute nonlymphocytic leukaemia in children. Pediatr Res 17:398–405

Weh HJ, Kabisch H, Landbeck G, Hossfeld DK (1986) Translocation (9;11)(p21;q23) in a child with acute monoblastic leukemia following 2 1/2 years after successful chemotherapy for neuroblastoma. J Clin Oncol 4:1518–1520

DNA Aneuploidy in Childhood Acute Lymphoblastic Leukemia: Relation to Clinical Determinants and Prognosis within Four Consecutive BFM Trials

W. Hiddemann[1], J. Harbott[2], W.-D. Ludwig[3], J. Ritter[4], A. Nehmer[5], A. Reiter[5], A. Kolkmeyer[6], T. Laing[6], and H. Riehm[5]

[1] Department of Internal Medicine, University of Göttingen, Robert Ko Ch Str. 40, W-3400 Göttingen, Fed. Rep. of Germany
[2] Department of Pediatrics, University of Gieβen, W-6300 Gieβen, Fed. Rep. of Germany
[3] Department of Internal Medicine, Klinikum Steglitz, Free University Berlin, W-1000 Berlin 45, Fed. Rep. of Germany
[4] Department of Pediatrics, University of Münster, W-4400 Münster, Fed. Rep. of Germany
[5] Department of Pediatrics, Medical School of Hannover, W-3000 Hannover, Fed. Rep. of Germany
[6] Department of Internal Medicine, University of Münster, Albert-Schweizer-Straβe 33, W-4400 Münster, Fed. Rep. of Germany

Introduction

The major breakthroughs in the treatment of childhood acute lymphoblastic leukemia (ALL) occurred in the late 1970s and early 1980s and came mainly from empirically designed treatment concepts (Riehm et al. 1980, 1990). Recent attempts to further improve the outcome in children with this disease have concentrated on unravelling the underlying pathogenetic mechanisms. They have provided the means to discriminate subgroups of patients with different biology, and prognosis, leading to the concept of a risk-adapted treatment stratification. Hence, various determinants derived from immunophenotype analysis (Greaves et al. 1981; Grist et al. 1989; Borowitz et al. 1990), flow cytometric determination of the cellular DNA content (Look et al. 1982; Hiddemann et al. 1986; Andreeff et al. 1986), and karyotype evaluations (Williams et al. 1982; Pui et al. 1990) have been shown to convey prognostic information. In particular, ploidy or chromosome number has proved to be a strong predictor of outcome with a favorable prognosis for patients with numerical aberrations who have more than 50 chromosomes. Structural abnormalities, on the other hand, were found to be associated with a higher frequency of relapses and a shorter remission duration (Williams et al. 1982; Pui et al. 1990; Secker-Walker 1984). Along this line, the detection of DNA aneuploidies by means of flow cytometric determination of the cellular DNA content also proved a powerful tool with prognostic implications. High-grade aneuploidy as defined by a DNA index ≥1.16 comprises an favorable prognostic factor which may turn out to be an

Recent Results in Cancer Research, Vol. 131

additional variable with independent prognostic significance (Look et al. 1985; Smets et al. 1985).

Here, we present a summary of the results of DNA measurements performed in children with ALL who were treated within the four consecutive Berlin-Frankfurt-Münster (BFM) ALL studies 79, 81, 83, and 86. In addition, the results of a comparative analysis of flow cytometric and karyotype evaluations are described.

Material and Methods

The current study comprises peripheral blood and bone marrow material from 860 children with newly diagnosed ALL who were treated within the BFM studies 79, 81, 83, and 86. Initial diagnostic work-up included conventional morphology and cytochemical staining as well as immunophentopye analysis and karyotype evaluations.

For measurements of the cellular DNA content, heparinized blood and/or bone marrow specimens were subjected to density gradient separation over Ficoll-Hypaque (density 1.078 g/ml) for 20 min at room temperature. The white cell layer was removed, resuspendend in Hank's balanced salt solution (HBSS), washed twice, and subsequently fixed in 96% ice-cold ethanol. Prior to staining the cells were centrifuged again at 1000 *g* for 10 min; the pellet was resuspended in a 0.5% pespsin HCl solution (Merck pepsin 1000 U/g) for 5–8 min and stained by ethidium bromide and mithramycin in combination. After 30 min of staining the cells were measured on a modified PAS 2 flow cytometer hooked up to a 1024-channel multichannel analyzer.

For the detection of DNA aneuploidies and for the determination of the DNA index all samples were mixed with diploid mononuclear cells from normal blood donors at two different concentrations. The appearance of a second $G_{0/1}$ peak and its variation according to the ratio between sample versus reference cells was considered to indicate a DNA aneuploidy. The degree of DNA aneuploidy was determined by the DNA index, defined as the relative DNA content of $G_{0/1}$ cells of the sample/relative DNA content of $G_{0/1}$ reference cells. (Barlogie et al. 1983; Hiddemann et al. 1984).

Statistical analyses included the modified chi-square test for groups of independent variables. Differences between mean values were calculated by the *t* test. The Kaplan-Meier method was used for the evaluation of life tables, with differences being assessed by the log-rank test.

Results

Measurements of the cellular DNA content were performed on 860 patients; in 401 cases results of cytogenetic analysis were available. DNA aneuploidies were identified in 318 cases (37%), DNA indices ranging from 0.52 to 2.16

with a median of 1.18. DNA aneuploidy in general was found to be associated with a low white blood cell count, pre-B-ALL immunophentoype, the expression of CD10, female gender, age between 2 and 10 years, and a low risk classification. These relations were most pronounced in children with DNA indices ≥1.16, as shown for immunophenotype and risk definition in Tables 1 and 2.

A combined analysis of all four BFM ALL studies indicates a significantly longer event-free interval in children with DNA indices ≥1.16 (Fig. 1) than in those with DNA <1.16, including cases without aneuploid DNA stemlines.

A separate analysis of each individual study confirmed the favorable outcome for children with DNA indices ≥1.16 in studies 79, 83, and 86. Furthermore, although DNA aneuploidy and DNA index ≥1.16 in particular were associated with low risk, a DNA index ≥1.16 may represent an additional and independent beneficial prognostic factor. Hence, in study BFM 83 a longer event-free interval was observed in children with DNA indices ≥1.16 in cases with low, standard, or high risk (Figs. 2–4).

A note of caution, however, emerges from the results of study BFM 81 in which, in contrast to the previous results, DNA aneuploidy and a DNA index ≥1.16 in particular were associated with an inferior prognosis (Fig. 5). Hence, a prospective study to define the relevance of DNA aneupolidy and DNA index ≥1.16 within the BFM trials seems clearly warranted.

Table 1. DNA aneuploidy and immunophenotype: BFM studies 81, 83, and 86

Immunological subgroup	DNA index					
	≤1.0		1.0–1.15		≥1.16	
	(*n*)	(%)	(*n*)	(%)	(*n*)	(%)
Pre-pre-B-ALL	28	88	1	3	3	9
Pre-B-ALL	38	80	3	6	7	14
Common-ALL	280	55	56	11	171	34
T-cell ALL	95	88	5	5	8	7

Table 2. DNA aneuploidy and risk definition: BFM studies 81, 83, and 86

Risk group	DNA index					
	≤1.0		1.0–1.15		≥1.16	
	(*n*)	(%)	(*n*)	(%)	(*n*)	(%)
RF <0.8	120	56	20	9	74	35
RF 0.8–1.2	143	57	35	14	72	39
RF ≥1.2	241	74	30	9	53	17

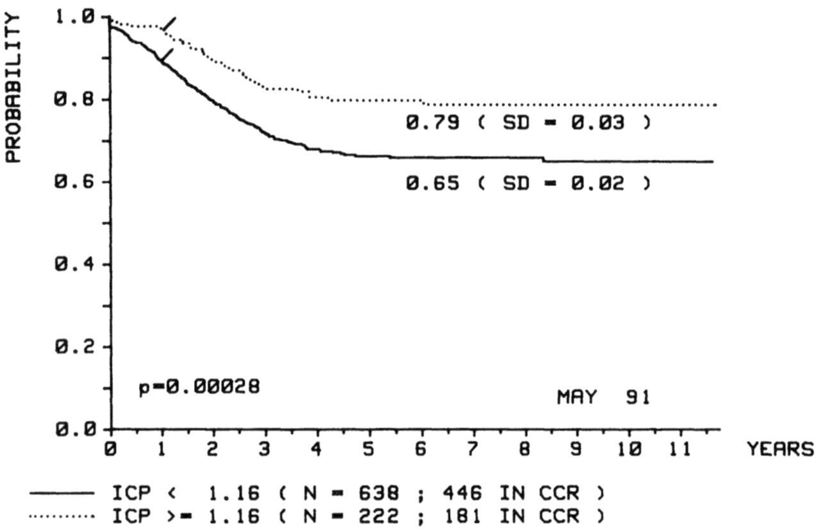

Fig. 1. Event-free survival of non-B-ALL cases in all four BFM ALL trials (79, 81, 83, 86). *ICP*, DNA index; *CCR*, continuous complete remission

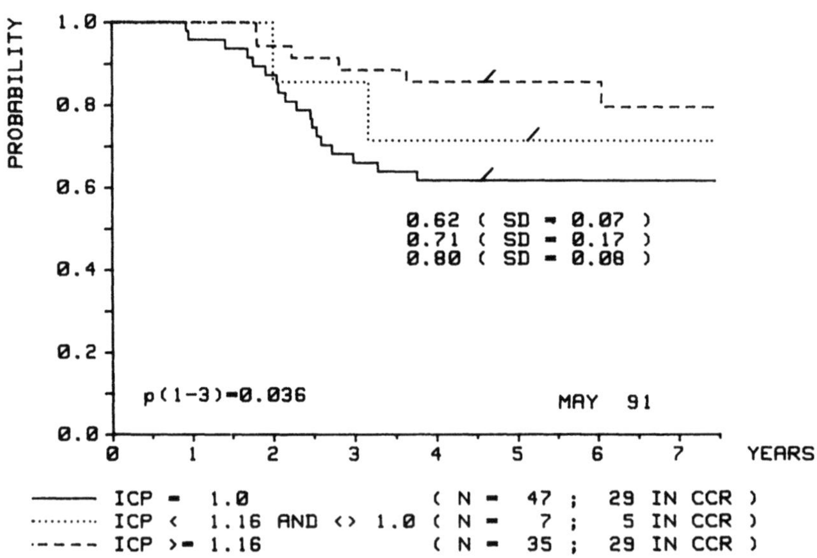

Fig. 2. Event-free survival of non-B-ALL cases with low risk (risk factor < 0.8) in BFM ALL trial 83

In a separate analysis DNA measurements were compared with the results of cytogenetic evaluations in 401 patients. As indicated by Table 3, aneuploid DNA stem lines were identified in 134 specimens (33%). Cytogenetic abnormalities were observed in 144 of 244 evaluable specimens (59%). In 157 patients (39%) karyotypes were not evaluable. In the latter

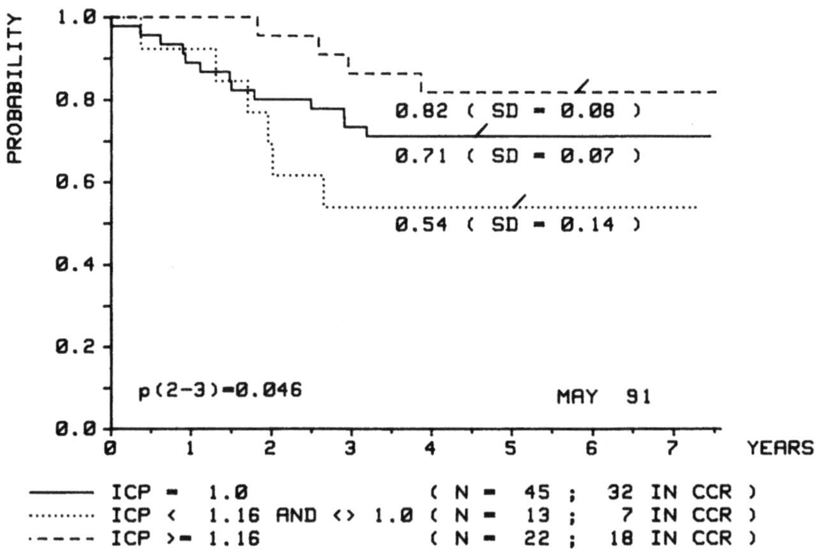

Fig. 3. Event-free survival of non-B-ALL cases with standard risk (risk factor 0.8–1.2) in BFM ALL trial 83

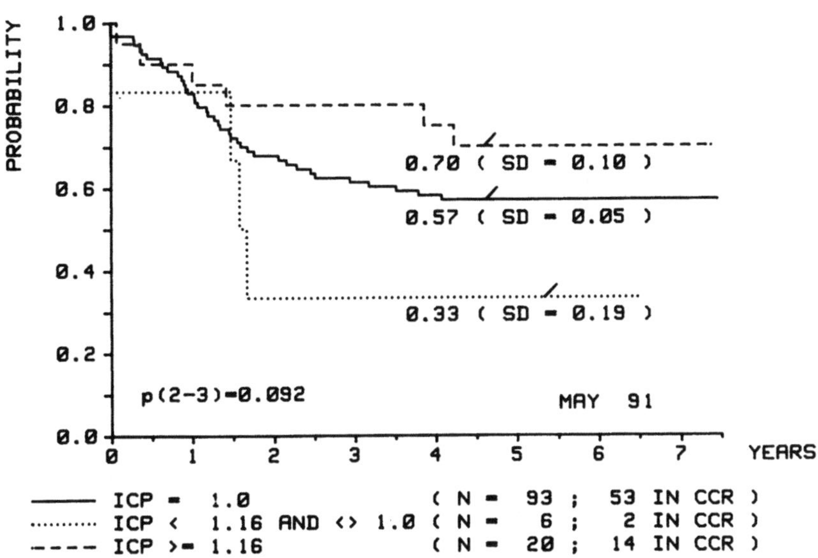

Fig. 4. Event-free survival of non-B-ALL cases with high risk (risk factor $\geqslant$ 1.2) in BFM ALL trial 83

group DNA aneuploidies were detected in 52 cases (33%). Remarkably, 16% of cases with normal cytogenetic findings revealed aneuploid DNA stem lines. While among patients with pseudodiploid karyotypes or numeric aberrations with one to three additional chromosomes aneuploid DNA stem lines were

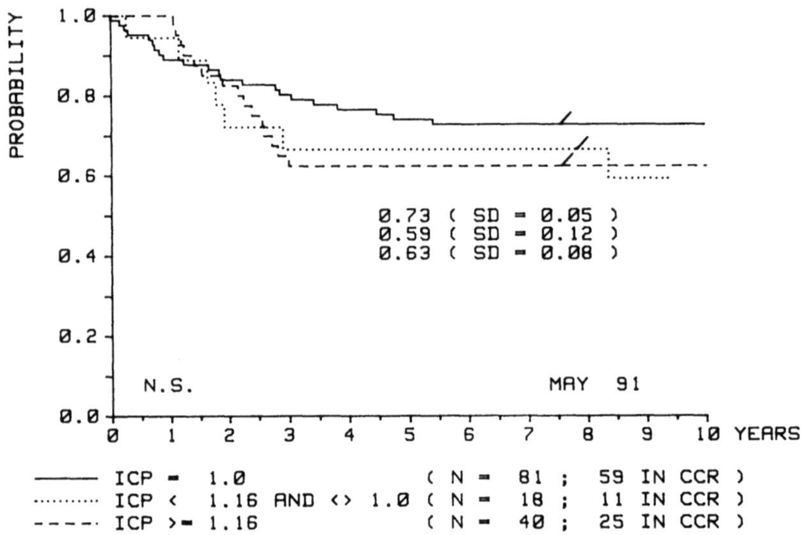

Fig. 5. Event-free survival of non-B-ALL cases in BFM ALL trial 81

Table 3. Flow cytometric DNA analysis

Karyotype analysis	Patients		DNA index ≠ 1.0		DNA index = 1.0	
	(*n*)	(%)	(*n*)	(%)	(*n*)	(%)
Karyotype not evaluable	157	39	105	67	52	33
Normal karyotype	100	25	84	84	16	16
Pseudodiploid karyotype	61	15	56	92	5	8
47–50 chromosomes	29	7	21	72	8	28
>50 chromosomes	54	14	1	2	53	98
Total	401	100	267	67	134	33

identified in only 8% and 28% of cases, a high correlation became evident in cases with numeric aberrations of more than three chromosomes, in whom 53 of 54 cases also had aneuploid DNA stem lines.

Discussion

When flow cytometry was first used for the investigation of hematological disorders by Büchner et al. in 1971 and shortly thereafter by Melamed and coworkers in 1972, it was the major goal of these and subsequent studies to assess the cell kinetics of these disorders and the impact of cytostatic therapy on the cell cycle. New developments in flow systems and improvements in cell preparation and staining techniques broadened the spectrum of application and provided the means for immunophenotyping by flow cytometry and for the detection of DNA aneuploidies, first described by Büchner et al. in 1971. Both parameters proved of clinical significance for the diagnostic classification of acute leukemias as well as for their prognosis, especially in children with ALL. Further studies indicated that in particular a DNA index ≥1.16 was associated with a favorable prognosis, corresponding to a better outcome for children with hyperdiploid karyotypes with >53 chromosomes (Williams et al. 1982; Pui et al. 1990; Secker-Walker 1984; Look et al. 1985; Smets et al. 1985). Although DNA index ≥1.16 is related to other low risk features such as low white blood cell count, a high proportion of cells in S phase, pre-B-ALL immunophenotype, and a low frequency of chromosomal translocations it was found to be an independent additional beneficial prognostic factor (Pui et al. 1990; Look et al. 1985; Smets et al. 1985). The results of the current investigations support these findings in part, in that overall children with DNA indices ≥1.16 had a longer event-free interval in three of the four consecutive BFM ALL studies in which DNA analyses were performed. In study BFM 83 in particular, where the largest number of patients was evaluated with a sufficiently long follow-up, DNA index ≥1.16 identified patients with a better outcome in the low- and standard- as well as high-risk categories. The results of study BFM 81, however, indicate the opposite relation and mean that caution is required in using a DNA index ≥1.16 for risk-adapted treatment stratification in the BFM studies at the present time. Prospective controlled studies are warranted to ultimately define the prognostic significance of DNA aneuploidy, which also represents an easily accessable parameter for multicenter trials.

The comparative evaluation of flow cytometric measurements and cytogenetic analyses emphasizes the values and limitations of both techniques. Hence, karyotypes were not evaluable in 39% of patient samples, while flow cytometric determinations were successful in 96% of samples. In 16% of children with normal karyotypes aneuploid DNA stem lines were identified, possibly indicating selection of normal cells for cytogenetic evaluations. On the other hand, the limitations of resolution power do not allow one to identify specific translocations or even numerical chromosomal aberrations with less than three chromosomes by flow cytometry. In the latter group, DNA aneuploidies could be detected in only 28% of cases. A high correlation between flow cytometric and karyotype analyses was evident, however, in cases with high numeric aberrations of more than three chromosomes; here, both techniques provided equivalent information in 53 of 54 cases. Hence, the two techniques should be used in a complementary way and should be added to the pretherapeutic analysis of children with ALL, possibly providing the means to discriminate prognostic subgroups and to improve the clinical management by introducing prospective risk-adapted stratification.

References

Andreeff M, Assing G, Cirrincione C (1986) Prognostic value of DNA/RNA flow cytometry in myeloblastic and lymphoblastic leukemia in adults: RNA content and S-phase predict remission duration and survival in multi-variate analysis. Ann N Y Acad Sci 468:387–406

Barlogie B, Raber MN, Schumann J, Johnson TS, Drewinko B, Swartzendruber D, Göhde W, Andreeff M (1983) Flow cytometry in clinical cancer research. Cancer Res 43:3982–3997

Borowitz MJ, Shuster JJ, Civin CI, Carroll AJ, Look AT, Behm FG, Land VJ, Pullen DJ, Crist WM (1990) Prognostic significance of CD34 expression in childhood B-precursor acute lymphocytic leukemia: a Pediatric Oncology Group study. J Clin Oncol 8:1389–1398

Büchner T, Dittrich W, Göhde W (1971) Die Impulscytophotometrie in der hämatologischen Cytologie. Klin Wochenschr 49:1090–1092

Crist W, Boyet J, Jackson J, Vietti T, Borowitz M, Chauvenet A, Winick N, Ragab A, Mahoney D, Head D, Iyer R, Wagner H, Pullen J (1989) Prognostic importance of the pre-B cell immunophenotype and other presenting features in B lineage childhood acute lymphoblastic leukemia. A Pediatric Oncology Group study. Blood 74:1251–1259

Greaves MF, Janossy G, Peto J, Kay H (1981) Immunologically defined subclasses of acute lymphoblastic leukemia in children: their relationship to presentation features and prognosis. Br J Haematol 48:179–189

Hiddemann W, Schumann J, Andreeff M, Barlogie B, Herman CJ, Leif RC, Mayall BH, Murphy RF, Sandberg AA (1984) Convention on nomenclature for DNA cytometry. Cytometry 5:445–446

Hiddemann W, Wörmann B, Ritter J, Thiel E, Göhde W, Lahme B, Henze G, Schellong G, Riehm H, Büchner T (1986) Frequency and clinical significance of DNA aneuploidy in acute leukemia. Ann N Y Acad Sci 468:227–240

Look AT, Melvin SL, Williams DL, Brodeur GM, Dahl GV, Kalwinsky DK, Murphy SH, Mauer AM (1982) Aneuploidy and percentage of S-phase cells determinded by flow cytomety correlate with cell phenotype in childhood acute leukemia. Blood 60:959–967

Look AT, Roberson PK, Williams DL, Rivera G, Bowman WP, Pui CH, Ochs J, Abromowitch M, Kalwinsky D, Dahl GV, George S, Murphy SB (1985) Prognostic importance of blast cell DNA content in childhood acute lymphoblastic leukemia. Blood 65:1079–1086

Melamed MR, Adams LR, Traganos F, Zimring A, Kamensky LA (1972) Acridine orange metachromasia for characterization of leukocytes in leukemia, lymphoma and other neoplasms. Cancer 29:1361–1368

Pui Ch, Crist WM, Look AT (1990) Biology and clinical significance of cytogenetic abnormalities in childhood acute lymphoblastic leukemia. Blood 76:1449–1463

Riehm H, Gadner H, Henze G, Langermann HJ, Odenwald E (1980) The Berlin childhood acute lymphoblastic leukemia therapy study, 1970–1976. Am J Pediatr Hematol Oncol 2:299–306

Riehm H, Gadner H, Henze G, Kornhuber B, Lampert F, Niethammer D, Reiter A, Schellong G (1990) Results and significance of six randomized trials in four consecutive ALL-BFM studies. In: Büchner T, Schellong G, Hiddemann W, Ritter J (eds) Acute leukemias – prognostic factors and treatment strategies II. Springer, Berlin Heidelberg New York, pp 439–450

Secker-Walker LM (1984) The prognostic implications of chromosomal findings in acute lymphoblastic leukemia. Cancer Genet Cytogenet 11:233–248

Smets LA, Slater RM, Behrendt H, Van't Veer MB, Homann-Blok J (1985) Phenotypic and karyotypic properties of hyperdiploid acute lymphoblastic leukaemia of childhood. Br J Haematol 61:113–123

Williams DL, Tsiatis A, Brodeur GM, Look AT, Melvin SL, Bowman WP, Klawinsky DK, Rivera G, Dahl GV (1982) Prognostic importance of chromosome number in 136 untreated children with acute lymphoblastic leukemia. Blood 60:864–871

Clinical Significance of Cytogenetic Studies in Childhood Acute Lymphoblastic Leukemia: Experience of the BFM Trials

J. Harbott[1], J. Ritterbach[1], W.-D. Ludwig[2], C.R. Bartram[3], A. Reiter[4], and F. Lampert[1]

[1] Oncocytogenetic Laboratory, Children's Hospital, University of Gießen, Feulgenstr. 12, 6300 Gießen, Fed. Rep. of Germany
[2] Klinikum Steglitz, Free University of Berlin, 1000 Berlin 45, Fed. Rep. of Germany
[3] Section of Molecular Biology, Department of Pediatrics II, University of Ulm, 7900 Ulm, Fed. Rep. of Germany
[4] Department of Pediatrics, Hannover Medical School, 3000 Hannover, Fed. Rep. of Germany

Introduction

During the past few years the number of cytogenetic analyses carried out on bone marrow and blood samples from children with acute lymphoblastic leukemia (ALL) has gradually increased, and as the number of patients found to have chromosomal aberrations in their leukemic cells rose, the clinical importance of these abnormalities became clearer. There is no doubt about the specificity of several chromosomal changes, e.g., t(8;14) in B-cell malignancies (Kaneko et al. 1980; Berger et al. 1985) or the translocations involving the band 14q11 (Williams et al. 1984; Harbott et al. 1986; Lampert et al. 1988), which can be helpful in leukemia diagnosis. The prognostic meaning of these typical aberrations, however, is not yet clear. Although most authors describe the chromosomal aberrations as an independent prognostic factor (Kaneko et al. 1981; Morse et al. 1983; Bloomfield et al. 1986; Williams et al. 1986; Yunis et al. 1986; Secker-Walker 1990), it has become evident during the last few years that their prognostic importance may be overcome by appropriate therapy (Fletcher et al. 1989; Secker-Walker 1990; Raimondi et al. 1990).

We analyzed bone marrow and blood samples from children who were treated by the protocol of one of the West German multicenter therapy studies, and the results were compared with the patients' clinical features and the outcome.

Material and Methods

From January 1984 to June 1991, 1841 bone marrow and blood samples of children with ALL (1364 at diagnosis and 473 at relapse) were sent in by 72

Recent Results in Cancer Research, Vol. 131

hospitals in the Federal Republic of Germany. Cytogenetic analysis was successful in 1030 cases (56%). Bone marrow samples, most frequently received by mail (90%–95%), were washed twice in RPMI 1640 and then either prepared directly and/or incubated in RPMI 1640 + 20% fetal calf serum (FCS) for a 24-h culture. The cell suspension was then brought into hypotonic solution (KCl, 15 min) and fixed in methanol–acetic acid (3:1). After being washed six to eight times, the cells were dropped onto a cold wet slide to spread the metaphases. G-banding was done after a trypsin pretreatment (10–15 s) 3–5 days later.

Results

Three hundred and seventy seven children (36%) showed a normal karyotype, while in the leukemic cells of nearly two thirds of the patients numerical and/or structural aberrations were found. The aberrant karyotypes were classified in four groups according to the modal chromosome number: while hypodiploidy was a rare event and found in only 37 children (4%), hyperdiploidy appeared more often. Most of these patients showed more than 50 chromosomes (n = 242; 24%), and only in 111 (11%) was the modal chromosome number between 47 and 50. The largest group of children had a pseudodiploid karyotype with 46 chromosomes and structural aberrations (n = 257; 25%).

The two hyperdiploid groups could be clearly distinguished by the cytogenetic results. In the metaphases of the group with more than 50 chromosomes a modal chromosome number of 54 dominated (Fig. 1a), and although nearly all chromosomes were involved in numerical changes in this group, extra copies of eight chromosomes were found in more than 60% of the patients: The chromosomes X, 4, 6, 10, 14, 17, and 18 were mostly found to be trisomic, whereas 21, which was involved in all but two patients, was very frequently tetrasomic and three times even pentasomic (Fig. 1b). Also, the structural aberrations differed from those of hyperdiploids with 47–50 chromosomes. Consistent chromosome aberrations, as described later, were only found in three patients with more than 50 chromosomes [1 × t(9;22); 2 × t(1;19)], and most rearrangements were random abnormalities, mostly involving the long arm of chromosome 1 at variant breakpoints (Fig. 1c).

The high specificity of numerical changes was not found in hypodiploids and hyperdiploids with 47–50 chromosomes, where the percentage of karyotypes with only numerical abnormalities was very small (2.7% in hypodiploids and 18.2% in hyperdiploids 47–50). The change in number very often arose by loss or duplication of one of the products of a reciprocal translocation. The structural abnormalities found in these groups were mainly consistent aberrations similar to those found in the pseudodiploid karyotypes. Because of the heterogeneity of the ploidy groups, a classification by the type of aberration is proposed and used in the following (Table 1).

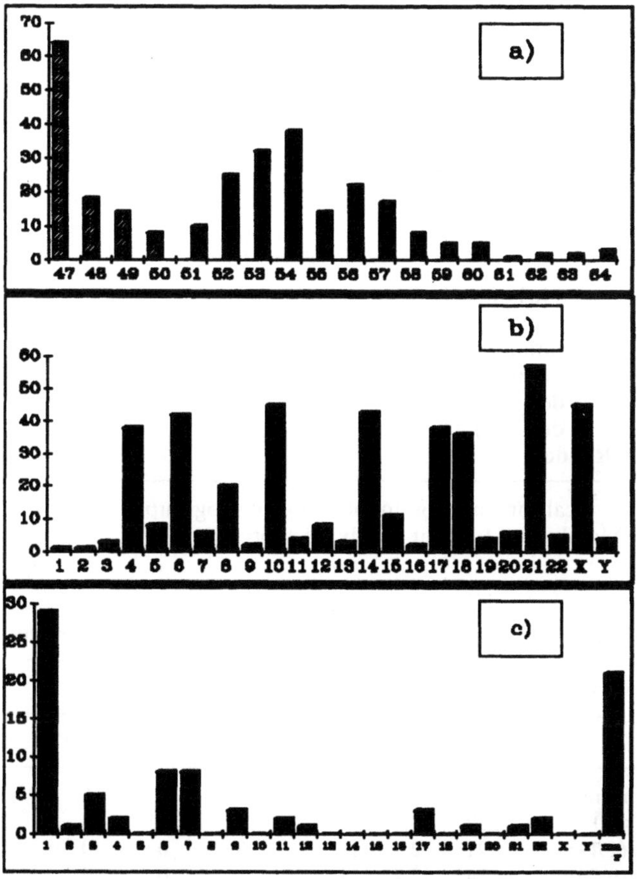

Fig. 1a–c. Cytogenetic features of hyperdiploid karyotypes with more than 50 chromosomes: **a** Frequency of modal chromosome number; **b** Frèquency of chromosomes involved in numerical abnormalities; and **c** structural aberrations (frequencies in absolute numbers)

The majority of consistent abnormalities was closely correlated to one immunophenotypic subgroup of ALL (Table 2). The t(8;14)(q24;q32), appearing in 16 patients, all with a B-cell ALL, was never found in any other immunological subgroup, and was nearly the only aberration of this group. The variant forms of this translocation, t(8;22) and t(2;8), did not appear in our series.

Aberrations involving the band q11 of chromosome 14 were the most frequent change in T-cell ALL (n = 14). Several chromosomes were found to be involved in 14q11-rearrangements, such as 11 (p13), 10 (q24), 1 (p32), 7 (p13?), and 21 (q22), and one patient showed an inversion of 14 [inv(14)(q11q32)]. Similar to t(8;14), this type of chromosomal abnormality

Table 1. Classification of karyotypes by the type of aberration

- Normal
- Aberrant
  - Consistent aberrations
    - Typical aberrations[a]
      - t(1;19)
      - t(4;11)
      - t(8;14)
      - t(9;22)
      - 14q11 aberrations
      - hyperdiploidy >50
    - Nonrandom aberrations[b]
      - del(6q)
      - der(9p)
      - der(12p)
  - Random aberrations

[a] Typical for one immunophenotypic subgroup.
[b] Mainly in ALL, but nearly all subtypes.

Table 2. Frequency of different karyotypes in children with ALL

Karyotype	Patients		Immunophenotype						
	(*n*)	(%)	Common	Pre-B	B	Pre-T/T	Pre-pre-B	Mixed	No data
normal	371	37.5	234	13	12	76	13	5	18
>50	237	24.0	207	25	0	1	1	0	3
t(1;19)	21	2.1	15	6	0	0	0	0	0
t(9;22)	24	2.4	21	2	0	0	1	0	0
t(4;11)	27	2.7	1	1	0	0	21	4	0
t(8;14)	16	1.6	0	0	16	0	0	0	0
der(14q11)	18	1.8	0	0	0	17	0	0	1
del(6q)	20	2.0	10	1	0	7	1	1	0
der(9p)	19	1.9	12	4	0	2	1	0	0
der(12p)	25	2.5	15	3	0	5	1	1	0
der(11q23)	12	1.2	4	2	0	1	2	1	2
random	199	20.1	124	13	2	32	14	4	10
Total	989	100	643	70	30	141	55	16	34
Percentage			65.0	7.1	3.0	14.3	5.6	1.6	3.4

was never found in another subtype of ALL. In T-cell ALL, however, several other chromosomal changes appeared: the nonrandom aberrations del(6q), der(9p), and der(12p), as well as the largest proportion of random aberrations (29%) and cells with normal karyotype (54%).

Translocations (4;11)(q21;q23) ($n = 27$) were specific for early defects of hematopoesis and were mainly recorded in pre-pre-B-cell ALL or mixed leukemias, but also in one patient with ALL M5 and two children with common/pre-B-cell ALL. t(4;11) appeared in nearly two thirds of all aberrant karyotypes of pre-pre-B-cell ALL, and other abnormalities were only found sporadically.

The other three typical chromosomal changes were found in common as well as in pre-B-cell ALL: t(9;22) in 24, t(1;19) in 21, and hyperdiploids with more than 50 chromosomes in 237 patients. The last-mentioned was very specific for common and pre-B-cell ALL and was only found twice in other immunosubtypes, T-cell and pre-pre-B-cell ALL, respectively. In 50.6% of all aberrant common ALL and 44% of pre-B-cell karyotypes, more than 50 chromosomes were found. The percentage of the nonrandom aberrations in common ALL was the lowest of all subgroups, ranging between 2% and 4%, and was only slightly higher in pre-B-cell ALL (1.7%–6.8%). Random aberrations were found in 30% and 23% of these two groups, respectively.

Although t(1;19) appeared only at a low frequency (3.7% in common ALL; 10.5% in pre-B-cell ALL), it was very specific and never found in any other subgroup. This is very similar to t(9;22), which was found in 5.1% of the aberrant karyotypes of common and 3.5% of pre-B-cell ALL. One patient with pre-pre-B-cell ALL was also diagnosed to have this aberration. Frozen bone marrow samples of ten Ph-positive patients were analyzed using the polymerase chain reaction (PCR) and a rearrangement of BCR-ABL was shown in all of them: nine had a breakpoint in the *m-bcr* region and only one child in the *M-bcr* region.

The nonrandom chromosome aberrations del(6q), der(9p), and der(12p) were found to be primary as well as secondary abnormalities, and they appeared in all subgroups but B-cell ALL. Because of the small number, however, a clear specifity was not seen, although del(6q) was found in 11% of all T-cell aberrations as the only abnormality.

Life-table analysis by the Kaplan–Meier method was performed for all patients with consistent aberrations who were treated by the protocol of the West German multicenter therapy studies ALL-BFM-83 and BFM-86 and whose bone marrow or blood was analyzed at the initial diagnosis of ALL. Whereas the therapy protocols in BFM-83 and -86 for patients with non-B ALL did not differ very much, there was an important change in the protocol for B-cell ALL.

Comparing the event-free survival (EFS) of children with t(8;14), a large difference was found: whereas all four children treated by BFM-83 relapsed within a period of 6 months, 80% of the BFM-86 patients were in continuous complete remission (CCR) after 50 months. A very poor prognosis was also seen for children with t(4;11) (probability of event-free survival, p_{EFS}, 0.327), whereas the aberrations of chromosome 14q11 were associated with a good prognosis (p_{EFS} about 0.8; Fig. 2a). Also, the nonrandom aberrations seem to have a good prognosis with a p_{EFS} of 0.701 for del(6q), 0.808 for der(9p), and a p_{EFS} of 1.0(!) for all patients with der(12p) ($n = 8$).

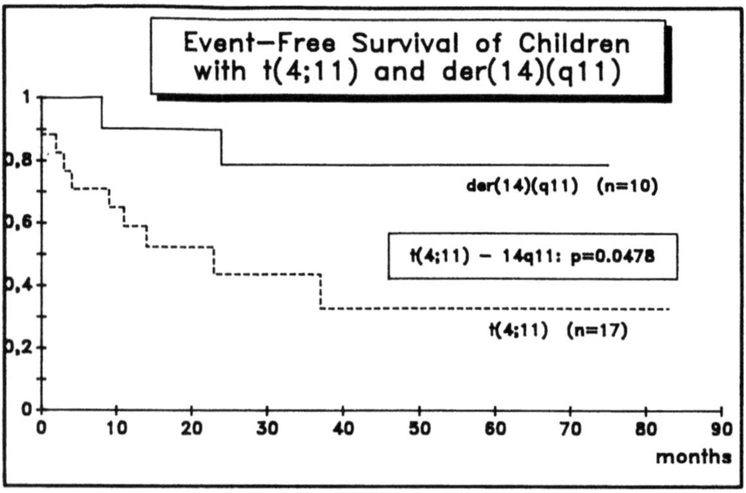

a

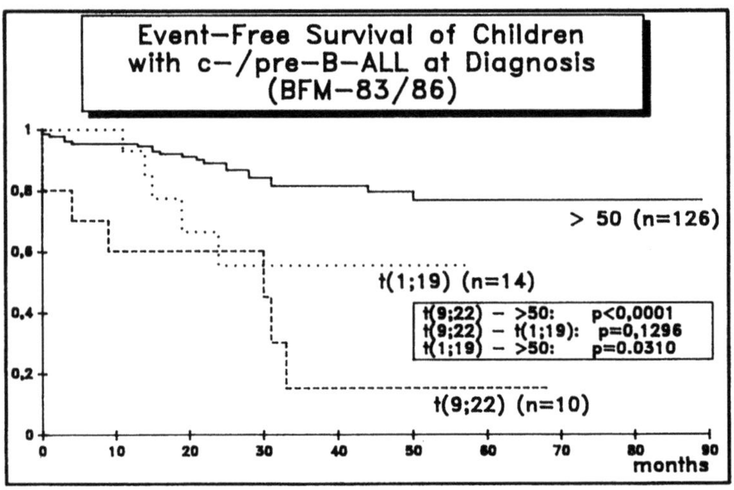

b

Fig. 2a,b. Life-table analysis by Kaplan–Meier method of children treated by the protocols BFM ALL 83 and 86. Outcome in patients **a** with t(4;11) and aberrations involving 14q11; and **b** with t(9;22), t(1;19), and hyperdiploid karyotype >50

Within the group of common/pre-B-cell ALL patients, there were different outcomes depending on the type of aberration (Fig. 2b): Whereas children with a hyperdiploid karyotype with more than 50 chromosomes had a good prognosis (p_{EFS} 0.767), the prognosis for Ph^1-positive children was very poor (p_{EFS} 0.150), and this difference was significant ($p < 0.0001$). The p_{EFS} for children with t(1;19) was intermediate (p_{EFS} 0.553), but differed significantly from that for hyperdiploidy >50 ($p = 0.0310$).

Discussion

The collaboration of physicians and specialized laboratories allowed several new methods to be evaluated to find prognostically meaningful subgroups of leukemia, resulting in a better, risk-adapted therapy to cure more children.

Cytogenetic methods showed that there were several chromosomal aberrations typical for a specific group of leukemia (Heerema 1990; Secker-Walker 1990; Heim and Mitelman 1987). The results of this study also show that in nearly three quarters of the patients with an aberrant karyotype only ten consistent abnormalities were registered. Six of them, the translocations t(1;19), t(4;11), t(8;14), and t(9;22), aberrations of chromosome 14q11, and karyotypes with more than 50 chromosomes, were each very specific for a single subtype of ALL. The others were also nonrandom, but appeared in all immunophenotypes with the exception of B-cell ALL.

This specifity of chromosome abnormalities is well known, as shown by several recent reviews (Heerema 1990; Secker-Walker 1990). In our series, however, t(1;19) was more often found in common than in pre-B-cell ALL, which was not described by others (Raimondi et al. 1990; Heerema 1990; Jackson et al. 1990; Smets et al. 1985).

The description of cytogenetic groups according to the modal chromosome number seems not to be sufficient to characterize prognostic subgroups, because they are too heterogeneous. In our study, only one of the 37 hypodiploid patients had only numerical changes, most of them showing consistent aberrations. In the group of hyperdiploid patients with 47–50 chromosomes, too, mainly consistent aberrations were found, and about three quarters had structural abnormalities. The numerical changes may be due to secondary events such as loss or doubling of one of the products of a reciprocal translocation.

We were able to show, however, that hyperdiploidy with more than 50 chromosomes is a separate group, not only regarding the chromosome number, but also regarding the type of numerical changes. A similar finding was also described by Secker-Walker (1990), who never found extra copies of chromosomes 4, 14, 17, and 18 in hyperdiploids 47–50, which are the most frequent trisomic chromosomes in the other hyperdiploid group. We therefore prefer a classification according to the type of aberration, which would be more convenient, especially for prognostic purposes.

As also reported by others (Secker-Walker 1990; Raimondi et al. 1990; Fletcher et al. 1989; Lampert et al. 1991), the prognostic significance of the cytogenetic features may depend on the alteration in therapy. In this series there was a poorer prognosis for patients with t(8;14) treated in the BFM-83 protocol than for those who were in BFM-86. This may be a result of the low numbers of patients, but was also described by other authors (Third International Workshop on Chromosomes in Leukemia 1983; Heim and Mitelman 1987; Berger et al. 1985). A change of prognosis was also described by Raimondi et al. (1990) for patients with t(1;19) in two different studies. The outcome for children with t(1;19) in this series corresponds with the results of the Total Therapy Study X (Raimondi et al. 1990).

While children with more than 50 chromosomes in the leukemic cells were found to have a good prognosis using several protocols (Jackson et al. 1990; Tsuchiya et al. 1990; Harbott et al. 1990b; Williams et al. 1982), patients with t(9;22) (Fletcher et al. 1989; Crist et al. 1990; Harbott et al. 1990b; Pullen et al. 1985) and t(4;11) have a very poor outcome (Pui et al. 1991; Arthur et al. 1982; Lampert et al. 1987).

In summary, among the large number of chromosomal aberrations in childhood ALL, only a few are nonrandom, typical for one immunophenotypic subgroup, and have prognostic significance, which may change by alteration in therapy.

Acknowledgements. This work was supported by the Kind-Philipp-Stiftung, the "Parents' Initiative Gießen", and the "Forschungshilfe Station Peiper".

References

Arthur DC, Bloomfield CD, Lindquist LL, Nesbit ME (1982) Translocation 4; 11 in acute lymphoblastic leukemia: clinical characteristic and prognostic significance. Blood 59:96–99

Berger R, Bernheim A (1985) Cytogenetics of Burkitt's lymphoma-leukaemia: a review. In: Lenoir G, O'Connor G, Olweny CLM (eds) Burkitt's lymphoma: a human cancer model. IARC Sci Publ 600:65–80

Bloomfield CD, Goldman AI, Alimena G, Borgström GH, Brandt L, Catovsky D, de la Chapelle A, Dewald GW, Garson OM, Garwicz S, Golomb HM, Hossfeld DK et al. (1986) Chromosomal abnormalities identify high-risk and low-risk patients with acute lymphoblastic leukemia. Blood 67:415–420

Crist WM, Carroll AJ, Shuster JJ, Jackson JF, Head DR, Borowitz MJ, Behm FG, Link MP, Steuber CP, Ragab AH, Hirt A, Brock B, Land VJ, Pullen DJ (1990) Philadelphia chromosome positive childhood acute lymphoblastic leukemia: Clinical and cytogenetic characteristics and treatment outcome. A Pediatric Oncology Group study. Blood 76:489–494

Fletcher JA, Kimball VM, Lynch EA, Donnelly M, Pavelka K, Gelber RD, Tantravahi R, Sallan SE (1989) Prognostic implications of cytogenetic studies in an intensively treated group of children with acute lymphoblastic leukemia. Blood 74:2130

Harbott J, Engel R, Gerein V, Schwamborn D, Rudolph R, Lampert F (1986) (11;14) translocation in three boys with acute lymphoblastic leukemia of T-cell immunophenotype. Blut 52:45–50

Harbott J, Ritterbach J, Janka-Schaub G, Ludwig WD, Reiter A, Riehm H, Lampert F (1990a) Cytogenetics of childhood ALL in German multicenter trials. Haematol Blood Transf US 33:451–459

Harbott J, Ritterbach J, Reiter A, Riehm H, Lampert F (1990b) Philadelphia positive acute lymphoblastic leukemia. An independent subgroup with poor prognosis. Klin Padiatr 202:289 (abstr)

Heerema NA (1990) Cytogenetic abnormalities and molecular markers of acute lymphoblastic leukemia. Hematol Oncol Clin North Am 4:795–820

Heim S, Mitelman F (1987) Cancer cytogenetics. Liss, New York

Jackson JF, Boyett J, Pullen DJ, Brock B, Patterson R, Land VJ, Borowitz MJ, Head DR, Crist WM (1990) Favorable prognosis associated with hyperdiploidy in children with acute lymphocytic leukemia correlates with extra chromosome 6: a Pediatric Oncology Group study. Cancer 66:1183–1189

Kaneko Y, Rowley JD, Check J, Variakojis D, Moohr JW (1980) The 14q+ chromosome in pre-B-ALL. Blood 56:782–785

Kaneko Y, Hayashi Y, Sakurai M (1981) Chromosomal findings and their correlation to prognosis in acute lymphocytic leukemia. Cancer Genet Cytogenet 4:227–235

Lampert F, Harbott J, Ludwig WD, Bartram CR, Ritter J, Gerein V, Neidhardt M, Mertens R, Graf N, Riehm H (1987) Acute Leukemia with chromosome translocation (4;11): 7 new patients and analysis of 71 cases. Blut 54:325–335

Lampert F, Harbott J, Ritterbach J, Ludwig WD, Fonatsch C, Schwamborn D, Stier B, Gnekow A, Gerein V, Stollmann B, Jobke A, Janka-Schaub G (1988) T-cell acute childhood lymphoblastic leukemia with chromosome 14q11 anomaly: a morphologic, immunologic, and cytogenetic analysis of 10 patients. Blut 56:117–123

Lampert F, Harbott J, Ritterbach J, Schellong G, Ritter J, Creutzig U, Riehm H, Reiter A (1991) Karyotypes in acute childhood leukemias may lose prognostic significance with more intensive and specific chemotherapy. Cancer Genet Cytogenet 54:277–279

Morse HG, Odom LF, Tubergen D, Hays T, Blake M, Robinson A (1983) Prognosis in acute lymphblastic leukemia of childhood as determined by cytogenetic studies at diagnosis. Med Pediatr Oncol 11:310–318

Pui CH, Frankel LS, Carroll AJ, Raimondi SC, Shuster JJ, Head DR, Crist WM, Land VJ, Pullen DJ, Steuber CP, Behm FG, Borowitz MJ (1991) Clinical characteristics and treatment outcome of childhood acute lymphoblastic leukemia with the t(4;11)(q21;q23): a collaborative study of 40 cases. Blood 77:440–447

Pullen DJ, Jackson JF, Crist WM, Caroll AJ, Boyett J, Borowitz MJ, Brock B, Iyer R, Buchanan G, Head DR, McWilliams N, Ragab AH (1985) Philadelphia chromosome positive (Ph+) acute lymphocytic leukemia (ALL) in children has clinical and biological features that predict poor prognosis and is cytogenetically and immunophenotypically heterogeneous. Blood 66:181

Raimondi SC, Behm FG, Roberson PK, Williams DL, Pui CH, Crist WM, Look AT, Rivera GK (1990) Cytogenetics of pre-B-cell acute lymphoblastic leukemia with emphasis on prognostic implications of the t(1;19). J Clin Oncol 8:1380–1388

Secker-Walker LM (1990) Prognostic and biological importance of chromosome findings in acute lymphoblastic leukemia. Cancer Genet Cytogenet 49:1–13.

Smets LA, Slater RM, Behrendt H, Van't Veer MB, Homan-Blok J (1985) Phenotypic and karyotypic properties of hyperdiploid acute lymphoblastic leukemia. Br J Haematol 61:113–123

Third International Workshop on Chromosomes in Leukemia (1983) Chromosomal abnormalities and their clinical significance in acute lymphoblastic leukemia. Cancer Res 43:868–873

Tsuchiya H, Matsuda I, Kaneko Y (1990) Why does childhood acute lymphoblastic leukemia with hyperdiploidy show a favorable prognosis? Cancer Genet Cytogenet 50:273–275

Williams DL, Tsiatis A, Brodeur GM, Look AT, Melvin SL, Bowman WP, Kalwinsky DK, Rivera GK, Dahl GV (1982) Prognostic importance of chromosome number in 136 untreated children with acute lymphoblastic leukemia. Blood 60:864–871

Williams DL, Look AT, Melvin SL, Roberson PK, Dahl GV, Flake T, Stass SA (1984) New chromosomal translocations correlate with specific immunophenotypes of childhood acute lymphoblastic leukemia. Cell 36:101–109

Williams DL, Harber J, Murphy SB, Look AT, Kalwinsky DK, Rivera GK, Melvin SL, Stass SA, Dahl GV (1986) Chromosomal translocations play a unique role

in influencing prognosis in childhood acute lymphoblastic leukemia. Blood 68: 205–212
Yunis JJ, Brunning RD (1986) Prognostic significance of chromosomal abnormalities in acute leucemias and myelodysplastic syndromes. Clin Haematol 15:597–620

Chromosomal Abnormalities in Adult Acute Lymphoblastic Leukemia: Results of the German ALL/AUL Study Group

H. Rieder[1], W.-D. Ludwig[2], W. Gassmann[3], E. Thiel[2], H. Löffler[3], D. Hoelzer[4], and C. Fonatsch[1]

[1] AG Tumorcytogenetik, Institut für Humangenetik, Medizinische Universität zu Lübeck, Ratzeburger Allee 160, W-2400 Lübeck, Fed. Rep. of Germany
[2] Abteilung für Innere Medizin, m.S. Hämatologie und Onkologie, Universitätsklinikum Steglitz, Hindenburgdamm 30, W-1000 Berlin 45, Fed. Rep. of Germany
[3] II. Medizinische Universitäts- und Poliklinik, Chemnitzstr. 33, W-2300 Kiel 1, Fed. Rep. of Germany
[4] Abteilung für Hämatologie, Zentrum der Inneren Medizin, Theodor-Stern-Kai 7, W-6000 Frankfurt am Main 70, Fed. Rep. of Germany

Introduction

The clinical and biologic significance of chromosomal aberrations has rendered cytogenetic investigations an indispensible tool in the diagnosis of acute lymphoblastic leukemia (ALL) (Secker-Walker 1990; Pui et al. 1990b). Among the chromosomal changes in adult ALL, the Ph translocation and the translocation t(4;11) are consistently found, and have been shown to identify patients with an extremely unfavorable prognosis. Moreover, the presence of any karyotypic alteration in adult ALL seems to imply a poor treatment outcome than in patients without chromosomal changes (Bloomfield et al. 1986, 1989). Therefore, not only the assessment of the frequency of well-known chromosomal rearrangements but also the identification of other karyotypic abnormalities is required, and the biologic and clinical importance of the cytogenetic findings must be evaluated in relation to clinical, morphologic, and immunologic parameters. In this report on chromosomal aberrations in adult ALL, some of these aspects will be touched upon within a discussion of specific chromosomal aberrations, including the possible significance of certain secondary aberrations in Ph-positive ALL.

Patients and Methods

All patients presented in this study were cytogenetically analyzed in the Arbeitsgruppe Tumorcytogenetik, Institut für Humangenetik, Medizinische Universität, Lübeck, in the course of the German multicenter therapy trial on acute lymphoblastic or undifferentiated leukemia of adults. Morphologic and/or immunologic diagnosis were established by central institutions (Kiel, Berlin); details have been published elsewhere (Löffler et al. 1987; Thiel et al. 1987). For cytogenetic analysis, bone marrow and/or blood samples were taken prior to therapy and sent by mail. Chromosomes were prepared and stained directly or after short-term cultivation, as described by Fonatsch et al. (1980). Chromosome abnormalities were designated according to the International System of Cytogenetic Nomenclature (ISCN 1985). Karyotypes of 100 patients have been investigated. Their ages ranged between 15.2 and 72.3 years (median 33.3, mean 37.5).

Results

Clonal chromosome aberrations were found in 62 (62%) of the cases, while only normal diploid karyotypes were detectable in 38 (38%).

Ploidy Groups. Figure 1 shows the distribution of the modal chromosome number of these 62 aberrant cases. The highest peak, at 46 chromosomes, represents pseudodiploid karyotypes in 35 cases. In seven patients hypodiploid metaphases were found with chromosome counts ranging from 36 to 45. Of the cases with a chromosome number higher than 46, 11 had chromosome counts up to 50, while nine showed hyperdiploidy with more than 50 chromosomes. Among the latter, two patients presented with a near-triploid and three with a near-tetraploid karyotype.

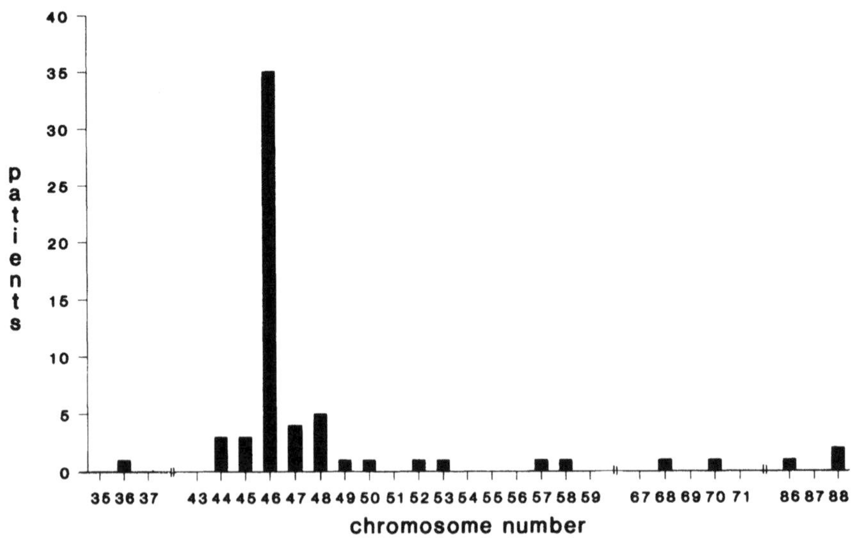

Fig. 1. Distribution of the modal chromosome numbers of 62 ALL patients with chromosomal abnormalities

Chromosomes 7 and 8 were involved most frequently in numerical changes. Gain of chromosome 8 was observed in three cases, always in addition to a Ph translocation. Loss of chromosome 7 occurred in three cases, accompanied by a Ph translocation in two cases and by a deletion of the short arm of chromosome 12 in one (Fig. 2).

Additional Structural Aberrations in Hypo- and Hyperdiploidy. Chromosomal rearrangements were found in hypo- and hyperdiploid adult ALL as well (Table 1), but most frequently in hypodiploid cases. The most consistent additional structural aberration was the translocation t(9;22)(q34;q11), which was also detected in two patients with hyperdiploid ALL, one with 53 and one with 58 chromosomes (Fig. 3). In one case, hypodiploidy resulted from the formation of a dicentric chromosome by a translocation tdic(19;20)(p13.3;q11.1) (Fig. 4).

Structural Chromosomal Changes. Of the 62 cases with an abnormal karyotype, 53 (85%) had structural rearrangements (Fig. 5). The long arms of chromosomes 9 and 22 were affected most frequently, this being due to the 20 cases with a Ph translocation. Ten patients showed involvement of

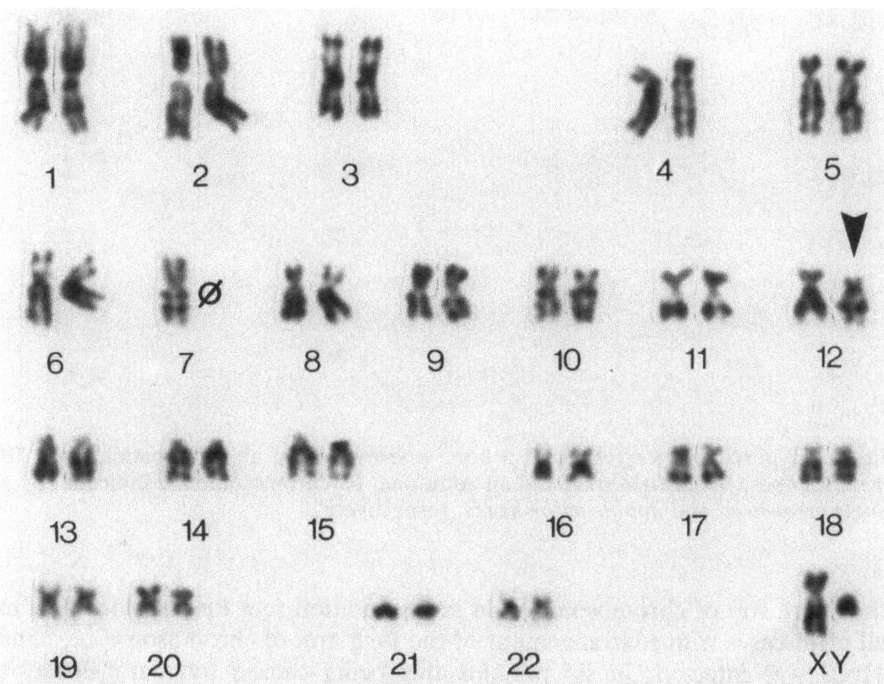

Fig. 2. Hypodiploid karyotype of a bone marrow cell of an ALL patient showing monosomy 7 and del(12)(p11.2) (*arrowhead*)

Table 1. Additional structural aberrations in hypo- and hyperdiploid cases

Chromosome count	Structural aberrations		Ph translocation	
	(*n*)	(%)	(*n*)	(%)
<46	6/7	85.7	3/7	42.9
47–50	8/11	72.7	4/11	36.4
>50	4/9	44.4	2/9	22.2

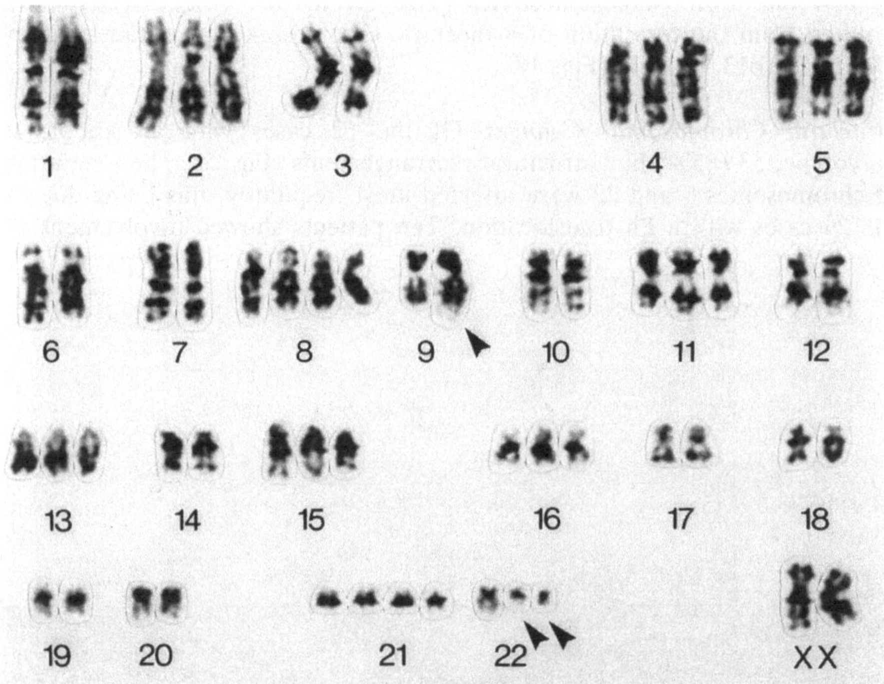

Fig. 3. Hyperdiploid karyotype of a bone marrow cell of an ALL patient with 58 chromosomes; t(9;22)(q34;q11) and an additional Ph-chromosome are indicated by a *single arrowhead* and *double arrowheads*, respectively

the short arm of chromosome 9, in six in addition to a Ph translocation. In all eight cases with rearrangement of the long arm of chromosome 11, band 11q23 was affected, in six patients this being caused by a translocation t(4;11)(q21;q23). One patient with B-cell ALL also showed involvement of 11q23 in a three-way translocation t(11;14;18)(q23;q32;q21) (Figs. 6, 7). The long arm of chromosome 1 was rearranged in five cases, leading to a

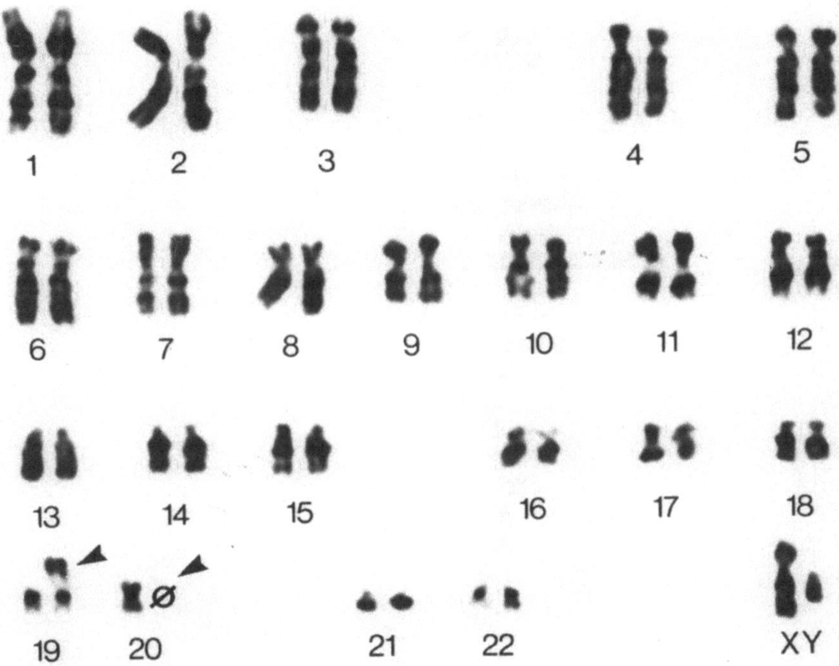

Fig. 4. Hypodiploid karyotype of a bone marrow cell of an ALL patient resulting from the formation of a dicentric translocation chromosome, tdic(19;20)(p13.3;q11.1) (*arrowhead*)

partial trisomy 1 by a duplication dup(1)(q23q32) in one patient and by an unbalanced translocation in two patients, in one patient in combination with a 14q+ marker chromosome. Out of five cases with rearrangement of the long arm of chromosome 2, two presented with an identical duplication of the segment 2q21q31 (Figs. 8, 9).

Correlation of Karyotype and Immunophenotype. The immunophenotype was established in 82 patients: 11 patients were classified as null ALL, 43 as common ALL, 11 as pre-B-cell ALL, 3 as B-cell ALL, and 15 as T-cell ALL, including three patients with a pre-T phenotype. As shown in Table 2, normal diploid cases were most frequent in T-cell ALL, whereas chromosomal abnormalities were detected in 70% of B-lineage ALL. Null and pre-B-cell ALL were preferentially associated with pseudodiploid karyotypes. Hyperdiploid karyotypes with chromosome numbers of 47–50 were only present in null and common ALL, whereas hyperdiploidy >50 was not found in null ALL but in common-, pre-B-cell, and in T-cell ALL.

In 44 immunophenotyped cases, structural chromosome aberrations were found (Fig. 10). A striking association of common and pre-B-cell ALL with

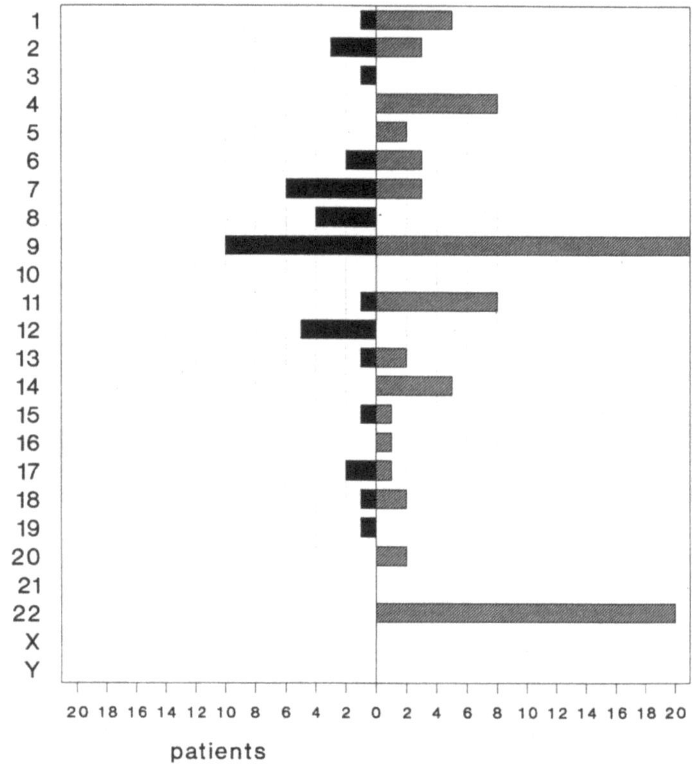

Fig. 5. Distribution of structural chromosomal rearrangements of 53 ALL patients according to the involvement of the short (p, *black bars*) and the long (q, *hatched bars*) chromosome arms

aberrations of chromosome 9 and 22 was detected. This is caused by the t(9;22) which was found in 13 cases of common ALL and five cases of pre-B-cell ALL. A translocation t(4;11) occurred in all five cases, with rearrangements of chromosomes 4 and 11 detected in null ALL.

Discussion

Structural Chromosomal Aberrations

The most consistent chromosomal aberrations were a translocation t(9;22)(q34;q11) detected in 20% of cases investigated and a translocation t(4;11)(q21;q23) found in 6%. This is in accordance to findings in other series, the Ph-translocation having been reported in 14.7%–25% and the t(4;11) in 3.2%–5.2% of adult ALL patients (Bloomfield et al. 1978; Third

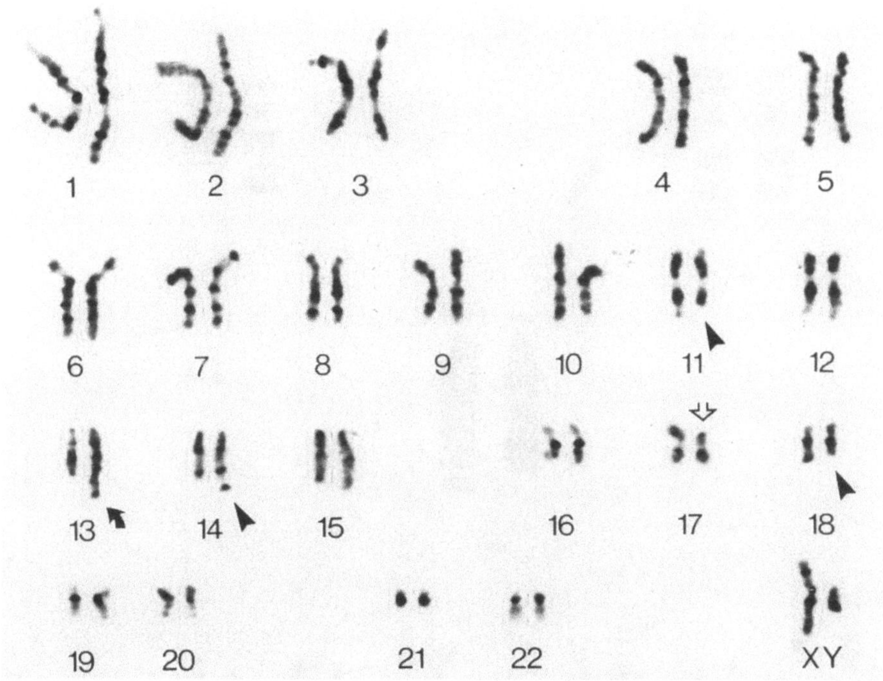

Fig. 6. G-banded karyotype of an unstimulated blood cell of a patient with B-cell ALL showing a three-way translocation t(11;14;18)(q23;q32;21) (*arrowheads*), a duplication of part of the long arm of chromosome 13, dup(13)(q14q34) (*arrow*), and a deletion of part of the short arm of chromosome 17, del(17)(p11) (*open arrow*)

International Workshop on Chromosomes in Leukemia 1981; Fenaux et al. 1988; Bloomfield et al. 1990; Hudis et al. 1990; Secker-Walker et al. 1991).

In 10% of cases the short arm of chromosome 9, 9p, was affected by structural rearrangements. Abnormalities of 9p leading to loss or rearrangement of genetic material were initially described as a cytogenetic subgroup of ALL by Kowalczyk and Sandberg (1983). So far, no data are available concerning the frequency of 9p aberrations in adult ALL from other studies. In childhood ALL, 9p anomalies have been found in 7%–10% of cases, in two thirds accompanied by other chromosome aberrations (Carroll et al. 1987; Murphy et al. 1989). In Ph-positive ALL, the nonrandom occurrence of abnormalities of 9p has been reported (Oshimura and Sandberg 1977; Sessarego et al. 1991; Rieder et al. 1991). As involvement of 9p is in general associated with lymphoid malignancies (Pollak and Hagemeijer 1987), the occurrence in Ph-positive ALL may directly be connected with the lymphatic phenotype of this leukemia.

Partial trisomy of the long arm of chromosome 1, 1q, was found in three patients (3%), in one patient together with a 14q+ marker chromosome. In

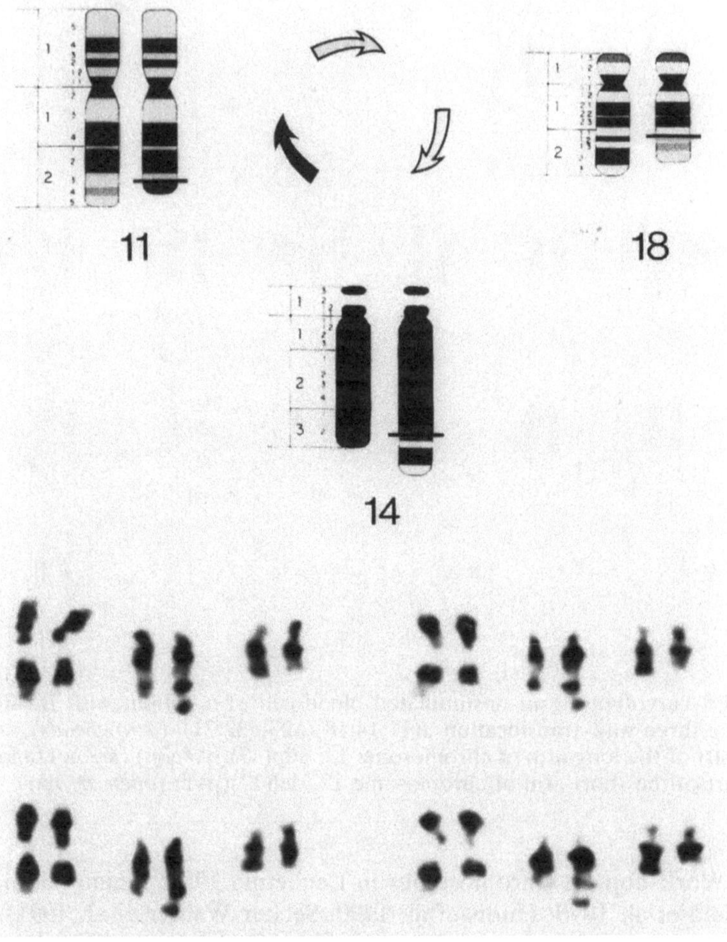

Fig. 7. Schematic presentation of the three-way translocation t(11;14;18)(q23,q32;q21) of Fig. 6 (*upper part*); four partial karyotypes demonstrating the normal and the translocation chromosomes (*lower part*)

Burkitt's type of acute lymphoblastic leukemia, this is a common secondary change (Berger et al. 1989), but it is also found in other subtypes of ALL as a result of unbalanced translocations and duplications of the long arm of chromosome 1, almost always in addition to other chromosomal changes (Mitelman 1988). Moreover, the translocation t(1;19)(q23;p13) in 68%–85% of cases (Raimondi et al. 1990; Lai et al. 1989) results in partial trisomy 1 with two normal chromosomes 1 and a derivative chromosome 19, der(19)t(1;19). Although the molecular changes of the t(1;19) have been characterized in detail (Mellentin et al. 1989, 1990; Kamps et al.

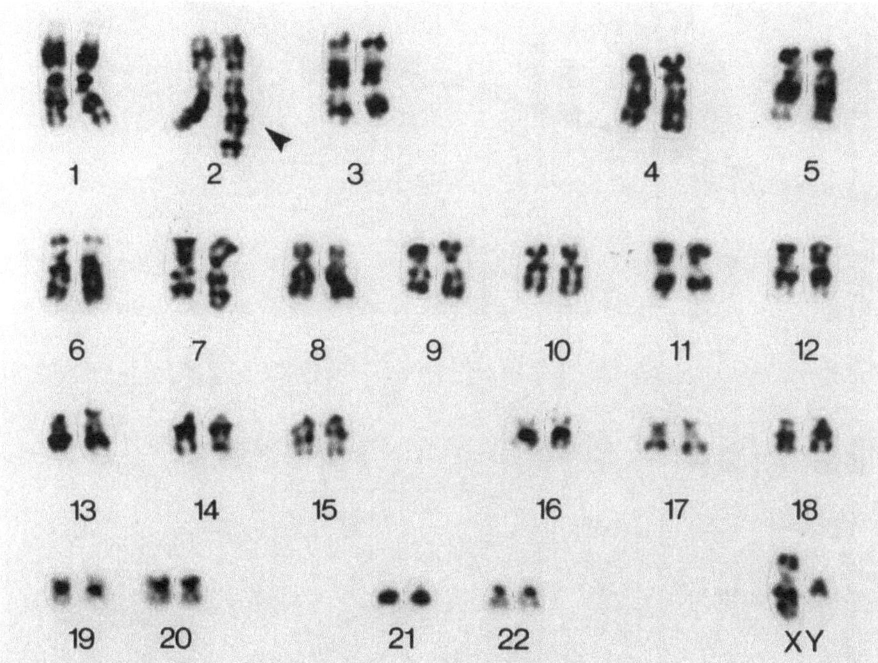

Fig. 8. G-banded karyotype of a bone marrow cell of a patient with common ALL showing a duplication dup(2)(q21q31) (*arrowhead*)

1990; Nourse et al. 1990; Hunger et al. 1991), an at least additional effect of the triple gene dosage of 1q to the leukemogenesis has to be taken into account. Support for trisomy 1q in ALL having an adverse prognostic impact can be taken from cytogenetic findings on relapse. Out of 11 ALL patients with karyotypic abnormalities first studied at relapse in our laboratory, two presented with a duplication of the long arm of chromosome 1 (data not shown).

A new recurring chromosome aberration, a duplication of the region q21–q31 of the long arm of chromosome 2, dup(2)(q21q31), was identified in two of our ALL patients. Since in one patient dup(2)(q21q31) was the sole cytogenetically detectable change, this is thought to represent a new primary chromosome aberration in ALL. Until now, only one other case with a duplication of the long arm of chromosome 2 has been reported (Pui et al. 1987), involving region q31q37 in childhood ALL. Thus, in addition, dup(2)(q21q31) may be specific for adult ALL.

Ploidy Groups

In this series of adult ALL, hypodiploid metaphases were found in 7% of the cases. Similar frequencies have been reported elsewhere, ranging from

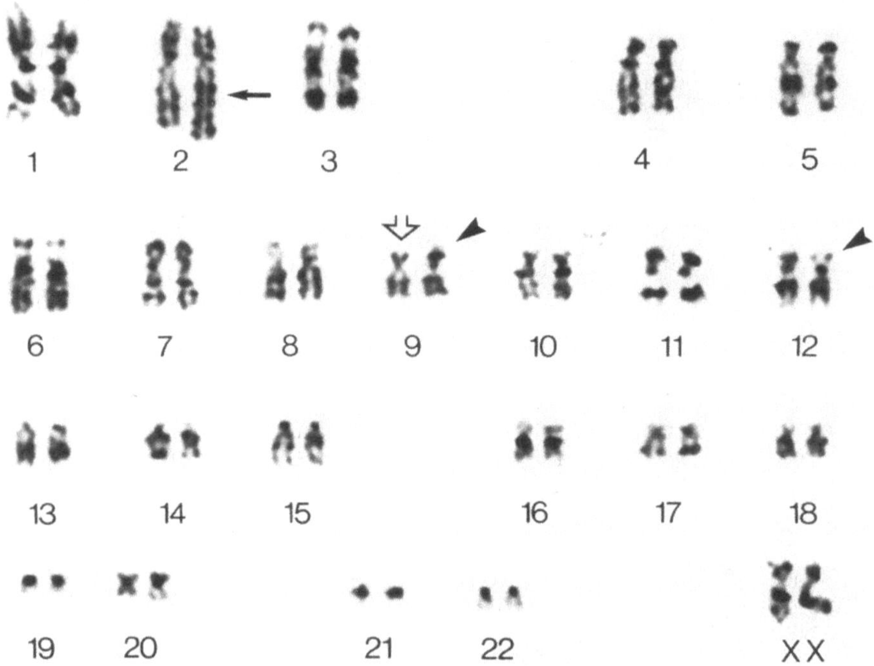

Fig. 9. G-banded karyotype of a bone marrow cell of a patient with common ALL demonstrating dup(2)(q21q31) (*arrow*), t(9;12)(p13;p11.2) (*arrowheads*), and del(9)(p22) (*open arrow*)

7.5%–8.4% (Third International Workshop on Chromosomes in Leukemia 1981; Secker-Walker 1984; Hudis et al. 1990). Additional structural aberrations were identified in all hypodiploid cases, except in a patient with a chromosome number of 36, the Ph translocation accounting for half of them. Moreover, the Ph translocation was associated with monosomy 7 in two cases, a combination which has already been reported to be associated with an extremely poor prognosis (Maddox et al. 1983; Futaki et al. 1989). In ALL, loss of chromosome 7 as the sole numerical chromosomal change – as was found in one of our patients – represents a very rare cytogenetic finding (Mitelman 1988; Michael et al. 1988). In the cases reported so far, monosomy 7 was associated with a prior history of mutagenic exposure, with a weak response to therapy, and an early relapse of the disease (Stricker and Linker 1983; Chan et al. 1985; Philip and Bjergaard-Pedersen 1988).

Hyperdiploid metaphases with chromosome counts of 47–88 were found in 20% of cases, 11% within the range 47–50 chromosomes and 9% with a chromosome number >50. This is in accordance with findings of Hudis et al. (1990) (>50, 9.4%) and of the Third International Workshop on Chromosomes in Leukemia (TIWC) (1981) (47–50, 12.7%; >50, 9.3%). The group

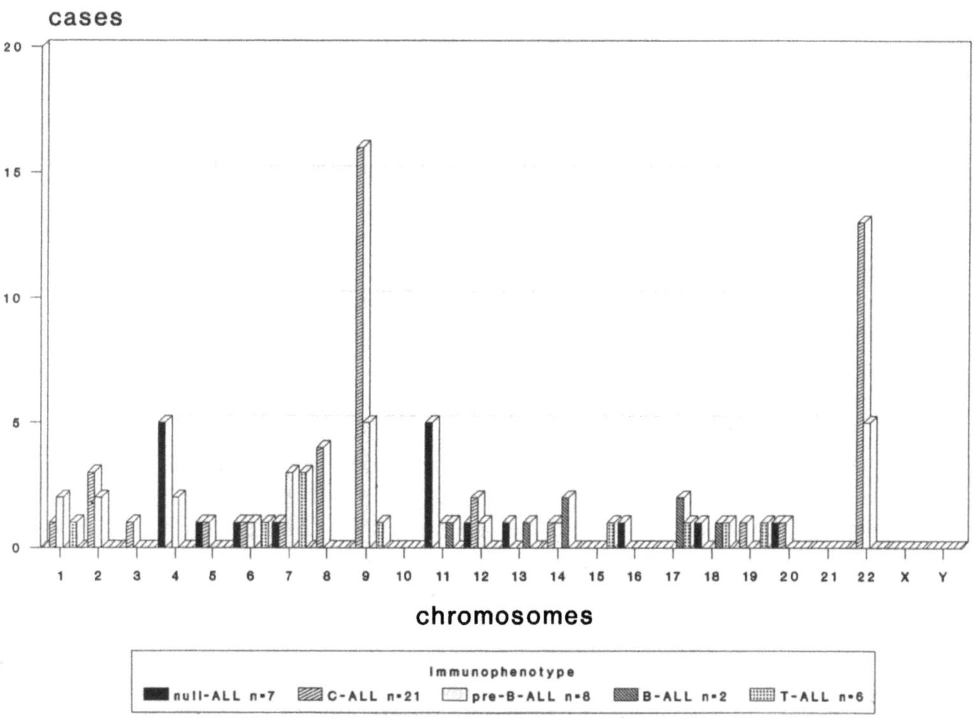

Fig. 10. Relation between chromosomal involvement in structural aberrations and the immunophenotype ($n = 44$)

Table 2. Relation between immunophenotype and ploidy groups ($n = 82$)

	Null ALL (n = 11)		Common ALL (n = 43)		Pre-B-cell ALL (n = 11)		T-cell ALL (n = 15)		B-cell ALL (n = 3)	
	(n)	(%)	(n)	(%)	(n)	(%)	(n)	(%)	(n)	(%)
Normal diploid	3	27.3	14	32.6	3	27.3	9	60.0	1	33.3
Pseudodiploid	5	45.5	13	30.2	6	54.5	4	33.3	2	66.7
Hypodiploid <46	2	18.2	4	9.3	0		0		0	
Hyperdiploid										
47–50	1	9.1	8	18.6	0		0		0	
>50	0		4	9.3	2	18.2	2	6.7	0	

consisting of hyperdiploid cases with >50 chromosomes was further subdivided by the TIWC into patients with 51–60 and patients with >60 chromosomes, accounting for 6.3% and 2.9% of the total, respectively. In our series, both subgroups were identified in slightly different proportions:

4% of the cases were in the range 50–60 and 5% had >60 chromosomes, the latter including two cases with near-triploid (2%) and three cases (3%) with near-tetraploid metaphases. Secker-Walker (1990) has already suggested that in adult ALL about 50% of the cases with hyperdiploidy >50 chromosomes are near-triploid or near-tetraploid. In this context, a recent study of childhood ALL might be of significance; the study suggests that patients with a near-tetraploid karyotype may have a more unfavorable prognosis than other patients with more than 50 chromosomes (Pui et al. 1990a).

The adverse influence of additional structural changes in hyperdiploidy with >50 chromosomes has also been demonstrated in childhood ALL (Pui et al. 1989). About half of the adult ALL patients with hyperdiploidy >50 in our series showed chromosomal rearrangements. The Ph translocation was found in two of these patients, suggesting that overall the Ph translocation occurs in about 22% of hyperdiploid ALL >50 chromosomes. An even higher frequency has been reported in the series of adult ALL patients who had been collected during the TWIC, five of 16 patients (31%) with hyperdiploidy >50 showing a Ph translocation (Third International Workshop on Chromosomes in Leukemia 1981; Secker-Walker 1984).

Karyotype and Immunophenotype

A close association of t(9;22) with common ALL and pre-B-cell ALL was found. The frequency was even higher in pre-B-cell ALL (45.5%) than in common ALL (30.2%). Therefore, it may be suggested that in adult ALL the Ph translocation is even more specific for pre-B-cell ALL than for common ALL. This is supported by the data of Secker-Walker et al. (1991), who found a Ph translocation in 15 of 55 adult patients with common ALL (27.3%) and in 5 of 12 patients with pre-B-cell ALL (41.7%).

In the same publication, five of 13 adult patients with null ALL were reported as having a t(4;11). Together with the findings of our series, in which t(4;11) was identified in 5 of 11 patients with null ALL (45%), the frequency of this chromosomal translocation in adult null ALL may be estimated at about 42%. As in other series, 11q23 rearrangements were not restricted to null ALL, but were also observed in one case with pre-B-cell and in one with B-cell All. In the former case, this was a t(4;11); the latter showed a three-way translocation t(11;14;18)(q23;q32;q21) in which apart from band 11q23, bands 18q21 and 14q32 were involved, chromosomal regions known to be rearranged in follicular non-Hodgkin's lymphoma (NHL) by the t(14;18)(q32;q21). In contrast, aberrations involving 11q23 are less common in NHL. Deletions in 11q23, a t(11;14)(q23;q32), and also a t(4;11)(q21;q23) with a t(14;18)(q32;q21) have been reported in single cases. As yet, however, neither in NHL nor in ALL has a three-way translocation been described involving 11q23, 18q21, and 14q32 (Levine et al. 1985; Kaneko et al. 1988; Mitelman 1988; Raimondi et al. 1989; Dyer et al. 1990).

Although the relation between the ploidy groups and the immunologic subgroups is obscured by the small number of cases, one finding should be briefly pointed out: The high frequency of normal diploid cases in T-cell ALL coincides with a significantly better prognosis of this immunologic subgroup compared to other immunophenotypes. This corresponds with the observation that adult ALL patients with only normal diploid or hyperdiploid metaphases are more likely to be cured than patients with pseudo- or hypodiploid metaphases, which, e.g., are found most frequently in null ALL, an immunologic subtype with a worse prognosis than T-cell ALL (Thiel et al. 1987; Bloomfield et al. 1989). Thus, the low frequency of chromosomal aberrations may contribute to the more favorable treatment outcome in T-cell ALL.

Conclusions

In this study, the high incidence of translocations t(9;22) and t(4;11) in adult ALL (26% of the cases investigated) has been confirmed. The possible prognostic and biologic significance of additional secondary aberrations and other primary, less frequently occurring chromosomal aberrations identified in our series, such as, near-triploidy, near-tetraploidy, partial trisomy 1q, and dup(2)(q21q31), has been discussed. The clinical relevance of these aberrations should be clarified when more adult ALL patients are cytogenetically investigated.

Acknowledgement. This study was supported in part by the Bundesministerium für Forschung und Technologie.

References

Berger R, Le Coniat M, Derré J, Vecchione D (1989) Secondary chromosomal abnormalities of band 13q34 in Burkitt lymphoma-leukemia. Genes Chromosomes Cancer 1:115–118

Bloomfield CD, Lindquist LL, Brunning RD, Yunis JJ, Coccia PF (1978) The Philadelphia chromosome in acute leukemia. Virchows Arch [B] 29:81–91

Bloomfield CD, Goldman AI, Alimena G, Berger R, Borgström GH, Brandt L, Catovsky D, de la Chapelle A, Dewald GW, Garson OM, Garwicz S, Colomb HM, Hossfeld DK, Lawler SD, Mitelman F, Nilsson P, Pierre RV, Philip P, Prigogina E, Rowley JD, Sakurai M, Sandberg AA, Secker-Walker LM, Tricot G, Van Den Berghe H, Van Orshoven A, Vuopio P, Whang-Peng J (1986) Chromosomal abnormalities identify high-risk and low-risk patients with acute lymphoblastic leukemia. Blood 67:415–420

Bloomfield CD, Secker-Walker LM, Goldman AI, Van Den Berghe H, de la Chapelle A, Ruutu T, Alimena G, Garson OM, Colomb HM, Rowley JD, Kaneko Y, Whang-Peng J, Prigogina E, Philip P, Sandberg AA, Lawler SD, Mitelman F (1989) Six-year follow-up of the clinical significance of karyotype in acute lymphoblastic leukemia. Cancer Genet Cytogenet 40:171–185

Bloomfield CD, Wurster-Hill D, Peng G, Le Beau M, Tantravahi R, Testa J, Davey FR, Ellison RR, Cuttner J, Schiffer C, Sobol RE, Lunghofer B, Carey M, Mick R, Arthur D (1990) Prognostic significance of the Philadelphia chromosome in adult acute lymphoblastic leukemia. In: Gale RP, Hoelzer D (eds) Acute lymphoblastic leukemia. Liss, New York, pp 101–109 (UCLA symposia on molecular and cellular biology, new series, vol 108)

Carroll AJ, Castleberry RP, Crist WM (1987) Lack of association between abnormalities of the chromosome 9 short arm and either "lymphomatous" features or T cell phenotype in childhood acute lymphoblastic leukemia. Blood 69: 735–738

Chan LC, Sheer D, Drysdale HC, Bevan D, Greaves MF (1985) Monosomy 7 and multipotential stem cell transformation. Br J Haematol 61:531–539

Dyer MJS, Fischer P, Nacheva E, Labastide W, Karpas A (1990) A new human B-cell non-Hodgkin's lymphoma cell line (Karpas 422) exhibiting both t(14;18) and t(4;11) chromosomal translocations. Blood 75:709–714

Fenaux P, Lai JL, Morel P, Nelken B, Taboureau O, Deminatti M, Bauters F (1988) Cytogenetics and their prognostic value in childhood and adult acute lymphoblastic leukemia (ALL) excluding L3. Hematol Oncol 7:307–317

Fonatsch C, Schaadt M, Kirchner H, Diehl V (1980) A possible correlation between the degree of karyotype aberrations and the rate of sister chromatid unchanges in lymphoma lines. Int J Cancer 26:749–756

Futaki M, Ito T, Inokuchi K, Yamada T, Ohki I, Kuwabara T, Dan K, Kuriya S, Nomura T, Shinohara T, Ohkawa Y (1989) Philadelphia-positive acute mixed leukemia with monosomy 7. Rinsho Ketsueki 30:1997–2001

Hudis C, Offit K, Jhanwar S, Schluger A, Berman E, Clarkson B, Chaganti R (1990) Prognostic significance of cytogenetic abnormalities in 126 adult patients with newly diagnosed lymphocytic leukemia. Proc Am Assoc Cancer Res 31:26

Hunger SP, Galili N, Carroll AJ, Crist WM, Link MP, Cleary M (1991) The t(1;19)(q23;p13) chromosomal translocation results in consistent fusion of E2A and PBX1 coding sequences in acute lymphoblastic leukemias. Blood 77:687–693

ISCN (1985) An international system for human cytogenetic nomenclature. Karger, Basel

Kamps MP, Murre C, Sun X-H, Baltimore D (1990) A new homeobox gene contributes the DNA binding domain of the t(1;19) translocation protein in pre-B ALL. Cell 60:547–555

Kaneko Y, Shikano T, Maseki N, Sakurai M, Takeda T, Hiyoshi Y, Mimaya J-I, Fujimoto T (1988) Clinical characteristics of infant acute leukemia with or without 11q23 translocations. Leukemia 2:672–676

Kowalczyk J, Sandberg AA (1983) A possible subgroup of ALL with 9p-. Cancer Genet Cytogenet 9:383–385

Lai JL, Fenaux P, Estienne MH, Huart JJ, Savary JB, Lepelley P, Jouet JP, Nelken B, Bauters F, Deminatti M (1989) Translocation t(1;19)(q23;p13) in acute lymphoblastic leukemia: a report on six new cases and an unusual t(17;19)(q11;q13), with special reference to prognostic factors. Cancer Genet Cytogenet 37:9–17

Levine EG, Arthur DC, Frizzera G, Peterson BA, Hurd DD, Bloomfield CD (1985) There are differences in cytogenetic abnormalities among histologic subtypes of the non-Hodgkin's lymphomas. Blood 66:1414–1422

Löffler H, Kayser W, Schmitz N, Thiel E, Hoelzer D, Büchner T, Urbanitz D, Spiegel K, Messerer D, Heinecke A (1987) Morphological and cytochemical classification of adult acute leukemias in two multicenter studies in the Federal Republic of Germany. In: Büchner T, Schellong G, Hiddemann W, Urbanitz D, Ritter J (eds) Haematology and blood transfusion: acute leukemias. Springer, Berlin Heidelberg New York, pp 21–27

Maddox A-M, Keating MJ, Trujillo J, Cork A, Youness E, Ahearn MJ, McCredie KB, Freireich EJ (1983) Philadelphia chromosome-positive adult acute leukemia with monosomy of chromosome number seven: a subgroup with poor response to therapy. Leuk Res 7:509–522

Mellentin JD, Murre C, Donlon TA, McCaw PS, Smith SD, Carroll AJ, McDonald ME, Baltimore D, Cleary ML (1989) The gene for enhancer binding proteins E12/E47 lies at the t(1;19) breakpoint in acute leukemias. Science 246:379–382

Mellentin JD, Nourse J, Hunger SP, Smith SD, Cleary ML (1990) Molecular analysis of the t(1;19) breakpoint cluster region in pre-B cell acute lymphoblastic leukemia. Genes Chromosomes Cancer 2:239–247

Michael PM,Garson OM, Tauro G, Rennie GC, Pilkington GR (1988) Prospective study of childhood acute lymphocytic leukemia: hematologic, immunologic, and cytogenetic correlations. Med Pediatr Oncol 16:153–161

Mitelman F (1988) Catolog of chromosome aberrations in cancer, 3rd edn. Liss, New York

Murphy SB, Raimondi SC, Rivera GK, Crone M, Dodge RK, Behm FG, Pui C-H, Williams DL (1989) Nonrandom abnormalities of chromosome 9p in childhood acute lymphoblastic leukemia: association with high-risk clinical features. Blood 74:409–415

Nourse J, Mellentin JD, Galili N, Wilkinson J, Stanbridge E, Smith SD, Cleary ML (1990) Chromosomal translocation t(1;19) results in synthesis of a homeobox fusion mRNA that codes for a potential chimeric transcription factor. Cell 60: 535–545

Oshimura M, Sandberg AA (1977) Chromosomes and causation of human cancer and leukemia XXV. Significance of the Ph1 (including unusual translocations) in various acute leukemias. Cancer 40:1149–1160

Philip P, Bjergaard-Pedersen J (1988) Cytogenetic, clinical, and cytologic characteristics of radiotherapy-related leukemias. Cancer Genet Cytogenet 31:227–236

Pollak C, Hagemeijer A (1987) Abnormalities of the short arm of chromosome 9 with partial loss of material in hematologic disorders. Leukemia 1:541–548

Pui C-H, Williams DL, Raimondi SC, Rivera GK, Look AT, Dodge RK, George SL, Behm FG, Crist WM, Murphy SB (1987) Hypodiploidy is associated with a poor prognosis in childhood acute lymphoblastic leukemia. Blood 70:247–253

Pui C-H, Raimondi SC, Dodge RK, Rivera GK, Fuchs LAH, Abromowitch M, Look AT, Furman WL, Crist WM, Williams DL (1989) Prognostic importance of structural chromosomal abnormalities in children with hyperdiploidy (>50 chromosomes) acute lymphoblastic leukemia. Blood 73:1963–1967

Pui C-H, Carroll AJ, Head D, Raimondi SC, Shuster JJ, Crist WM, Link MP, Borowitz MJ, Behm FG, Land VJ, Nash MB, Pullen DJ, Look AT (1990a) Near-triploid and near-tetraploid acute lymphoblastic leukemia of childhood. Blood 76:590–596

Pui C-H, Crist WM, Look AT (1990b) Biology and clinical significance of cytogenetic abnormalities in childhood acute lymphoblastic leukemia. Blood 76:1449–1463

Raimondi SC, Peiper SC, Kitchingman GR, Behm FG, Williams DL, Hancock ML, Mirro J Jr (1989) Childhood acute lymphoblastic leukemia with chromosomal breakpoints at 11q23. Blood 73:1627–1634

Raimondi SC, Behm FG, Roberson PK, Williams DL, Pui C-H, Crist WM, Look AT, Rivera GK (1990) Cytogenetics of pre-B-cell acute lymphoblastic leukemia with emphasis on prognostic implications of the t(1;19). J Clin Oncol 8:1380–1388

Rieder H, Freund M, Fonatsch C (1991) Abnormalities of the short arm of chromosome 9 – a nonrandom secondary aberration in Philadelphia chromosome-positive acute lymphoblastic leukemia (ALL). Cancer Genet Cytogenet 53:139–142

Secker-Walker LM (1984) The prognostic implications of chromosomal findings in acute lymphoblastic leukemia. Cancer Genet Cytogenet 11:233–248

Secker-Walker LM (1990) Prognostic and biological importance of chromosome findings in acute lymphoblastic leukemia. Cancer Genet Cytogenet 49:1–13

Secker-Walker LM, Craig JM, Hawkins JM, Hoffbrand AV (1991) Philadelphia positive acute lymphoblastic leukemia in adults – age distribution, BCR breakpoint and prognostic significance. Leukemia 5:196–199

Sessarego M, Defferrari R, Fugazza G, Comelli A, Salvidio E, Ajmar F (1991) Involvement of the short arm of the derivative chromosome 9 in Philadelphia-positive acute lymphoblastic leukemia. Cancer Genet Cytogenet 52:43–49

Stricker RB, Linker CA (1983) Acute lymphoblastic leukemia with monosomy 7 in a Hiroshima survivor 37 years after the bomb. JAMA 250:640–641

Thiel E, Hoelzer D, Dörken B, Löffler H, Messerer C, Huhn D (1987) Clinical relevance of blast cell immunophenotype as determined with monoclonal antibodies in acute lymphoblastic leukemia of adults. In: Büchner T, Schellong G, Hiddemann W, Urbanitz D, Ritter J (eds) Haematology and blood transfusion: acute leukemias. Springer, Berlin Heidelberg New York, pp 95–103

Third International Workshop on Chromosomes in Leukemia (1981) Clinical significance of chromosomal abnormalities in acute lymphoblastic leukemia. Cancer Genet Cytogenet 4:111–137

IV. Minimal Residual Disease in Acute Leukemias: Detection and Immunotherapeutic Strategies

Molecular Genetic Techniques for Detection of Minimal Residual Disease in Acute Lymphoblastic Leukemia: Possibilities and Limitations

C.R. Bartram

Section of Molecular Biology, Department of Pediatrics II, University of Ulm, W-7900 Ulm, Fed. Rep. of Germany

Introduction

Despite impressive advances in the treatment of acute lymphoblastic leukemia (ALL), disease relapse following successful remission induction still poses a significant clinical problem (Champlin and Gale 1989). Since most recurrences originate from neoplastic cells escaping the therapeutic intervention, the development of methods to monitor individual responses of patients, to detect impending relapses prior to clinical manifestation, or to determine the quality of a bone marrow scheduled for autologous transplantation represents a major challenge of today's oncology.

Until recently, the methods used for the identification of residual disease, including Southern blot analysis, have not been sensitive enough to demonstrate less than 1%–10% neoplastic cells in a sample being examined, a detection level also achieved by morphological examination. However, the use of double-color immunofluorescence and polymerase chain reaction (PCR) strategies has opened new avenues to the analysis of minimal residual leukemia by allowing the identification of as few as 10^{-6} malignant cells (Campana et al. 1990a; Saiki et al. 1988). In the following, I will briefly summarize our experience with the application of PCR methods in diagnosis and monitoring of ALL Patients.

Clonospecific T-Cell Receptor δ Probes

The genes encoding immunoglobulin (Ig) and T-cell receptor (TCR) chains are all assembled from multiple segments which recombine during B- and T-cell differentiation. Accordingly, leukemia cells of every ALL patient exhibit a distinct immunogenotype that can readily be demonstrated by Southern blot analysis. Based on the unique pattern of Ig and/or TCR gene rearrangements, a variety of PCR methods have been proposed for the

Recent Results in Cancer Research, Vol. 131

evaluation of therapeutic efficacy (D'Auriol et al. 1989; Hansen-Hagge et al. 1989; Yamada et al. 1989). A strategy developed in our laboratory proceeds from the immunogenotypic characterization of 497 ALL patients enrolled in the German multicenter ALL trials BFM (children) and BMFT (adults). This study revealed that a TCRδ rearrangement and/or deletion is present in 97% of T-cell acute lymphoblastic leukemia (T-ALL) cases and also in 88% of common cell acute lymphoblastic leukemia (cALL) cases (Hansen-Hagge et al. 1989; Yokota et al. 1991). Even more remarkable is the observation of a preferential recombination pattern depending on the immunophenotype. Thus in T-ALL a prevalence of $V_{\delta1}DJ_{\delta1}$ (29%), $V_{\delta2}DJ_{\delta1}$ (11%), and $D_{\delta2}J_{\delta1}$ (19%) recombinations contrasts with a predominant rearrangement of $V_{\delta2}D_{\delta3}$ (52%) and $D_{\delta2}D_{\delta3}$ (16%) in B-precursor leukemias.

Despite this limited repertoire of recombination events occurring in ALL, the respective TCRδ loci show enormous junctional diversity due to imprecise joining and insertion of N-region nucleotides. The amplification of TCRδ junctional regions thus leads to the generation of clonospecific probes which can be used for the identification of minimal residual leukemia. The detection limit of each probe varies (Table 1), but they allow the identification of 10^{-4}–10^{-6} neoplastic cells in the vast majority of cases. In the frew exceptions, sequence analyses of the junctional regions and subsequent synthesis of oligonucleotide probes finally provided us with tools of sufficient sensitivity.

Thus far we have analyzed bone marrow (BM) or peripheral blood (PB) samples obtained from 52 pediatric and 11 adult ALL patients, including 40 cALL and 23 T-ALL cases (Table 2). Since PB samples contained significantly fewer residual cells in all instances where both PB and BM specimens from a patient were tested, only data from the latter source are presented. In a group of 47 patients studied during complete clinical/hematological remission, bone marrow samples obtained during consolidation therapy exhibited remaining neoplastic cells at a level of 10^{-2} to 10^{-4} in most cases (Table 2). Remarkably, a significant number of patients still showed minimal residual leukemia at frequencies of 10^{-3}–10^{-6} during the phase of maintenance therapy. By contrast, patients generally lacked evidence of ALL cells after termination of treatment. However, it is important to note that the result obtained from a single PCR analysis bears only limited prognostic relevance. More important appears to be the determination of the kinetic behavior of a neoplastic cell population through serial PCR analyses. Thus, a steady increase of blasts may indicate an imminent relapse, while a continuous, albeit prolonged decline of neoplastic cells may

Table 1. Detection level of 63 clonospecific TCRδ probes

Number of ALL cells	$10^{-2/-3}$	$10^{-3/-4}$	10^{-4}	10^{-5}	10^{-6}
Number of cases	3	4	21	27	8

Table 2. PCR analyses in 63 ALL patients using clonospecific TCRδ probes

A. 47 ALL patients in complete remission

Therapeutic phase	Months after diagnosis	No. of samples[a]	PCR status	
			pos.	neg.
Consolidation	1–6	14	10	4
Maintenance	7–24	30	9	21
Termination	>24	32	1[b]	31

B. Serial PCR analysis[a] in 16 ALL patients before relapse

$n = 12$	Persistance/increase of leukemic cells 6–12 months prior to clinical manifestation
$n = 3$	Detection of residual leukemia only 3–6 weeks before relapse
$n = 1$	Failure to identify relapse due to continuing TCRδ rearrangement

[a] Evaluation of 76 (A) and 49 (B) bone marrow samples obtained during complete clinical/hematological remission, respectively.
[b] Patient relapsed 8 months after PCR analysis.

be associated with a favorable course (Fig. 1). It is interesting that the dynamic disparities in the reduction of leukemic cells observed in our series did not correlate with known risk factors and may therefore identify a novel component of the individual response to chemotherapy. Similar results have recently been reported by other groups (Maclntyre et al. 1990; Yamada et al. 1990).

A complementary set of data stems from PCR analysis of 16 ALL patients who experienced a relapse during the course of the disease (Table 2). In most instances a steady increase in residual neoplastic cells was observed several months prior to clinical manifestation of the disease (Fig. 1). In three cases PCR analysis failed to detect leukemia cells in multiple BM specimens obtained uring maintenance therapy but scored positive a few weeks before clinical relapse. It remains a possibility that this late detection was caused by the focal nature of residual blasts.

In this context, another limitation of PCR analysis should be considered. Any subpopulation of leukemia cells undergoing further rearrangements at the loci represented in a clonospecific probe would escape detection. In fact, we experienced this pitfall in one patient (Table 2). Clonal variations at rearranged TCRδ genes might occur in 10% of cases according to our preliminary data. This proportion is relatively low compared to secondary rearrangements affecting IgH loci, which occur in approximately 30% of

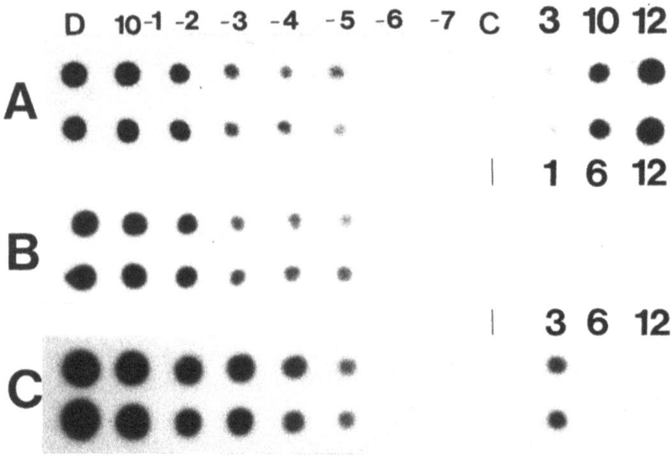

Fig. 1. Detection of minimal residual disease in three ALL patients by clonospecific TCRδ probes. DNAs of leukemia cells at diagnosis (*D*) were diluted into peripheral blood cell DNA of three healthy individuals (*C*) at 10^{-1}–10^{-7} and established a detection limit of approximately 10^{-5} leukemia cells in all cases. Bone marrow DNA samples obtained during the patients' complete clinical/hematological remission were also included (*numbers* indicate months after diagnosis). Sample 12 from patient A was obtained at the time of clinical relapse. Upon amplification, the corresponding DNA fractions (20 ng) were spotted onto nylon filters and hybridized to the clonospecific probes. Note the considerable differences in the kinetic behavior of residual leukemia among the three patients

ALL patients (Raghavachar et al. 1987), posing a major problem for PCR strategies based on this marker system.

BCR-ABL Rearrangements

The Philadelphia (Ph) translocation was originally discovered in chronic myelocytic leukemia (CML), but it is also observed in acute leukemias. Cytogenetically the Ph chromosomes are indistinguishable between different leukemia entities. On the molecular level, however, two distinct subtypes have been defined (Kurzrock et al. 1988). While the breakpoints of CML patients have been mapped almost exclusively to the major breakpoint cluster region (*M-bcr*) on chromosome 22, the majority of Ph-positive ALL patients exhibit a rearrangement in the minor breakpoint cluster region (*m-bcr*) of the BCR gene. In a recent study including 314 ALL cases a BCR-ABL rearrangement, the molecular hallmark of the Ph translocation, was observed in 55% of adult cALL patients, in contrast to only 6% and 17% of children with primary and recurrent neoplasias, respectively (Maurer et al. 1991). This analysis also confirmed the poor prognosis associated with BCR-

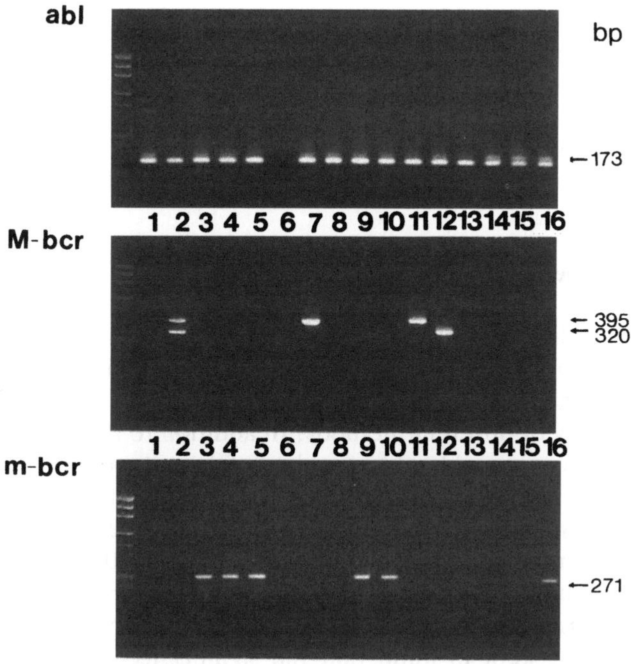

Fig. 2. PCR analysis of 13 adult cALL patients. Two Ph-positive leukemias with known *m-bcr* or *M-bcr* breakpoints (*lanes 5, 7*) and a water sample (*lane 6*) were included as positive and negative controls, respectively. Following the generation of complementary (c)DNA from RNA samples, three equal volumes were amplified by use of oligomers detecting either normal ABL fragments (173 bp) or chimeric BCR-ABL products indicating breakpoints in *M-bcr* (395 bp or 320 bp) or *m-bcr* (271 bp). BCR-ABL rearrangements are observed in eight of the 13 ALL patients. Note the presence of two chimeric fragments in one case with a *M-bcr* breakpoint (*lane 2*). The intensity of *m-bcr*-specific signals is consistently weaker than of *M-bcr* or normal ABL amplification products, since only single rounds of PCR were performed in *m-bcr* analyses

ABL-positive ALL. In view of the high frequency of Ph-positive ALL in adults the detection of chimeric BCR-ABL genes by PCR apparently constitutes a useful approach to monitor minimal residual disease. Thus far we have analyzed 17 BM and 12 PB samples obtained from 12 Ph-positive ALL patients during complete clinical/hematological remission 3–14 months after initial diagnosis. Interestingly, nine specimens, including BM samples from three patients, scored PCR-negative. These preliminary data suggest that currently available chemotherapeutic regimens can decrease the number of Ph-positive cells below the detection level of PCR in at least some patients. This result should encourage a prospective evaluation of this issue.

However, because of the shortcomings of PCR, particularly the risk of false positives, the combined use of several methods may be required to achieve accurate identification of residual neoplastic cells. Along this line, we have studied the remission status of nine adult Ph-positive ALL patients by concurrent PCR analyses using the TCRδ and BCR-ABL markers, respectively. All patients were in complete remission at the time of investigation. Six cases were PCR-positive and three PCR-negative. The respective data obtained by both approaches matched in each case.

Prospects

The clinical significance of detecting as few as 10^{-6} residual leukemia cells is far from being settled. It should be emphasized, however, that the issue of minimal residual disease can nowadays be approached successfully by a variety of different methods. In addition to the two PCR strategies discussed above, a considerable number of hematopoietic neoplasias with a known molecular basis of associated chromosomal defects have recently become accessible to PCR analysis. An alternative technique is the use of multicolor immunophenotyping (Campana et al. 1990b). Since all approaches bear limitations and advantages, the use of several methods will be necessary to confirm and complement results derived from a single technique. It should also be kept in mind that the significance of minimal residual disease has most likely to be established individually for different leukemia entitites and treatment modalities.

Acknowledgements. I thank my coworkers T.E. Hansen-Hagge, J.W.G. Janssen, M. Schmidtberger, C. Tell, and S. Yokota, who have performed the molecular genetic analyses summarized above. I gratefully acknowledge the fruitful cooperation with A. Biondi and D. Campana as well as the participants of the multicenter ALL trials for children (BFM) and adults (BMFT), namely D. Hoelzer, W.-D. Ludwig, H. Riehm, and E. Thiel. Supported by grants from the Deutsche Forschungsgemeinschaft, Deutsche Krebshilfe, and Förderkreis für tumor- und leukämiekranke Kinder Ulm.

References

Campana D, Coustan-Smith E, Janossy G (1990a) The immunologic detection of residual disease in acute leukemia. Blood 76:163–171

Campana D, Yokota S, Coustan-Smith E, Hansen-Hagge TE, Janossy G, Bartram CR (1990b) The detection of residual acute lymphoblastic leukemia cells with immunologic methods and polymerase chain reaction: a comparative study. Leukemia 4:609–614

Champlin R, Gale RP (1989) Acute lymphoblastic leukemia: recent advances in biology and therapy. Blood 73:2051–2066

D'Auriol L, MacIntyre E, Galibert E, Sigaux (1989) In vitro amplification of T cell γ gene rearrangements: a new tool for the assessment of minimal residual disease in acute lymphoblastic leukemias. Leukemia 3:155–158

Hansen-Hagge TE, Yokota S, Bartram CR (1989) Detection of minimal residual disease inacute lymphoblastic leukemia by in vitro amplification of rear-ranged T-cell receptor δ chain sequences. Blood 74:1762–1767

Kurzrock R, Gutterman JU, Talpaz M (1988) The molecular genetics of Philadelphia chromosome-positive leukemias. N Engl J Med 319:990–998

Maclntyre EA, d'Auriol L, Duparc C, Leverger G, Galibert F, Sigaux F (1990) Use of oligonucleotide probes directed against T cell antigen receptor gamma delta variable-(diversity)-joining juncitonal sequences as a general method for detecting minimal residual disease in acute lymphoblastic leukemias. J Clin Invest 86: 2125–2135

Maurer J, Janssen JWG, Thiel E, van Denderen J, Ludwig WD, Aydemir Ü, Heinze B, Fonatsch C, Harbott J, Reiter A, Riehm H, Hoelzer D, Bartram CR (1991) Detection of chimeric BCR-ABL genes in acute lymphoblastic leukaemia by polymerase chain reaction. Lancet 337:1055–1058

Raghavachar A, Thiel E, Bartram CR (1987) Analyses of phenotype and genotype in acute lymphoblastic leukemias at first presentation and in relapse. Blood 70:1079–1083

Saiki RK, Gelfand DH, Stoffel S, Scharf SJ, Higuchi R, Horn GT, Mullis KB, Erlich HA (1988) Primer-directed enzymatic amplification of DNA with a thermostable DNA polymerase. Science 239:487–491

Yamada M, Hudson S, Tournay O, Bittenbender S, Shane SS, Lange B, Tsujimoto Y, Caton AJ, Rovera G (1989) Detection of minimal disease in hematopoietic malignancies of the B-cell lineage by using third-complementarity-determining region (CDR-III) specific probes. Proc Natl Acad Sci USA 86:5123–5127

Yamada M, Wasserman R, Lange B, Reichard BA, Womer RB, Rovera G (1990) Minimal residual disease in childhood B-lineage lymphoblastic leukemia. Persistence of leukemia cells during the first 18 months of treatment. N Engl J med 323:488–495

Yokota S, Hansen-Hagge TE, Ludwig WD, Reiter A, Raghavachar A, Kleihauer E, Bartram CR (1991) The use of polymerase chain reactions to monitor minimal residual disease in acute lymphoblastic leukemia patients. Blood 77:331–339

Immunophenotypic and Immunogenotypic Detection of Minimal Residual Disease in Acute Lymphoblastic Leukemia

J.J.M. van Dongen, T.M. Breit, H.J. Adriaansen, A. Beishuizen, and H. Hooijkaas

Department of Immunology, University Hospital Dijkzigt/Erasmus University, P.O. Box 1738, 3000 DR Rotterdam, The Netherlands

Introduction

Despite major improvements in the treatment of patients with acute lymphoblastic leukemias (ALL) during the last two decades, still 20%–30% of children with ALL and 60%–75% of adult ALL patients will develop a relapse (Hoelzer et al. 1984; Linker et al. 1987; Riehm et al. 1990; Veerman et al. 1990; Ellison et al. 1991). Apparently, the current treatment protocols are not capable of killing all leukemic cells in these patients, although they seemed to be in complete remission according to cytomorphological criteria. Since the detection limit of cytomorphological techniques is 1%–5% leukemic cells, it is obvious that such techniques can only provide superficial information about the effectiveness of leukemia treatment. More sensitive techniques for the detection of low numbers of leukemic cells are needed to obtain better insight into the reduction of tumor mass during induction treatment and further eradication of the leukemic cells during maintenance treatment.

During the past decade several methods for the detection of minimal residual disease (MRD) have been developed and evaluated, such as cytomorphology, cytogenetics, cell culture systems, immunological marker analysis and molecular-biological techniques (Sonta and Sandberg 1977; Van Dongen et al. 1986; Wright et al. 1987; Estrov and Freedman 1988; Hittelman et al. 1990; Campana et al. 1990a; Bartram et al. 1990; Van Dongen and Wolvers-Tettero 1991a). In most studies the detection limits of these techniques were 1%–5% malignant cells. However, depending on the immunophenotype or the genotype of the leukemia, immunological marker analysis and the polymerase chain reaction (PCR) technique are able to detect lower frequencies of leukemic cells, as low as 10^{-4}–10^{-5} (10–1 leukemic cells per 100000 normal cells) (Van Dongen et al. 1984a, 1986, 1992; Bartram et al. 1990; Campana et al. 1990b). In the PCR technique leukemia-specific nucleotide sequences are used for MRD detection, such as

Recent Results in Cancer Research, Vol. 131

junctional regions of rearranged immunoglobulin (lg) and T-cell receptor (TcR) genes as well as breakpoint fusion regions of chromosome aberrations.

In this manuscript we will discuss the possibilities and limitations of immunological marker analysis, PCR analysis of junctional regions, and PCR analysis of breakpoint fusion regions for the detection of MRD in ALL patients.

Immunological Marker Analysis

ALL cells are generally regarded as the malignant counterparts of cells in immature stages of normal lymphopoiesis. Most ALL cells indeed have immunophenotypes comparable to normal immature lymphoid cells, which implies that the presence of these normal cells limits the immunological detectability of the leukemic cells. Therefore, immunological markers only allow the detection of malignant cells if the "positive cells" occur at higher frequencies than in normal cell samples. For most markers this results in detection limits, which are not lower than 1%–10% (10^{-2}–10^{-1}) (Van Dongen et al. 1986; Smith and Kitchens 1989; Campana et al. 1990a). Despite this limitation, several possibilities remain.

In our experience one of the best approaches for detecting MRD by immunological marker analysis is the detection of positive cells outside their normal breeding sites and "homing areas" (Janossy et al. 1980, 1981; Van Dongen et al. 1986; Smith and Kitchens 1989; Campana et al. 1990a). Leukemic cells with an "aberrant" phenotype (e.g., cross-lineage marker expression) may also allow the detection of MRD (Campana et al. 1990a). Several of these possibilities will be discussed.

Normal Immature Lymphoid Cells in Blood and Bone Marrow

The nuclear enzyme terminal deoxynucleotidyl transferase (TdT) is expressed by immature lymphoid cells of the B-cell lineage (precursor B cells) and T-cell lineage (cortical thymocytes) (Janossy et al. 1981; Campana et al. 1985, 1987; Van Dongen et al. 1985; Smith and Kitchens 1989). TdT^+ cells are reliably detectable on cytocentrifuge preparations by fluorescence microscopy due to the typical TdT staining pattern. The detailed immunophenotype of these cells can easily be studied by double immunofluorescence (IF) stainings for cell membrane or intracellular markers and TdT (Fig. 1) (Campana et al. 1985, 1987; Van Dongen et al. 1985; Smith and Kitchens 1989). The results of such double IF stainings have demonstrated that the far majority of TdT^+ cells in bone marrow (BM) and peripheral blood (PB) represent precursor B cells, which express the B-cell markers CD19 and/or CD22 on their cell membrane and in part also the CD10 antigen (Janossy et al. 1980; Campana et al. 1985; Smith and Kitchens 1989). The frequency of

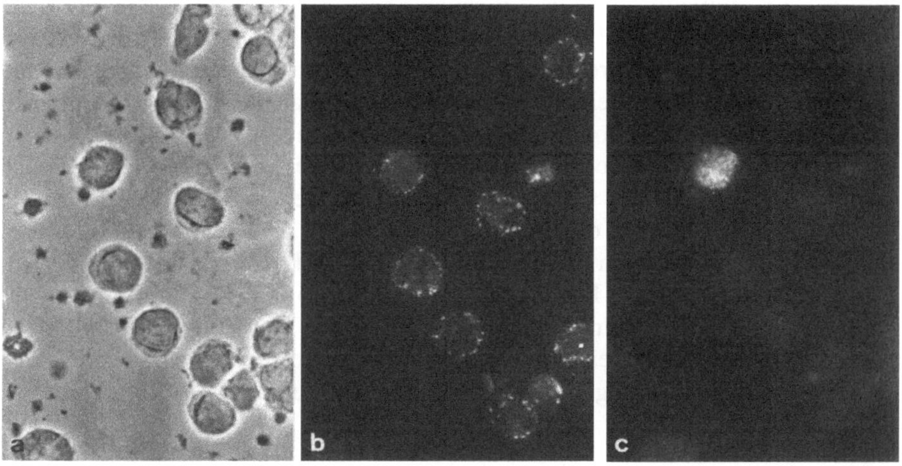

Fig. 1a-c. Double IF staining for the T-cell marker CD4 and TdT on PB cells from a T-ALL patient in an early phase of relapse. **a** Phase contrast morphology; **b** $CD4^+$ cells (rhodamine labeled); **c** TdT^+ cells (fluorescein labeled). One TdT^+ cell expresses the CD4 antigen, while the other $CD4^+$ cells are TdT^-. The $CD4^+/TdT^+$ cell most probably represents a T-ALL cell (Van Dongen et al. 1986)

the TdT^+ cells in normal PB is <0.4%, but in BM their frequency can be as high as 10%–15% (Van Dongen et al. 1986). Especially in regenerating BM, high frequencies of TdT^+ precursor B cells can be found (Van Dongen et al. 1986).

Detection of Malignant Precursor B Cells

The background of normal TdT^+ precursor B cells in BM and PB will hamper the detection of malignant TdT^+ precursor B cells (precursor-B-ALL). Nevertheless, in patients with a $CD10^+$ precursor-B-ALL (common ALL or pre-B-ALL), double IF stainings for the CD10 antigen and TdT may be used for discrimination between a homogeneous $CD10^+/TdT^+$ leukemic cell population and a normal heterogeneous precursor B cell population, which consists of a mixture of $CD10^-/TdT^+$ cells, $CD10^+/TdT^+$ cells, and $CD10^+/TdT^-$ cells (Van Dongen et al. 1986; Smith and Kitchens 1989; Knulst et al. 1993). This approach may be useful for the early diagnosis of smoldering ALL in patients with a suspected hypoplastic bone marrow, the early diagnosis of a lymphoid blast crisis in chronic myeloid leukemia, and the discrimination between regenerating BM and a relapse in an early phase (Van Dongen et al. 1984b, 1986; Smith and Kitchens 1989; Knulst et al. 1993).

It has been suggested that double IF staining for cytoplasmic expression of Igμ heavy chain (Cyμ) and TdT could be used for detection of MRD in pre-B-ALL patients, because normal Cyμ$^+$/TdT$^+$ pre-B cells are rare in BM (Janossy et al. 1980; Campana et al. 1985, 1990a). However, the expression of Cyμ in pre-B-ALL is variable with respect to intensity and percentage of positive cells. Therefore, we feel that the proposed double IF staining is not suitable for routine MRD detection.

Approximately 10% of precursor-B-ALL express a myeloid marker such as CD13, CD14, CD15, CD33, or CD_w65 (Drexler et al. 1991). This cross-lineage myeloid marker expression may be useful to detect MRD by use of double IF stainings for a myeloid marker and TdT (Campana et al. 1990a), since myeloid marker$^+$/TdT$^+$ cells are rare in normal BM and not detectable in normal PB (Adriaansen et al. 1990a,b). However, one should be aware that the cross-lineage expression of myeloid markers in precursor-B-ALL is often weak and generally concerns a subpopulation of the ALL cells (Drexler et al. 1991).

Single Ig Light Chain Expression in B-Cell ALL

B-lineage ALL with surface membrane Ig (SmIg) expression, the so-called B-ALL, represents a small special subgroup of ALL (1%–2% of ALL), which is generally characterized by the presence of a Burkitt-type chromosome translocation (Pui et al. 1990). Since B lymphocytes express only one type of Ig light chain (Igκ or Igλ), it is possible to use this single Ig light chain expression for the detection of low numbers of SmIg$^+$ B-ALL cells (Smith et al. 1984; Letwin et al. 1990). In our experience the most accurate approach is the determination of the Igκ versus Igλ distribution (κ/λ ratio) within the B-cell population by use of double IF stainings for Ig light chain and B-cell marker expression. In particular, the B-cell markers CD19 and CD20 appear to be useful for this purpose. The κ/λ ratio of normal B-cell populations, as determined by use of SmIg/B-cell marker double IF stainings, varies between 0.8 and 2.5. It is obvious that the size of the normal B-cell population in BM and PB influences the detectability of B-ALL cells. Due to this background of normal cells, the detection limit of routinely performed SmIg/B-cell marker double IF staining in BM and PB is 10^{-1}–10^{-2}.

Detection of MRD in ALL of the T-Cell Lineage

Nearly all T-cell ALL (T-ALL) express TdT as well as the pan-T-cell markers CD2, cytoplasmic CD3 (CyCD3), CD5, and CD7 (Greaves 1986; Campana et al. 1987; Van Dongen et al. 1988a,b). Many of them express additional T-cell markers such as CD1, CD4, and/or CD8 (Greaves 1986; Van Dongen et al. 1988a,b). In healthy individuals this T-cell marker$^+$/TdT$^+$ phenotype is expressed by most cortical thymocytes (Janossy et al.

1981; Campana et al. 1987; Van Dongen 1988a), but in extrathymic locations like BM and PB such cells are absent or rare (<0.3% in BM and <0.02% in PB) (Janossy et al. 1981; Van Dongen et al. 1984a, 1985; Campana et al. 1987; Smith and Kitchens 1989). If they occur, they generally only express the CD2 and/or CD7 antigens, but not other T-cell markers (Van Dongen et al. 1984a, 1985; Campana et al. 1987).

In a series of seven dilution experiments we demonstrated that routinely performed T-cell marker/TdT double IF stainings have a detection limit of 10^{-4}–10^{-5} (Van Dongen et al. 1984a; Ryan and Van Dongen 1988). Therefore, we used the double IF staining technique for detection of MRD in BM and/or PB samples of 26 T-ALL patients during follow-up. In this 8-year follow-up study, 10 of the 26 T-ALL patients developed one or two relapses (a total of 12 relapses). All BM relapses except one were detected 4–21 weeks (median 15 weeks) earlier than by use of conventional cytomorphology. In these patients the percentages of $CD5^+/TdT^+$ cells in PB appeared to parallel those in BM, indicating that T-ALL patients can most probably be monitored by analysis of their PB only. The follow-up data from two relapsed T-ALL patients in our study are summarized in Figs. 2

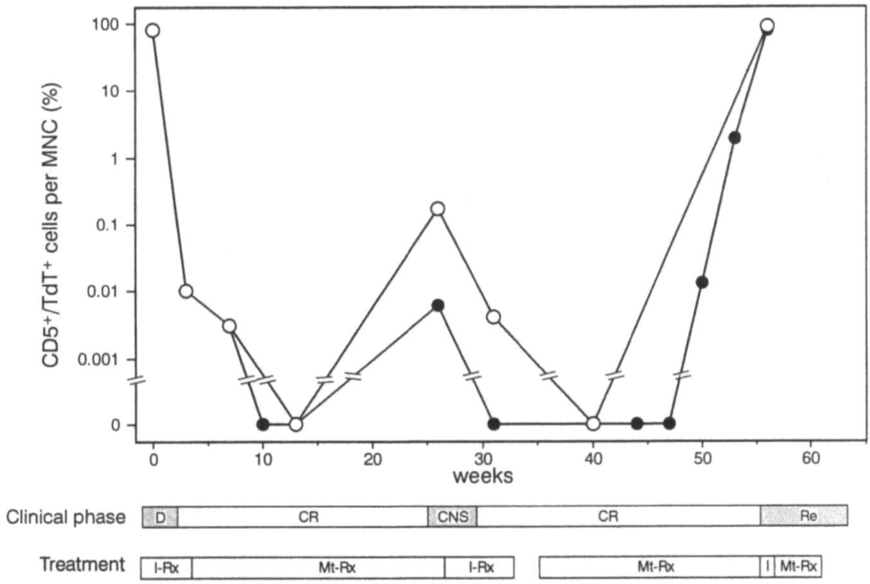

Fig. 2. Follow-up of T-ALL patient JT (5 years, female) by use of CD5/TdT double IF stainings. Symbols: •—•, PB samples; o—o, BM samples. Abbreviations: *D*, diagnosis; *CR*, complete remission; *CNS*, central nervous system leukemia; *Re*, relapse; *I-Rx* or *I*, induction treatment; *Mt-Rx*, maintenance treatment; *MNC*, mononuclear cells. In the period of CNS leukemia, T-ALL cells were detected in both PB and BM. The systemic relapse was detected 6 weeks earlier than by conventional cytomorphology

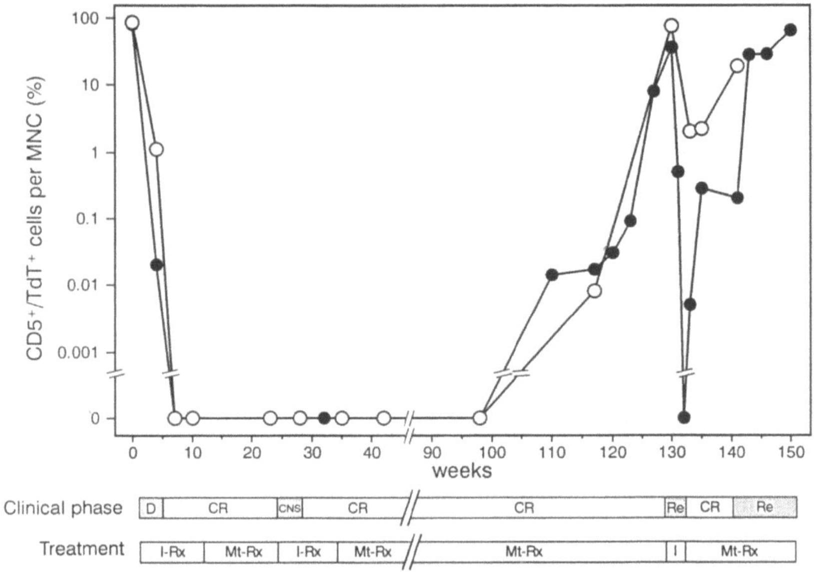

Fig. 3. Follow-up of T-ALL patient MZ (6 years, female) by use of CD5/TdT double IF stainings. Symbols: •—•, PB samples; o—o, BM samples. Abbreviations: *D*, diagnosis; *CR*, complete remission; *CNS*, central nervous system leukemia; *Re*, relapse; *I-Rx* or *I*, induction treatment; *Mt-Rx*, maintenance treatment; *MNC*, mononuclear cells. The first relapse was detected 20 weeks earlier than by conventional cytomorphology

and 3. One BM relapse was not predicted, probably because no BM or PB samples were analyzed during the 15-week period before relapse. In the BM and PB samples of the other 16 T-ALL patients, no $CD5^+/TdT^+$ cells were detected during a follow-up period of 1–101 months (median 43 months). These patients are still in remission according to cytomorphological and clinical criteria. Our follow-up study indicates that the T-cell marker/TdT double IF staining represents a sensitive and specific technique for the detection of MRD and prediction of relapse in T-ALL patients.

Detection of Central Nervous System Leukemia

Normal TdT^+ cells can be found in BM, PB, and some other locations, but we have never found TdT^+ cells in cerebrospinal fluid (CSF) without blood contamination (Hooijkaas et al. 1989). Therefore, the TdT-IF assay is useful for the early detection of central nervous system (CNS) involvement in patients with a TdT^+ leukemia, especially if no leukemic blasts are detectable upon cytomorphological analysis (Bradstock et al. 1980; Casper et al. 1983; Hooijkaas et al. 1989). Due to the high sensitivity of the TdT-IF assay, CNS leukemia is detectable at diagnosis in 15%–25% of ALL patients (Hooijkaas et al. 1989; Homans et al. 1990), a much higher frequency than the commonly reported 5% based on cytomorphological criteria (Lampert et al. 1984; Editorial 1985). Our 7-year experience with the TdT-IF assay on CSF samples (without blood contamination) from children with ALL indicates that the presence of TdT^+ cells in CSF at diagnosis is a high-risk factor for the development of CNS leukemia despite standard CNS prophylaxis. Also, during follow-up, the TdT-IF assay is a sensitive technique for the early detection of CNS leukemia as well as for the exclusion of CNS leukemia in patients with a reactive lymphocytic infiltrate in their CSF (Hooijkaas et al. 1989). Therefore, we feel that the TdT-IF assay should be added to the routine diagnostic work-up (cytomorphology and cell counting) of CSF samples in ALL patients at diagnosis and during follow-up.

Phenotypic Shifts

The value of immunological marker analysis for the detection of MRD may be limited by the occurrence of changes in the immunophenotype of the leukemic cells (Pui et al. 1986; Campana et al. 1990a). Such phenotypic shifts may lead to false-negative results with the above-described methods, especially if loss of TdT expression occurs. However, loss of TdT expression has not been observed frequently in ALL.

Detection of MRD by Use of the PCR Technique

Basic Principles of the PCR Technique

The PCR technique allows the selective amplification of a particular DNA region while it is still incorporated in the total genomic DNA (Ehrlich et al. 1988; White et al. 1989). Knowledge of the precise nucleotide sequences which flank the DNA region of interest is a prerequisite for the PCR technique. Based on this information, two synthetic oligonucleotides are prepared which can hybridize to the flanking sequences of opposite strands (primer annealing), if the DNA has been denatured to single-stranded DNA. The two oligonucleotides serve as primers for the *Taq* polymerase-mediated DNA synthesis (primer extension), which proceeds across the DNA region of interest using this region as template. The PCR process involves temperature-regulated cycles of DNA denaturation (~94°C), primer annealing (55°–60°C), and primer extension (~72°C). Because the extension product of one primer can serve as template for the other primer in a subsequent cycle, each successive PCR cycle essentially doubles the number of PCR products. Continuation of the PCR for 20–30 cycles theoretically results in 2^{20}–2^{30} times amplification of the DNA region of interest. The PCR products obtained can easily be detected in a dot-blot or Southern blot by use of a probe which specifically hybridizes to the amplified DNA fragment. Also, messenger (m)RNA can be used as target for the PCR technique, after the mRNA has been transcribed into complementary (c)DNA by use of reverse transcriptase (Todd et al. 1987; White et al. 1989).

Detection of MRD Via PCR-Mediated Amplification of Leukemia-Specific Sequences

If the target DNA or mRNA sequences are tumor-specific, it is possible to detect a few malignant cells in between many normal cells. Several studies indicate that the detection limit of the PCR technique is 10^{-4}–10^{-5} (Lee et al. 1987; Crescenzi et al. 1988; Bartram et al. 1990; Campana et al. 1990b; Van Dongen et al. 1992). In the initial PCR studies on the detection of MRD, well-defined chromosome translocations were used as tumor-specific markers (Lee et al. 1987; Crescenzi et al. 1988; Gabert et al. 1989; Morgan et al. 1989). Recent studies indicate that it is also possible to detect MRD by use of PCR-mediated amplification of junctional regions of rearranged Ig and TcR genes (D'Auriol et al. 1989; Hansen-Hagge et al. 1989; Yamada et al. 1989, 1990; Jonsson et al. 1990; Macintyre et al. 1990; Yokoto et al. 1991b; Neale et al. 1991; Van Dongen et al. 1992).

False-Positive Results Due to Carry-Over of PCR Products

One of the main pitfalls of the PCR technique is the chance of carry-over of PCR products via equipment, reagents, pipets, and aerosolization. This cross-contamination of PCR products will easily lead to false-positive results, because the highly sensitive PCR technique in principle can detect a single PCR product (Kwok and Higuchi 1989; White et al. 1989). All possible precautionary measures should be taken to prevent carry-over of PCR products between patient samples. Procedures to minimize the chance of this cross-contamination are: physical separation of pre-PCR and post-PCR tubes, aliquoting of reagents sufficient for one PCR, modification of laboratory guidelines (changing gloves frequently, spinning of tubes before opening, minimization of sample handling, use of UV light for decontamination, etc.), and careful selection of positive and negative controls (Kwok and Higuchi 1989; White et al. 1989; Sarkar and Sommer 1990). If possible, the PCR products obtained from each leukemia patient sample should be checked by use of a patient-specific oligonucleotide probe (see below).

Junctional Regions of Rearranged Ig and TcR Genes

Junctional Regions as Leukemia-Specific PCR Targets

The use of junctional regions of rearranged Ig and TcR genes as tumor-specific markers is based on the fact that these junctional regions vary enormously due to the joining of different variable (*V*), diversity (*D*), and joining (*J*) gene segments as well as the random insertion and deletion of nucleotides at the joining sites (Van Dongen and Wolvers-Tettero 1991a). This implies that the junctional regions are different in each lymphocyte or clone of lymphocytes. Therefore, it is assumed that the junctional regions of rearranged Ig and TcR genes in leukemias are unique and represent specific markers for each individual leukemia.

Based on the above assumption, it has been suggested that Ig heavy chain (IgH) gene junctional regions as well as junctional regions of rearranged TcRγ and TcRδ genes could be used as targets for MRD PCR analysis, using *V* and *J* gene-specific oligonucleotides as primers (D'Auriol et al. 1989; Yamada et al. 1989; Hansen-Hagge et al. 1989; Macintyre et al. 1990; Jonsson et al. 1990; Yokoto et al. 1991b; Neale et al. 1991). In principle, PCR analysis of junctional regions of rearranged Ig light chain genes, TcRα genes and TcRβ genes may also be applicable for detection of MRD. The choice of primers is dependent on the type of Ig or TcR gene as well as the rearranged *V* and *J* gene segments. It may be possible to design general primers which recognize (virtually) all *V* or *J* gene segments of a particular Ig or TcR gene complex, or specific primers which recognize individual *V* or *J* gene segments or families of *V* or *J* gene segments (D'Auriol et al. 1989; Yamada et al. 1989; Hansen-Hagge et al. 1989; Deane and Norton 1990). Examples of such primers for *V* and *J* gene segments of the TcRγ gene are given in Fig. 4 (Breit et al. 1991). The junctional region PCR products

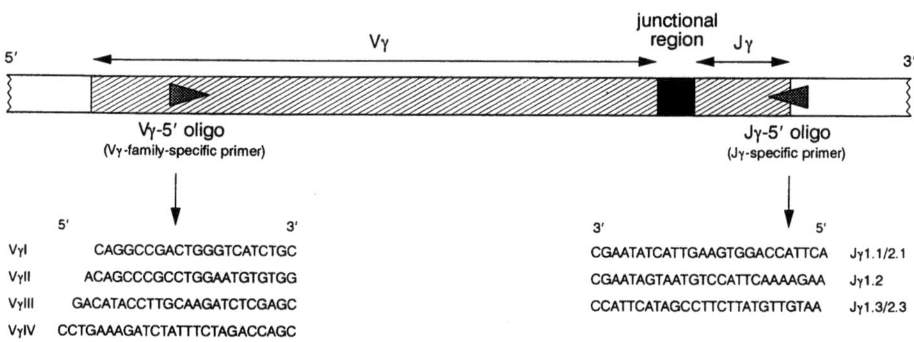

Fig. 4. Schematic diagram of a *Vγ* gene segment joined to a *Jγ* gene segment via a fictitious junctional region, which generally contains additional nucleotides. The positions of the *Vγ*-family-specific primers and the *Jγ*-specific primers are indicated. The sequences of the presented primers and the PCR technique for amplification of *Vγ*–*Jγ* junctional regions are described by Breit et al. (1991)

obtained can subsequently be analyzed in a dot-blot or Southern blot by use of a leukemia-specific junctional region probe in order to discriminate between the leukemia-derived junctional region and junctional regions from normal cells which have rearranged the same (or comparable) *V* and *J* gene segments as the leukemic cells. For each leukemia one should determine which junctional region(s) can be used as targets for the MRD PCR analysis and which primers are optimal for this purpose. Also, the leukemia-specific junctional region probes have to be designed for each individual patient (D'Auriol et al. 1989; Yamada et al. 1989; Hansen-Hagge et al. 1989; Macintyre et al. 1990; Jonsson et al. 1990; Yokoto et al. 1991b; Neale et al. 1991; Van Dongen et al. 1992).

Detection Limit of the MRD PCR Technique

The theoretical detection limit of the MRD PCR technique is approximately 10^{-6}. This is based on the assumption that one cell contains approximately 10 pg DNA and that one PCR tube can contain maximally 10 µg DNA. To determine the detection limit of the MRD PCR technique, we have diluted T-ALL cells in PB mononuclear cells of a healthy individual. This T-ALL contained a *Vδ1–Jδ1* rearrangement on one allele and a *Vδ2–Jδ1* rearrangement on the other allele. Direct sequencing of the junctional region PCR products revealed that the *Vδ1–Jδ1* junctional region consisted of 37 nucleotides. This allowed the design of a highly specific junctional region probe which was capable of detecting very low frequencies of leukemic cells in the dilution experiment, down to 10^{-6} (Fig. 5).

Frequency of Ig and TcR Gene Rearrangements in ALL

Rearrangements of Ig and/or TcR genes occur at high frequency in ALL. Approximately 98% of precursor-B-ALL have rearranged or deleted IgH

Fig. 5A,B. Dilution experiment in which T-ALL cells with a *Vδ1–Jδ1* rearrangement were diluted in PB mononuclear cells from a healthy individual. The accuracy of the dilution experiment was checked by use of CD1/TdT double IF stainings (**A**), which could follow the dilution down to ~0.001% (10^{-5}). Using the *Vδ1–3'* and *Jδ1–5'* oligonucleotides as primers, Vδ1–J*δ1* PCR products were obtained, which were run in an agarose gel (**B**, *top*) and blotted to a nylon membrane. The filter was hybridized with the ^{32}P-labeled leukemia-specific junctional region probe, which was designed according to the sequence data of the *Vδ1–JΔ1* junctional region (37 bp). Methods and primers are described by Breit et al. (1991). Leukemia-specific-junctional-region PCR products were still detectable in the 10^6-fold dilution sample (**B**, *bottom*). This figure illustrates that the leukemia-derived *Vδ1–Jδ1* PCR products are easily detectable between the many different *Vδ1–Jδ1* PCR products from normal cells

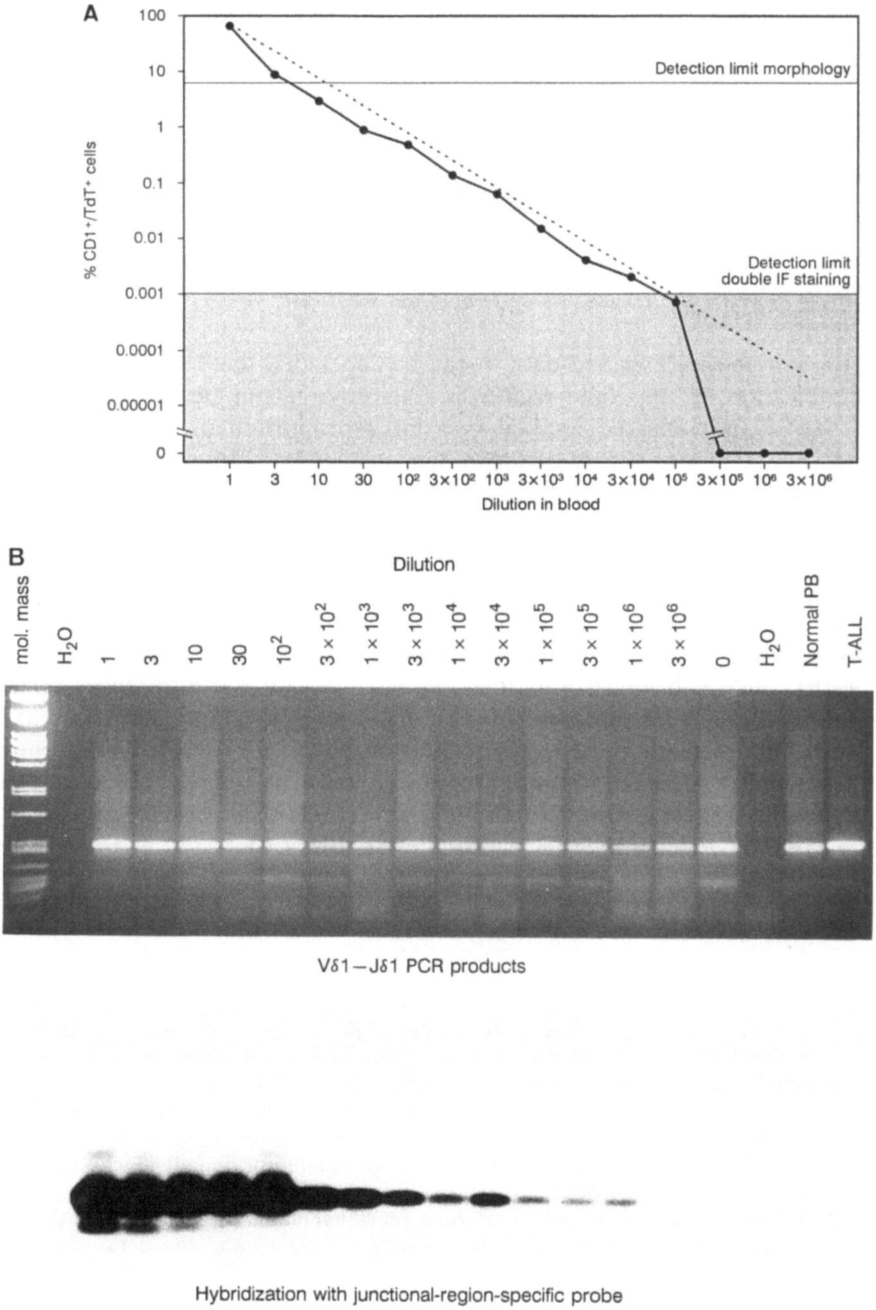
A
100
10
1
0.1
0.01
0.001
0.0001
0.00001
0
% CD1+/TdT+ cells
Detection limit morphology
Detection limit double IF staining
1 3 10 30 10² 3×10² 10³ 3×10³ 10⁴ 3×10⁴ 10⁵ 3×10⁵ 10⁶ 3×10⁶
Dilution in blood
B
Dilution
mol. mass
H2O
1
3
10
30
10²
3 × 10²
1 × 10³
3 × 10³
1 × 10⁴
3 × 10⁴
1 × 10⁵
3 × 10⁵
1 × 10⁶
3 × 10⁶
0
H2O
Normal PB
T-ALL
Vδ1—Jδ1 PCR products
Hybridization with junctional-region-specific probe

genes, whereas rearrangements and/or deletions of TcRγ and TcRδ genes are found in 91% and 96% of T-ALL, respectively (Van Dongen and Wolvers-Tettero 1991b). Although rearranged Ig and TcR genes are expressed only in B and T lymphocytes, respectively, cross-lineage Ig and TcR gene rearrangements occur at relatively high frequencies. This especially concerns TcRγ and TcRδ gene rearrangements in precursor-B-ALL (Van Dongen and Wolvers-Tettero 1991b). The frequencies of the various Ig and TcR gene rearrangements in precursor-B-ALL and T-ALL are summarized in Table 1 (Felix et al. 1990; Van Dongen and Wolvers-Tettero 1991b; Beishuizen et al. 1991b).

Pitfalls of MRD PCR Analysis of Junctional Regions

From the above-described data, it can be concluded that the PCR-mediated amplification of junctional regions is a sensitive technique for the detection of MRD which can be applied in a large proportion of ALL. However, one should realize that this technique has several pitfalls (Table 2). For example, a necessary condition for this application is the stability of the leukemia-specific junctional region during follow-up. In ~40% of precursor-B-ALL, multiple IgH gene rearrangements are found at diagnosis (Fig. 6) (Kitchingman et al. 1986; Bird et al. 1988; Katz et al. 1989; Beishuizen et al. 1991b). These are probably caused by continuing rearrangement processes, which lead to subclone formation (Bird et al. 1988; Beishuizen et al. 1991b). Such subclone formation may also explain the differences in IgH gene rearrangement patterns between diagnosis and relapse, which occur in ~50% of precursor-B-ALL cases (Beishuizen et al. 1991a). This form of oligoclonality at diagnosis and clonal evolution at relapse will frequently cause false-negative results, if the IgH gene junctional regions are used for the MRD PCR technique (Beishuizen et al. 1991a,b).

Table 1. Frequencies (%) of Ig and TcR gene rearrangements in ALL

	IgH		Igκ		Igλ	TcRβ	TcRγ	TcRδ	
	R	D	R	D	R	R	R	R	D
Precursor-B-ALL[a]	95	3	28	17	20	33	55	54	26
T-ALL[b]	14	0	0	0	0	89	91	68	28

R, one or both alleles rearranged; D, both alleles deleted or one allele with the other allele in germline configuration.

[a] Data concerning IgH gene and TcR gene rearrangements in precursor-B-ALL are derived from Van Dongen and Wolvers-Tettero (1991b) and the data concerning the Igκ and Igλ gene rearrangements are derived from Felix et al. (1990) and Beishuizen et al. (1991b).

[b] Data derived from Van Dongen and Wolvers-Tettero (1991b).

Table 2. Pitfalls of MRD PCR analysis of junctional regions

1. Occurrence of oligoclonality and clonal progression at Ig or TcR gene level (e.g., IgH gene level in precursor-B-ALL).
2. Background of normal cells with the same rearranged gene segments (e.g., *Vδ1-Jδ1* rearrangements in 0.1%–10% of normal PB lymphocytes or *Vγ1-Jγ2.3* rearrangements in large proportion of PB T lymphocytes).
3. Type of rearrangement and size of junctional region (e.g., *Vδ-Jδ* rearrangements with large junctional regions, but *Dδ-Dδ* rearrangements with short junctional regions).
4. Theoretically, normal cells may have junctional regions that are identical to those in leukemic cells.
5. Hybridization conditions, washing stringency, and exposure time influence the specificity and sensitivity of the MRD PCR technique.

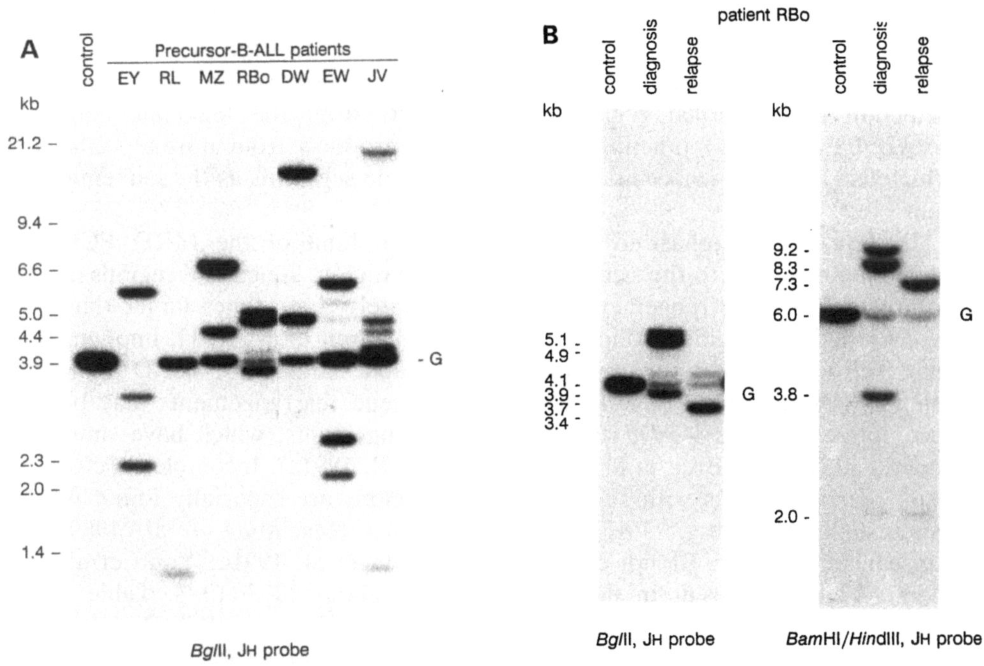

Fig. 6A,B. Southern blot analysis of IgH genes in precursor-B-ALL at diagnosis (**A**) and relapse (**B**). Control DNA and DNA from precursor-B-ALL cell samples were digested with *Bgl*II or *Bam*HI and *Hin*dIII, size separated, and blotted to a nylon membrane, which was hybridized with the ^{32}P-labeled J_H probe (Van Dongen and Wolvers-Tettero 1991a). Molecular mass markers or the size of the rearranged bands as well as the size of the germline bands (*G*) are indicated in kilobases (*kb*) in the *left margin* of each part. In several precursor-B-ALL at diagnosis (**A**) more than two rearranged bands are present, most of them differing in density. In patient *RBo* obvious differences in IgH gene rearrangement patterns were found between diagnosis and relapse in both restriction enzyme digests (**B**)

Multiple TcRγ and TcRδ gene rearrangements caused by subclone formation are rare (Van Dongen and Wolvers-Tettero 1991b). Changes in TcRγ and TcRδ gene rearrangement patterns at relapse occur in 40% of cases, but generally concern only one allele (Beishuizen et al. 1993). Therefore, the junctional regions of rearranged TcRγ and TcRδ genes probably represent a more reliable target for the MRD PCR technique in acute leukemias than the junctional regions of IgH genes. An additional advantage of using TcRγ and TcRδ junctional regions as target for the MRD PCR technique is the fact that the TcRγ and TcRδ genes contain only a few *V* and *J* gene segments (Lefranc 1988; Loh et al. 1988; Takihara et al. 1988, 1989; Van Dongen and Wolvers-Tettero 1991a), whereas the junctional regions of complete *V-(D-)J* rearrangements are extensive (Loh et al. 1988; Takihara et al. 1989; Macintyre et al. 1989, 1990; Neale et al. 1991; Breit et al. 1991). This implies that only a restricted number of oligonucleotide primers are necessary, while the leukemia-specific junctional region probes will differ extensively between the leukemias. The high specificity of the leukemia-specific junctional region probe allows the detection of junctional region PCR products from the leukemic cells between the (many) junctional region PCR products from normal cells, which use the same (or comparable) *V* and *J* gene segments as the leukemic cells.

It should be emphasized that the detection limit of the MRD PCR technique is related to the size of the junctional region. Junctional regions of complete *Vδ-Jδ* rearrangements are approximately three times larger than *Vγ-Jγ* junctional regions (Macintyre et al. 1990; Breit et al. 1991), implying that TcRδ junctional regions are more suitable targets for MRD PCR analysis (Breit et al. 1991). However, TcRδ gene rearrangements may be incomplete, such as *Vδ-Dδ* and *Dδ-Dδ* rearrangements, which have short junctional regions (Breit et al. 1991; Yokota et al. 1991a). Incomplete TcRδ gene rearrangements with short junctional regions are especially found in precursor-B-ALL, e.g., *Vδ2-Dδ3* and *Dδ2-Dδ3* (Macintyre et al. 1989; Loiseau et al. 1989; Biondi et al. 1990; Yokota et al. 1991a; Yano et al. 1991). This may result in detection limits of about 10^{-3}–10^{-4}. Table 3 summarizes the allelic frequencies of the different types of TcRδ gene rearrangements (Breit et al. 1993), and Table 4 summarizes the diversity of TcRδ and TcRγ gene junctional regions, i.e., the number of randomly inserted and deleted nucleotides at the *V-(D-)J* joining sites.

In the case of short junctional regions, it may theoretically happen that normal cells occur which have junctional regions that are identical to those in leukemic cells. Finally, it should be emphasized that the specificity and sensitivity of the junctional region MRD PCR technique is influenced by the hybridization conditions, washing stringency, and film exposure time of the junctional region specific probe. These should be carefully determined to obtain reproducible results.

Table 3. Allelic frequencies of different types of TcRδ gene rearrangements in ALL (from T.M. Breit et al., unpublished results)

Type of rearrangement	Allelic frequencies (%)			
	Precursor B ALL (n=91)	$CD3^-$ T-ALL (n=73)	$TcR\gamma\delta^+$ T-ALL (n=25)	$TcR\alpha\beta^+$ T-ALL (n=40)
Vδ1-Jδ1	0%	14%	54%	3%
Vδ2-Jδ1	0%	7%	6%	4%
Vδ3-Jδ1	0%	3%	8%	1%
Dδ2-Jδ1	0%	6%	14%	1%
Dδ2-Dδ3	3%	3%	0%	0%
Vδ2-Dδ3	24%	3%	4%	0%
Other rearrangements	6%	25%	10%	10%
Deleted	45%	25%	4%	81%
Germline	23%	14%	0%	0%

Table 4. Junctional region diversity of TcRγ and TcRδ rearrangements and fusion region diversity of *tal-1* deletions in ALL

Rearrangement (no. of alleles analyzed)	Size of junctional/fusion region		No. of deleted nucleotides	
	mean	range	mean	range
TcRδ gene rearrangements[a]				
Vδ-Jδ (n = 45)	28.3	5–47	5.0	0–20
Vδ-Dδ (n = 12)	4.8	0–11	3.8	0–9
Dδ-Jδ (n = 10)	20.7	10–40	12.1	0–29
TcRγ gene rearrangements[b]				
Vγ-Jγ (n = 30)	7.3	0–25	9.1	1–27
tal-1 region deletion[c]				
type 1 (n = 36)	7.3	0–17	6.0	0–24
type 2 (n = 4)	10.0	6–15	5.5	3–10

[a] Data from Macintyre (1989, 1990), Yokota et al. (1991a), and Breit et al. (1991, 1993).
[b] Data from Macintyre (1990) and Breit et al. (1991, 1993).
[c] Data from Brown et al. (1990), Bernard et al. (1991), and Breit et al. (1993).

Despite the above-mentioned limitations, the preliminary results of the first clinical MRD PCR studies on junctional regions in precursor-B-ALL and T-ALL are promising (Macintyre et al. 1990; Yokoto et al. 1991b; Neale et al. 1991; Bartram et al. 1992). These initial results have demonstrated that during the first half year of treatment residual leukemic cells were present in most BM samples. During further maintenance treatment, ~30% of the BM samples were still positive, but after termination of treatment virtually no positivity was found using the MRD PCR technique (Yokoto et al. 1991b; Bartram et al. 1992). Prospective studies on large series of patients are needed to evaluate the prognostic value of the junctional region MRD PCR technique.

Chromosome Aberrations as Leukemia-Specific PCR Targets

In the initial MRD PCR studies well-defined chromosome translocations were used as tumor-specific markers, e.g., t(14;18)(q32;q21) and t(9;22)(q34;q11) (Lee et al. 1987; Crescenzi et al. 1988; Gabert et al. 1989; Morgan et al. 1989). For this purpose, oligonucleotide primers were designed to recognize sequences at opposite sides of the breakpoint recombination area so that the PCR product represented the tumor-specific hybrid sequences. In routinely performed MRD PCR analysis, the PCR products should not exceed ~2 kilobases (kb) (Erlich et al. 1988; White et al. 1989). Therefore, PCR-mediated amplification of DNA sequences can only be used for chromosome aberrations in which the breakpoints cluster in a small area (total breakpoint area <2 kb), such as in t(14;18) where the *bcl-2* gene is juxtaposed to one of the *J* gene segments of the IgH genes (Bakhshi et al. 1987; Cotter et al. 1990). Other examples are the T-ALL-associated aberrations t(1;14)(p34;q11), t(10;14)(q24;q11) and a specific 90-kb deletion involving the *tal-1* gene (Chen et al. 1990; Kagan et al. 1990; Brown et al. 1990).

Specific Deletion in the **tal-1** *Gene Region in T-ALL*

Recent reports indicate that 10%–25% of T-ALL have a specific deletion of ~90 kb on chromosome 1 (Brown et al. 1990; Jonsson et al. 1991; Bernard et al. 1991; Breit et al. 1993). These deletions occur in the region of the so-called *tal-1* gene, which is also involved in t(1;14)(p34;q11) (Chen et al. 1990; Brown et al. 1990). Two types of *tal-1* deletions have been described, both of which are not detectable by routine cytogenetic analysis, but easily detectable by Southern blotting or PCR analysis (Brown et al. 1990; Jonsson et al. 1991; Bernard et al. 1991). This is due to the fact that both deletions are mediated via specific heptamer sequences, which are homologous to the heptamers in the recombination sequences of Ig and TcR genes (Brown et al. 1990; Bernard et al. 1991) (Fig. 7). These specific deletions enable the application of the MRD PCR technique by use of primers flanking the

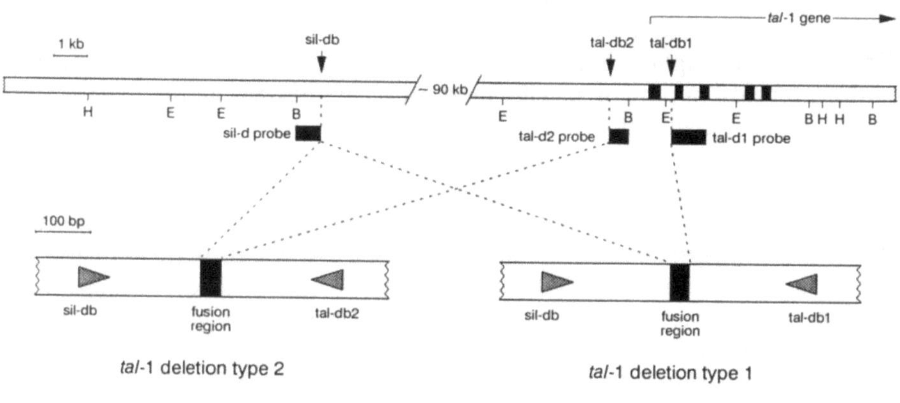

Fig. 7. Schematic diagram of the two types of *tal-1* deletions. The normal germline configuration of the *tal-1* gene locus and the 90 kb upstream region of the *sil* locus are indicated (*top*). The *three arrows* indicate the type 1 *tal-1* deletion breakpoint (*tal-db*1), the type 2 *tal-1* deletion breakpoint (*tal-db2*), and the *sil* locus deletion breakpoint (*sil-db*). The relevant restriction sites (*B*, *Bam*HI; *E*, *Eco*RI; *H*, *Hin*dIII) and the relevant probes for the Southern blot detection of the two types of *tal-1* deletions are given (*top*). The fusion regions of the two types of *tal*-1 deletions and the positions of the primers for PCR analysis of the breakpoint fusion regions are indicated at the *bottom*

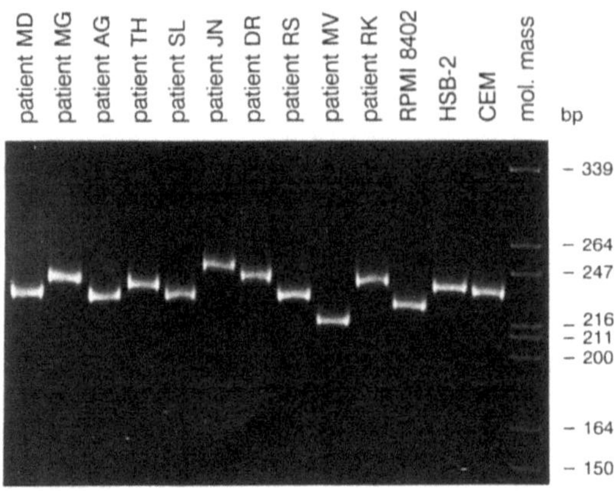

Fig. 8. Polyacrylamide gel electrophoresis of *tal-1* deletion PCR products of ten T-ALL and three T-cell lines (RPMI 8402, HSB-2, and CEM). PCR-mediated amplification of the *tal-1* deletion regions was performed by use of the C and D oligonucleotide primers. Primers and methods are described by Jonsson et al. (1991) and Breit et al. (1991, 1993), respectively. The ethidium bromide-stained gel illustrates the differences in the sizes of the PCR products, indicating that the fusion region of the *tal-1* deletion breakpoints is different in each leukemia.

deleted genomic segment (Brown et al. 1990; Bernard et al. 1991) (Fig. 7). Sequencing of *tal-1* deletion regions has revealed that the fusion region of the deletion break-points is different in each leukemia due to random insertion and deletion of nucleotides, comparable to the junctional regions in rearranged Ig and TcR genes (Jonsson et al. 1991; Bernard et al. 1991) (Table 4). This implies that the *tal-1* deletion is not only a leukemia-specific marker, but also a patient-specific marker, if one designs an oligonucleotide probe which specifically recognizes the fusion region of the *tal-1* deletion breakpoints (Table 4).

We have analyzed 85 cases of T-ALL by Southern blotting and found a type 1 *tal-1* deletion in 10 cases (12%) and a type 2 *tal-1* deletion in one case (1%). PCR analysis and direct sequencing of the fusion regions of the 10 type 1 *tal-1* deletions revealed that the fusion regions differed in size and nucleotide sequence (Fig. 8) (Breit et al. 1993). Bernard et al. (1991) demonstrated that also in the case of type 2 *tal-1* deletion the breakpoint fusion region is different in each patient. The *tal-1* deletions are therefore important targets for the MRD PCR technique in T-ALL, especially in T-ALL cases which have deleted both TcRδ gene alleles, e.g., the majority of TcRαβ$^+$ T-ALL (Tables 1, 3).

Leukemia-Specific Hybrid mRNA as PCR Target

In most translocations the breakpoints are spread over much larger areas than 2 kb. This implies that the precise breakpoint recombination area has

Table 5. Techniques for the detection of MRD in BM and PB of ALL patients

Type of leukemia	Immunological marker analysis by double IF staining		PCR analysis of junctional regions of Ig or TcR genes[a]		PCR analysis of chromosome aberrations[b]		
	Type of double staining	Frequency of applicability[c] (%)	Ig or TcR gene	Frequency of applicability[c] (%)	Aberration	Frequency of applicability[c] (%)	Target[d] (mRNA or DNA)
Precursor-B-ALL (80%–85% of ALL)	CD10/TdT (detection limit 10^{-1}–10^{-2})	90	IgH	98	t(9;22)(q34;q11)	childhood: 5–8 adult: 30–40	*bcr-abl* (mRNA)
			TcRγ	55	t(1;19)(q23;p13)	5–8	*E2A-Pbx*1 (mRnA)
	myeloid marker/TdT (detection limit 10^{-4}–10^{-5})	10	TcRδ	54	t(4;11)(q21;q23)	~3	?
B-ALL (1%–2% of ALL)	SmIg/B-cell marker (detection limit 10^{-1}–10^{-2})	100	IgH	100	t(8;14)(q24;q32)	~90	c-*myc*-IgH (?)
					t(8;22)(q24;q11)	~5	c-*myc*-Igλ (?)
					t(2;8)(q12;q24)	~2	Igκ-c-*myc* (?)
T-ALL (15%–20% of ALL)	T-cell marker/TdT (detection limit 10^{-4}–10^{-5})	>95	TcRγ	91	deletion in *tal-1* gene	10–25	del (*tal-1*) (DNA)
			TcRδ	68	t(1;14)(p34;q11)	1–3	*tal-1*-TcRδ (DNA)
			IgH	14	t(10;14)(q24;q11)	1–3	*tcl-3*-TcRδ (DNA)
					t(11;14)(p13;q11)	5–10	T-ALL^{bcr}-TcRδ (?)

[a] The detection limit of PCR analysis of junctional regions of rearranged Ig and TcR genes varies from 10^{-3} to 10^{-6} and is dependent on the size of the junctional region.
[b] The detection limit of PCR analysis of chromosome aberrations is 10^{-5}–10^{-6}.
[c] The indicated percentages represent frequencies within each type of ALL. The frequencies of the specific chromosome aberrations are derived from Ahuja and Cline (1988), Boehm and Rabbitts (1989), and Pui et al. (1990).
[d] For several well-known chromosome aberrations the precise PCR target (at mRNA or DNA level) is indicated, but for some other well-known aberrations the targets are not yet identified.

to be determined for each individual patient, which is a laborious and time-consuming effort (Hermans et al. 1987). However, in several leukemias it has been found that, as a consequence of the translocation, a new leukemia-specific hybrid gene has been created, which is transcribed into a leukemia-specific hybrid mRNA. This hybrid mRNA can be used as target for the MRD PCR analysis after reverse transcription into cDNA. Examples are: *bcr-abl* mRNA in the case of t(9;22) (Biennerhasett et al. 1988; Hermans et al. 1988; Maurer et al. 1991), *dek-can* mRNA in the case of t(6;9) (Von Lindern et al. 1990), *PML-RARa* mRNA in the case of t(15;17) (De Thé et al. 1990; Longo et al. 1990; Biondi et al. 1991), and *E2A-Pbx*1 mRNA in most cases of t(1;19) (Hunger et al. 1991; Kamps et al. 1990, 1991).

One should be aware that PCR products obtained via a leukemia-specific hybrid mRNA are not patient specific. Therefore, false-positive results due to cross-contamination of PCR products between samples from different patients are difficult to recognize. This is in contrast to the PCR products obtained from junctional regions of rearranged TcRγ and TcRδ genes or from breakpoint fusion regions of *tal-1* deletions, which can be checked by use of patient-specific oligonucleotide probes (Table 4).

An advantage of using specific chromosome translocations as tumor-specific markers is their stability during the disease course. Only 10%–15% of ALL, however, have a specific, microscopically detectable chromosome translocation and in a large part of these aberrations the precise breakpoints are not (yet) known (Table 5) (Ahuja and Cline 1988; Boehm and Rabbitts 1989; Pui et al. 1990; Jonsson et al. 1991).

Conclusion

The information summarized above indicates that immunological marker analysis as well as the PCR technique are valuable for the detection of MRD in ALL. However, one should realize that each of these techniques has its own limitations and pitfalls.

Immunological marker analysis is a relatively simple and cheap technique, which enables quantification of MRD due to the evaluation of the IF stainings at the single-cell level. This technique gives excellent results in T-ALL, but is limited in ALL of B-cell lineage (Table 5).

MRD PCR analysis using junctional regions of rearranged Ig and TcR genes seems to be a promising technique, which can be applied in a large proportion of ALL cases (Table 5). However, one should be aware that subclone formation and clonal evolution at the IgH gene level are frequent events in precursor-B-ALL, which will cause false-negative results. Changes in TcR gene rearrangement patterns may also occur. In addition, the size of the junctional region will influence the detection limit of the technique. This especially concerns the incomplete TcRδ gene rearrangements, which represent the most frequent rearrangements in precursor-B-ALL (Table 3).

MRD PCR analysis using chromosome aberrations has the advantage that these aberrations are most probably directly related to the oncogenic event and therefore represent stable tumor-specific markers. The main limitation of this technique is the fact that in the majority of ALL cases no chromosome aberrations with well-defined breakpoints have been found so far (Table 5).

Carry-over of PCR products represents a major cause of false-positive results with the MRD PCR techniques. In case of MRD PCR detection via junctional regions of rearranged TcRγ and TcRδ genes or breakpoint fusion regions of *tal-1* deletions, a leukemia-specific/patient-specific oligonucleotide probe will only recognize PCR products from the same patient. This prevents false-positive results due to carryover of PCR products between samples from different patients. However, in the case of MRD PCR detection via leukemia-specific mRNA from a translocation-mediated hybrid gene, false-positive results due to cross-contamination are very difficult to identify. Therefore, one should consider the possibility of raising specific antibodies against the protein products of leukemia-specific hybrid genes, such as the *bcr-abl* protein (Van Denderen et al. 1989), since such an approach may allow detection of leukemic cells at the single-cell level.

It is obvious from Table 5 that the three MRD techniques described are optimally applicable in T-ALL. However, prospective studies on large groups of acute leukemia patients using the three different techniques in parallel are needed to evaluate which technique is most efficient and reliable for each patient group. In the future, the MRD technique of choice will probably depend on the immunophenotype of the leukemia, the presence of rearranged Ig and/or TcR genes, and the presence of a chromosome aberration with well-defined breakpoints, as well as on the chance of immunophenotypic shifts and changes in Ig/TcR gene rearrangement patterns. The origin of the cell sample (BM, PB, or CSF), its volume, and its cellularity will influence the choice as well.

Acknowledgements. We gratefully acknowledge Professor Dr R. Benner for his continuous support and advice, Mr. T.M. van Os for his assistance in the preparation of the figures, and Mrs. A.D. Korpershoek for secretarial support. We thank Drs. K. Hählen, F.G.A.J. Hakvoort-Cammel, W.J.D. Hofhuis, C. van der Heul, A.C.J.M. Holdrinet, M.C. Kappers-Klunne, B. Löwenberg, I.M. Risseeuw-Appel, C.G. Tromp, M. van Marwijk Kooij, M.B. van 't Veer, and G.E. van Zanen for collecting the many cell samples of ALL patients at diagnosis and during follow-up.

References

Adriaansen HJ, Hooijkaas H, Kappers-Klunne MC, Hählen K, Van 't Veer MB, Van Dongen JJM (1990a) Double marker analysis for terminal deoxynucleotidyl transferase and myeloid antigens in acute nonlymphocytic leukemia patients and healthy subjects. Haematol Blood Transfus 33:41–49

Adriaansen HJ, Van Dongen JJM, Kappers-Klunne MC, Hählen K, Van 't Veer MB, Wijdenes-De Bresser JHFM, Holdrinet ACJM, Harthoorn-Lasthuizen EJ, Abels J, Hooijkaas H (1990b) Terminal deoxynucleotidyl transferase positive subpopulations occur in the majority of ANLL: implications for the detection of minimal disease. Leukemia 4:404–410

Ahuja H, Cline MJ (1988) Genetic and cytogenetic changes in acute lymphoblastic leukemia. Med Oncol Tumor Pharmacother 5:211–222

Bakhshi A, Wright JJ, Graninger W, Seto M, Owens J, Cossman J, Jensen JP, Goldman P, Korsmeyer SJ (1987) Mechanism of the t(14;18) chromosomal translocation: structural analysis of both derivative 14 and 18 reciprocal partners. Proc Natl Acad Sci USA 84:2396–2400

Bartram CR, Yokota S, Hansen-Hagge TE, Janssen JWG (1990) Detection of minimal residual leukemia by polymerase chain reactions. Bone Marrow Transplant 6s:4–8

Bartram CR, Yokota S, Biondi A, Janssen JWG, Hansen-Hagge TE (1992) Detection of minimal residual disease in acute lymphoblastic leukemia patients by polymerase chain reaction. In: Hiddemann W, Büchner T, Plunkett W, Keating M, Wörmann B, Andreeff M (eds) Acute leukemias III. Pharmacokinefics and management of relapse in refractory disease. Springer, Berlin Heidelberg New York, pp 171–177

Beishuizen A, Hählen K, Van Wering ER, Van Dongen JJM (1991a) Detection of minimal residual disease in childhood leukemia with the polymerase chain reaction. N Engl J Med 324:772–773

Beishuizen A, Hählen K, Hagemeijer A, Verhoeven M-AJ, Hooijkaas H, Adriaansen HJ, Wolvers-Tettero ILM, Van Wering ER, Van Dongen JJM (1991b) Multiple rearranged immunoglobulin genes in childhood acute lymphoblastic leukemia of precursor-B-cell origin. Leukemia 5:657–667

Beishuizen A, Verhoeven M-AJ, Hählen K, Van Wering ER, Van Dongen JJM (1993) Differences in immunoglobulin and T-cell receptor gene rearrangement patterns in acute lymphoblastic leukemia between diagnosis and relapse. Haematol Blood Transfus (in press)

Bernard O, Lecointe N, Jonveaux P, Souyri M, Mauchauffé, Berger R, Larsen CJ, Mathieu-Mahul D (1991) Two site-specific deletions and t(1;14) translocation restricted to human T-cell acute leukemias disrupt the 5′ part of the tal-1 gene. Oncogene 6:1477–1488

Biondi A, Di Celle PF, Rossi V, Casorati G, Matullo G, Giudici G, Foa R, Migone N (1990) High prevalence of T-cell receptor Vδ2-(D)-Dδ3 or Dδ1/2-Dδ3 rearrangements in B-precursor acute lymphoblastic leukemias. Blood 75:1834–1840

Biondi A, Rambaldi A, Alcalay M, Pandolfi PP, Lo Coco F, Diverio D, Rossi V, Mencarelli A, Longo L, Zangrilli D, Masera G, Barbui T, Mandelli F, Grignani F, Pelicci PG (1991) RAR-α-gene rearrangements as a genetic marker for diagnosis and monitoring in acute promyelocytic leukemia. Blood 77:1418–1422

Bird J, Galili N, Link M, Stites D, Sklar J (1988) Continuing rearrangement but abscence of somatic hypermutation in immunoglobulin genes of human B cell precursor leukemia. J Exp Med 168:229–245

Blennerhassett GT, Furth ME, Anderson A, Burns JP, Chaganti RSK, Blick M, Talpaz M, Dev VG, Chan LC, Wiedemann LM, Greaves MF, Hagemeijer A, Van der Plas D, Skuse G, Wang N, Stam K (1988) Clinical evaluation of a DNA probe assay for the Philadelphia (Ph[1]) translocation in chronic myelogenous leukemia. Leukemia 2:648–657

Boehm T, Rabbitts TH (1989) A chromosomal basis of lymphoid malignancy in man. Eur J Biochem 185:1–17

Bradstock KF, Papageorgiou ES, Janossy G, Hoffbrand AV, Willoughby ML, Roberts RD, Bollum FJ (1980) Detection of leukaemic lymphoblasts in CSF by immunofluorescence for terminal transferase. Lancet i:1144

Breit TM, Wolvers-Tettero ILM, Hählen K, Van Wering ER, Van Dongen JJM (1991) Extensive junctional diversity of γδ T-cell receptors expressed by T-cell acute lymphoblastic leukemias: implications for the detection of minimal residual disease. Leukemia 5:1076–1086

Breit TM, Mol EJ, Wolvers-Tettero ILM, Ludwig W-D, Van Wering ER, Van Dongen JJM (1993) Site-specific deletions involving the *tal*-1 and *sil* genes are restricted to cells of the T-cell receptor αβ lineage: T-cell receptor δ gene deletion mechanism affects multiple genes. J Exp Med (in press)

Brown L, Cheng J-T, Chen Q, Siciliano MJ, Crist W, Buchanan G, Baer R (1990) Site-specific recombination of the tal-1 gene is a common occurrence in human T cell leukemia. EMBO J 9:3343–3351

Campana D, Janossy G, Bofill M, Trejdosiewicz LK, Ma D, Hoffbrand AV, Mason DY, Lebacq A-M, Forster HK (1985) Human B cell development: I. Phenotypic differences of B lymphocytes in the bone marrow and peripheral lymphoid tissue. J Immunol 134:1524–1530

Campana D, Thompson JS, Amlot P, Brown S, Janossy G (1987) The cytoplasmic expression of CD3 antigens in normal and malignant cells of the T lymphoid lineage. J Immunol 138:648–655

Campana D, Coustan-Smith E, Janossy G (1990a) The immunologic detection of minimal residual disease in acute leukemia. Blood 76:163–171

Campana D, Yokota S, Coustan-Smith E, Hansen-Hagge TE, Janossy G, Bartram CR (1990b) The detection of residual acute lymphoblastic leukemia cells with immunologic methods and polymerase chain reaction: a comparative study. Leukemia 4:609–614

Casper JT, Lauer SJ, Kirchner PA, Gottschall JL, Camitta BM (1983) Evaluation of cerebrospinal fluid mononuclear cells obtained from children with acute lymphocytic leukemia: advantages of combining cytomorphology and terminal deoxynucleotidyl transferase. Am J Clin Pathol 80:666–670

Chen Q, Cheng J-T, Tsai L-H, Schneider N, Buchanan G, Carroll A, Crist W, Ozanne B, Siciliano MJ, Baer R (1990) The tal gene undergoes chromosome translocation in T cell leukemia and potentially encodes a helix-loop-helix protein. EMBO J 9:415–424

Cotter F, Price C, Zucca E, Young BD (1990) Direct sequence analysis of the $14q^+$ and $18q^-$ chromosome junctions in follicular lymphoma. Blood 76:131–135

Crescenzi M, Seto M, Herzig GP, Weiss PD, Griffith RC, Korsmeyer SJ (1988) Thermostable DNA polymerase chain amplification of t(14;18) chromosome breakpoints and detection of minimal residual disease. Proc Natl Acad Sci USA 85:4869–4873

D'Auriol L, Macintyre E, Galibert F, Sigaux F (1989) In vitro amplification of T cell γ gene rearrangements: a new tool for the assessment of minimal residual disease in acute lymphoblastic leukemias. Leukemia 3:155–158

Deane M, Norton JD (1990) Immunoglobulin heavy chain variable region family usage is independent of tumor cell phenotype in human B lineage leukemias. Eur J Immunol 20:2209–2217

De Thé H, Chomienne C, Lanotte M, Degos L, Dejean A (1990) The t(15;17) translocation of acute promyelocytic leukaemia fuses the retinoic acid receptor α gene to a novel transcribed locus. Nature 347:558–561

Drexler HG, Thiel E, Ludwig W-D (1991) Review of the incidence and clinical relevance of myeloid antigen-positive acute lymphoblastic leukemia. Leukemia 5:637–645

Ellison RR, Mick R, Cuttner J, Schiffer CA, Silver RT, Henderson ES, Woliver T, Royston I, Davey FR, Glicksman AS, Bloomfield CD, Holland JF (1991) The effects of postinduction intensification treatment with cytarabine and daunorubicin in adult acute lymphocytic leukemia: A prospective randomized clinical trial by cancer and leukemia group B. J Clin Oncol 9:2002–2015

Editorial (1985) Leukaemia and the central nervous system. Lancet i:1196–1198

Erlich HA, Gelfand DH, Saiki RK (1988) Specific DNA amplification. Nature 331:461–462

Estrov Z, Freedman MH (1988) Growth requirements for human acute lymphoblastic leukemia cells: Refinement of a clonogenic assay. Cancer Res 48:5901–5907

Felix CA, Poplack DG, Reaman GH, Steinberg SM, Cole DE, Taylor BJ, Begley CG, Kirsch IR (1990) Characterization of immunoglobulin and T-cell receptor gene patterns in B-cell precursor acute lymphoblastic leukemia of childhood. J Clin Oncol 8:431–442

Gabert J, Lafage M, Maraninchi D, Thuret I, Carcassonne Y, Mannoni P (1989) Detection of residual bcr/abl translocation by polymerase chain reaction in chronic myeloid leukaemia patients after bone-marrow transplantation. Lancet ii:1125–1128

Greaves MF (1986) Differentiation-linked leukemogenesis in lymphocytes. Science 234:697–704

Hansen-Hagge TE, Yokota S, Bartram CR (1989) Detection of minimal residual disease in acute lymphoblastic leukemia by in vitro amplification of rearranged T-cell receptor δ chain sequences. Blood 74:1762–1767

Hermans A, Heisterkamp N, Von Lindern M, Van Baal S, Meijer D, Van der Plas D, Wiedemann LM, Groffen J, Bootsma D, Grosveld G (1987) Unique fusion of bcr and c-abl genes in Philadelphia chromosome positive acute lymphoblastic leukemia. Cell 51:33–40

Hermans A, Selleri L, Gow J, Wiedemann L, Grosveld G (1989) Molecular analysis of the Philadelphia translocation in chronic myelogenous and acute lymphocytic leukemia. Cancer Cells 7:21–26

Hittelman WN, Tigaud J-D, Estey E, Vadhan-Raj S (1990) Premature chromosome condensation in the study of minimal residual disease. Bone Marrow Transplant 6:9–13

Hoelzer D, Thiel E, Löffler H, Bodenstein H, Plaumann L, Büchner T, Urbanitz D, Koch P, Heimpel H, Engelhardt R, Müller U, Wendt F-C, Sodomann H, Rühl H, Herrmann F, Kaboth W, Dietzfelbinger H, Pralle H, Lunscken Ch, Hellriegel K-P, Spors S, Nowrousian RM, Fischer J, Fülle H, Mitrou PS, Pfreundschuh M, Görg Ch, Emmerich B, Queisser W, Meyer P, Labedzki L, Essers U, König H, Mainzer K, Herrmann R, Messerer D, Zwingers T (1984) Intensified therapy in acute lymphoblastic and acute undifferentiated leukemia in adults. Blood 64:38–47

Homans AC, Barker BE, Forman EN, Cornell CJ Jr, Dickerman JD, Truman JT (1990) Immunophenotypic characteristics of cerebrospinal fluid cells in children with acute lymphoblastic leukemia at diagnosis. Blood 76:1807–1811

Hooijkaas H, Hählen K, Adriaansen HJ, Dekker I, Van Zanen GE, Van Dongen JJM (1989) Terminal deoxynucleotidyl transferase (TdT)-positive cells in cerebrospinal fluid and development of overt CNS leukemia: a 5-year follow-up study in 113 children with a TdT-positive leukemia or non-Hodgkin's lymphoma. Blood 74:416–422

Hunger SP, Galili N, Carroll AJ, Crist WM, Link MP, Cleary ML (1991) The t(1;19)(q23;p13) results in consistent fusion of E2A and PBX1 coding sequences in acute lymphoblastic leukemias. Blood 77:687–693

Janossy G, Bollum FJ, Bradstock KF, Ashley J (1980) Cellular phenotypes of normal and leukemic hemopoietic cells determined by analysis with selected antibody combinations. Blood 56:430–441

Janossy G, Tidman N, Papageorgiou ES, Kung PC, Goldstein G (1981) Distribution of T lymphocyte subsets in the human bone marrow and thymus: an analysis with monoclonal antibodies. J Immunol 126:1608–1613

Jonsson OG, Kitchens RL, Scott FC, Smith RG (1990) Detection of minimal residual disease in acute lymphoblastic leukemia using immunoglobulin hypervariable region specific oligonucleotide probes. Blood 76:2072–2079

Jonsson OG, Kitchens RL, Baer RJ, Buchanan GR, Smith RG (1991) Rearrangements of the tal-1 locus as clonal markers for T cell acute lymphoblastic leukemia. J Clin Invest 87:2029–2035

Kagan J, Finger LR, Besa E, Croce CM (1990) Detection of minimal residual disease in leukemic patients with the t(10;14) (q24;q11) chromosomal translocation. Cancer Res 50:5240–5244

Kamps MP, Murre C, Sun X, Baltimore D (1990) A new homeobox gene contributes the DNA binding domain of the t(1;19) translocation protein in pre-B ALL. Cell 60:547–555

Kamps MP, Look AT, Baltimore D (1991) The human t(1;19) translocation in pre-B ALL produces multiple nuclear E2A-Pbx1 fusion proteins with differing transforming potentials. Genes Dev 5:358–368

Katz F, Ball L, Gibbons B, Chessells J (1989) The use of DNA probes to monitor minimal residual disease in childhood acute lymphoblastic leukemia. Br J Haematol 73:173–180

Kitchingman GR, Mirro J, Stass S, Rovigatti U, Melvin SL, Williams DL, Raimondi SC, Murphy SB (1986) Biologic and prognostic significance of the presence of more than two μ heavy-chain genes in childhood acute lymphoblastic leukemia of B precursor cell origin. Blood 67:698–703

Knulst AC, Adriaansen HJ, Hählen K, Stigter JCM, Van den Beemd MWM, Hagemeijer A, Van Dongen JJM, Hooijkaas H (1993) Early diagnosis of smoldering acute lymphoblastic leukemia using immunological marker analysis. Leukemia (in press)

Kwok S, Higuchi R (1989) Avoiding false positives with PCR. Nature 339:237–238

Lampert F, Henze G, Langermann H-J, Schellong G, Gadner H, Riehm H-J (1984) Acute lymphoblastic leukemia: current status of therapy in children. In: Thiel E, Thierfelder S (eds) Leukemia. Recent developments in diagnosis and therapy. Springer, Berlin Heidelberg New York, pp 159–81 (Recent results in cancer research, vol 93)

Lee M-S, Chang K-S, Cabanillas F, Freireich EJ, Trujillo JM, Stass SA (1987) Detection of minimal residual cells carrying the t(14;18) by DNA sequence amplification. Science 237:175–178

Lefranc M-P (1988) The human T-cell rearranging gamma (TRG) genes and the gamma T-cell receptor. Biochimie 70:901–908

Letwin BW, Wallace PK, Muirhead KA, Hensler GL, Kashatus WH, Horan PK (1990) An improved clonal excess assay using flow cytometry and B-cell gating. Blood 75:1178–1185

Linker CA, Levitt LJ, O'Donnell M, Ries CA, Link MP, Forman SJ, Farbstein MJ (1987) Improved results of treatment of adult acute lymphoblastic leukemia. Blood 69:1242–1248

Loh EY, Cwirla S, Serafini AT, Phillips JH, Lanier LL (1988) Human T-cell-receptor δ chain: genomic organization, diversity, and expression in populations of cells. Proc Natl Acad Sci USA 85:9714–9718

Loiseau P, Guglielmi P, Le Paslier D, Macintyre E, Gessain A, Bories J-C, Flandrin G, Chen Z, Sigaux F (1989) Rearrangements of the T cell receptor δ gene in T acute lymphoblastic leukemia cells are distinct from those occurring in B lineage acute lymphoblastic leukemia and preferentially involve one Vδ gene segment. J Immunol 142:3305–3311

Longo L, Pandolfi PP, Biondi A, Rambaldi A, Mencarelli A, Lo Coco F, Diverio D, Pegoraro L, Avanzi G, Tabilio A, Zangrilli D, Alcalay M, Donti E, Grignani F, Pelicci PG (1990) Rearrangements and aberrant expression of the retinoic acid receptor α gene in acute promyelocytic leukemias. J Exp Med 172:1571–1575

Macintyre EA, D'Auriol L, Amesland F, Loiseau P, Chen Z, Boumsell L, Galibert F, Sigaux F (1989) Analysis of junctional diversity in the preferential Vδ1-Jδ1 rearrangement of fresh T-acute lymphoblastic leukemia cells by in vitro gene amplification and direct sequencing. Blood 74:2053–2061

Macintyre EA, D'Auriol L, Duparc N, Leverger G, Galibert F, Sigaux F (1990) Use of oligonucleotide probes directed against T cell antigen receptor gamma delta variable-(diversity)-joining junctional sequences as a general method for detecting minimal residual disease in acute lymphoblastic leukemias. J Clin Invest 86:2125–2135

Maurer J, Janssen JWG, Thiel E, Van Denderen J, Ludwig W-D, Aydemir Ü, Heinze B, Fonatsch C, Harbott J, Reiter A, Riehm H, Hoelzer D, Bartram CR (1991) Detection of chimeric BCR-ABL genes in acute lymphoblastic leukemia by the polymerase chain reaction. Lancet 337:1055–1058

Morgan GJ, Janssen JWG, Guo A-P, Wiedemann LM, Hughes T, Gow J, Goldman JM, Bartram CR (1989) Polymerase chain reaction for detection of residual leukaemia. Lancet i:928–929

Neale GAM, Menarguez J, Kitchingman GR, Fitzgerald TJ, Koehler M, Mirro J Jr, Goorha RM (1991) Detection of minimal residual disease in T-cell acute lymphoblastic leukemia using polymerase chain reaction predicts impending relapse. Blood 78:739–747

Pui C-H, Raimondi SC, Behm FG, Ochs J, Furman WL, Bunin NJ, Ribeiro RC, Tinsley PA, Mirro J (1986) Shifts in blast cell phenotype and karyotype at relapse of childhood lymphoblastic leukemia. Blood 68:1306–1310

Pui C-H, Crist WM, Look AT (1990) Biology and clinical significance of cytogenetic abnormalities in childhood acute lymphoblastic leukemia. Blood 76:1449–1463

Riehm H, Gadner H, Henze G, Kornhuber B, Lampert F, Niethammer D, Reiter A, Schellong G (1990) Results and significance of six randomized trials in four consecutive ALL-BFM studies. Haematol Blood Transfus 33:439–450

Ryan DH, van Dongen JJM (1988) Detection of residual disease in acute leukemia using immunological markers, In: Bennett JM, Foon KA (eds) Immunologic approaches to the classification and management of lymphomas and leukemias. Nijhoff, Dordreclit, pp 173–207

Sarkar G, Sommer SS (1990) Shedding light on PCR contamination. Nature 343:27

Smith RG, Kitchens RL (1989) Phenotypic heterogeneity of TdT^+ cells in the blood and bone marrow: implications for surveillance of residual leukemia. Blood 74:312–319

Smith BR, Weinberg DS, Robert NJ, Towle M, Luther E, Pinkus GS, Ault KA (1984) Circulating monoclonal B lymphocytes in non-Hodgkin's lymphoma. N Eng J Med 311:1476–1481

Sonta S, Sandberg AA (1977) Chromosomes and causation of human cancer and leukemia: XXVIII. Value of detailed chromosome studies on large numbers of cells in CML. Am J Hematol 3:121–126

Takihara Y, Tkachuk D, Michalopoulos E, Champagne E, Reimann J, Minden M, Mak TW (1988) Sequence and organization of the diversity, joining, and constant region genes of the human T-cell δ-chain locus. Proc Natl Acad Sci USA 85:6097–6101

Takihara Y, Reimann J, Michalopoulos E, Ciccone E, Moretta L, Mak TW (1989) Diversity and structure of human T cell receptor δ chain genes in peripheral blood γ/δ-bearing T lymphocytes. J Exp Med 169:393–405

Todd JA, Bell JI, McDevitt HO (1987) HLA-DQ$_{\beta}$gene contributes to susceptibility and resistance to insulin-dependent diabetes mellitus. Nature 329:599–604

Van Denderen J, Hermans A, Meeuwsen T, Troelstra C, Zegers N, Boersma W, Grosveld G, Van Ewijk W (1989) Antibody recognition of the tumor-specific bcr-abl joining region in chronic myeloid leukemia. J Exp Med 169:87–98

Van Dongen JJM, Wolvers-Tettero ILM (1991a) Analysis of immunoglobulin and T cell receptor genes. Part I: Basic and technical aspects. Clin Chim Acta 198:1–91

Van Dongen JJM, Wolvers-Tettero ILM (1991b) Analysis of immunoglobulin and T cell receptor genes. Part II: possibilities and limitations in the diagnosis and management of lymphoproliferative diseases and related disorders. Clin Chim Acta 198:93–174

Van Dongen JJM, Hooijkaas H, Hählen K, Benne K, Bitter WM, Van der Linde-Preesman AA, Tettero ILM, Van de Rijn M, Hilgers J, Van Zanen GE, Hagemeijer A (1984a) Detection of minimal residual disease in TdT positive T cell malignancies by double immunofluorescence staining. In: Löwenberg B, Hagenbeek A (eds) Minimal residual disease in acute leukemia. Nijhoff, The Hague, pp 67–81

Van Dongen JJM, Hooijkaas H, Hagemeijer A, Hählen K, Van Zanen GE, Lansdorp PM (1984b) Characterization and monitoring of the malignant cells in the blastic and chronic phase of chronic myeloid leukemia. In: Peeters H (ed) Protides of the biological fluids. Pergamon, Oxford pp 711–714

Van Dongen JJM, Hooijkaas H, Comans-Bitter WM, Hählen K, De Klein A, Van Zanen GE, Van 't Veer MB, Abels J, Benner R (1985) Human bone marrow cells positive for terminal deoxynucleotidyl transferase (TdT), HLA-DR, and a T cell marker may represent prothymocytes. J Immunol 135:3144–3150

Van Dongen JJM, Hooijkaas H, Adriaansen HJ, Hählen K, Van Zanen GE (1986) Detection of minimal residual acute lymphoblastic leukemia by immunological marker analysis: possibilities and limitations. In: Hagenbeek A, Löwenberg B (eds) Minimal residual disease in acute leukemia 1986. Nijhoff, Dordrecht, pp 113–133

Van Dongen JJM, Krissansen GW, Wolvers-Tettero ILM, Comans-Bitter WM, Adriaansen HJ, Hooijkaas H, Van Wering ER, Terhorst C (1988a) Cytoplasmic expression of the CD3 antigen as a diagnostic marker for immature T-cell malignancies. Blood 71:603–612

Van Dongen JJM, Adriaansen HJ, Hooijkaas H (1988b) Immunophenotyping of leukemias and non-Hodgkin's lymphomas: immunological markers and their CD codes. Neth J Med 33:298–314

Van Dongen JJM, Breit TM, Adriaansen HJ, Beishuizen A, Hooijkaas H (1992) Detection of minimal residual disease in acute leukemia by immunological marker analysis and polymerase chain reaction. Leukemia 6S1:47–59

Veerman AJP, Hählen K, Kamps WA, Van Leeuwen EF, De Vaan GAM, Van Wering ER, Van der Does-Van den Berg A, Solbu G, Suciu S (1990) Dutch childhood leukemia study group: early results of study ALL VI (1984–1988). Hematol Blood Transfus 33:473–477

Von Lindern M, Poustka A, Lerach H, Grosveld G (1990) The (6;9) chromosome translocation, associated with a specific subtype of nonlymphocytic leukemia, leads to aberrant transcription of a target gene on 9q34. Mol Cell Biol 10:4016–4026

White TJ, Arnheim N, Erlich HA (1989) The polymerase chain reaction. Trends Genet 5:185–189

Wright JJ, Poplack DG, Bakhshi A, Reaman G, Cole D, Jensen JP, Korsmeyer SJ (1987) Gene rearrangements as markers of clonal variation and minimal residual disease in acute lymphoblastic leukemia. J Clin Oncol 5:735–741

Yamada M, Hudson S, Tournay O, Bittenbender S, Shane SS, Lange B, Tsujimoto Y, Caton AJ, Rovera G (1989) Detection of minimal disease in hematopoietic malignancies of the B-cell lineage by using third-complementarity-determining region (CDR-III)-specific probes. Proc Natl Acad Sci USA 86:5123–5127
Yamada M, Wasserman R, Lange B, Reichard BA, Womer RB, Rovera G (1990) Minimal residual disease in childhood B-lineage lymphoblastic leukemia: persistence of leukemic cells during the first 18 months of treatment. N Engl J Med 323:448–455
Yano T, Pullman A, Andrade R, Uppenkamp M, De Villartay JP, Reaman G, Crush-Stanton S, Cohen DI, Raffeld M, Cossman J (1991) A common Vδ2-Dδ2-Dδ3 T cell receptor gene rearrangement in precursor B acute lymphoblastic leukaemia. Br J Haematol 79:44–49
Yokota S, Hansen-Hagge TE, Bartram CR (1991a) T-cell receptor δ gene recombination in common acute lymphoblastic leukemia: Preferential usage of Vδ2 and frequent involvement of the Jα cluster. Blood 77:141–148
Yokota S, Hansen-Hagge TE, Ludwig W-D, Reiter A, Raghavachar A, Kleihauer E, Bartram CR (1991b) Use of polymerase chain reactions to monitor minimal residual disease in acute lymphoblastic leukemia patients. Blood 77:331–339

Detection of Aberrant Antigen Expression in Acute Myeloid Leukemia by Multiparameter Flow Cytometry

B. Wörmann[1], M. Safford[2], S. Könemann[1], T. Büchner[3], W. Hiddemann[1], and L.W.M.M. Terstappen[2]

[1] University of Göttingen, Department of Internal Medicine, W-3400 Göttingen, Fed. Rep. of Germany,
[2] Becton Dickinson Immunocytometry Systems, 2350 Qume Drive, San José, CA 95131, USA,
[3] University of Münster, Department of Internal Medicine A, W-4400 Münster, Fed. Rep. of Germany

Introduction

Acute leukemias are conventionally diagnosed by light microscopical evaluation of bone marrow aspirates or biopsies. Distinction between acute lymphoblastic (ALL) and acute myeloid leukemia (AML) is supported by cytochemistry and is well reproducible between experienced hematologists and/or pathologists (Bennett et al. 1976; MIC Classification 1988). Disagreement can arise within the myeloid lineage, e.g. in the distinction of "de novo" and "secondary" leukemias, in the distinction of myelodysplastic syndromes (MDS) in advanced stages (RAEB-T), and in the distinction of benign myeloproliferative disease in infants. All these exceptions comprise far less than 5% of all cases. The largest discrepancies arise in the subclassification of AML using the FAB classification (Argyle et al. 1989). The usefulness of additional diagnostic tools in the routine of leukemia diagnosis must be judged based on their ability to provide the correct diagnosis in disputed cases, to identify clinically relevant subpopulations for early treatment stratification, and to detect residual leukemic cells in hematological complete remission for postremission therapy monitoring. Since today, only patients within one subset of AML, the acute promyelocytic leukemia APL, FAB M3, may receive different induction therapy (Castaigne et al. 1990; Warrell et al. 1991), the lack of concordance between different hematocytologists has little significance for the patients. This may change, when more subpopulations with distinctly different prognosis are identified.

The most widely used additional tool in leukemia diagnostics is immunophenotyping. Its major role in initial diagnosis lies in the subdivision of ALL according to the differentiation of normal lymphoid precursors (Greaves et al. 1981; Foon et al. 1986; Neame et al. 1986; Ludwig et al. 1989). Within AML, immunophenotyping has little immediate impact on treatment. Although an extensive body of literature is available which relates prognosis to antigen expression of the leukemia, there is no general

Recent Results in Cancer Research, Vol. 131

consensus. Studies have focused on the expression of single markers such as the progenitor cell antigen CD34 (Tucker et al. 1990; Geller et al. 1990; Ball et al. 1990) or the MDR protein (Ito et al. 1989; Sato et al. 1990), and on the expression of lymphoid markers on myeloid leukemia (Sperling et al. 1991).

More recently, the significance of aberrant antigen expression on leukemic cells has been stressed. Its major use may be the detection of residual leukemic cells in AML patients in complete remission, where the sensitivity of light microscopy is limited to 5%. Campana et al. (1990), Delwel et al. (1988), and Terstappen and Loken (1988) described different patterns of aberrant coexpression. Technical prerequisites for the unequivocal identification of aberrant antigen expression are the initial identification of the leukemic cell population based on light scatter properties using laser-equipped flow cytometric instruments, automated multiparameter analysis, and directly conjugated monoclonal antibodies with two or three different fluorescence dyes (Terstappen et al. 1991b). The chance of detecting a combination of antibodies which distinguishes the leukemic cell population from normal hematopoietic progenitors increases with the number of antibodies tested. In order to keep this approach technically and economically feasible, we have analyzed the usefulness of a fixed combination of commercially available monoclonal antibodies using two-color immunofluorescence in a prospective study of 100 patients with newly diagnosed AML. The set detects lymphoid- and myeloid-lineage associated antigens, and is designed to distinguish acute leukemias of B, T, and myeloid lineage. We focused on the informative antibody combinations for aberrant antigen expression in patients with AML using multiparameter flow cytometry.

Material and Methods

Samples. Bone marrow aspirates from 100 patients with the new clinical diagnosis of AML were analyzed. All patients were admitted to the Department of Internal Medicine A of the University of Münster. Diagnosis and classification were based on light microscopy of Pappenheim stained slides, and on cytochemical reaction with periodic acid–Schiff (PAS), myeloperoxidase, and esterase.

Cell Preparation. Bone marrow aspirates of the patients were prepared for flow cytometric analysis using erythrocyte lysis. One volume of bone marrow was diluted with 14 volumes of the lysing solution ($10^{-4}\,M$ EDTA, $10^{-3}\,M$ $KHCO_3$, $0.17\,M$ NH_4Cl in H_2O, pH 7.3) and gently mixed. Cells were lysed for 3–5 min at room temperature, and then centrifuged at 200 *g* for 5 min at room temperature. The pellet was resuspended in a volume of RPMI 1640 (Whittaker, Walkersville, MD, USA) 14 times larger than the original bone marrow volume and centrifuged at 200 *g* for 5 min at 4°C. This washing step was repeated twice and the cells were finally resuspended in phosphate-buffered saline (PBS) containing 1% bovine serum albumin and 20 m*M* HEPES (pH 7.3). The cell concentration was adjusted to 1×10^7 cells/ml.

Monoclonal Antibodies. Monoclonal antibodies against T-cell antigens were used as internal standards for setup of the instrument: anti-CD3 (Anti-HumanLeu4 FITC), anti-CD4 (Anti-HumanLeu3 PE), and anti-CD8 (Anti-HumanLeu2 FITC). The following antibodies were used for identification and distinction of myeloid leukemic cells: anti-CD5 (Anti-HumanLeu1 PE), anti-CD7 (Anti-HumanLeu9 FITC), anti-CD10 (Anti-Human CALLA FITC), anti-CD13 (Anti-HumanLeuM7 PE), anti-CD14 (Anti-HumanLeuM3 PE), anti-CD19 (Anti-HumanLeu12 PE), anti-CD33 (Anti-HumanLeuM9 PE), anti-CD34 (8G12 FITC), anti-CD38 (Anti-HumanLeu17 PE), anti-CD45 (Anti-HumanHLe-1 FITC), and anti-HLA-DR (FITC). Controls included irrelevant, fluorescence-labeled, isotype-matched monoclonal antibodies.

Flow Cytometry. Flow cytometric analysis was performed on a FACScan (BDIS). Data acquisition was performed using the FACScan Research Software (BDIS). The instrument setup was standardized using T lymphocytes as reference. This was achieved by gating on the fluorescence intensity of $CD3^+$ lymphocytes, followed by an adjustment of the light scattering detectors to locate the $CD3^+$ lymphocytes in a standard position in the correlative display of forward light scattering and orthogonal light scattering. The fluorescence detectors were adjusted using a tight-light scattering gate, obtained from the light scattering of the $CD3^+$ lymphocytes, followed by adjustment of the two fluorescence detectors of an unstained sample. Adjustment of the crossover of fluorescence signals of FITC and PE into other than the assigned detectors was obtained by compensation of samples stained with CD4 FITC and CD8 PE respectively. The forward light scattering and orthogonal light scattering signals and the two fluorescence signals were determined for each cell and data of 30000 events were stored in list-mode data files.

Data Analysis. The analysis of the four-dimensional data was performed with the Consort 30 software (BDIS).

Results

Light Scatter

Light scatter allows identification of the leukemic cell population in the majority of cases. Different profiles can be distinguished, which show some correspondence to the FAB classification, as previously published (Terstappen

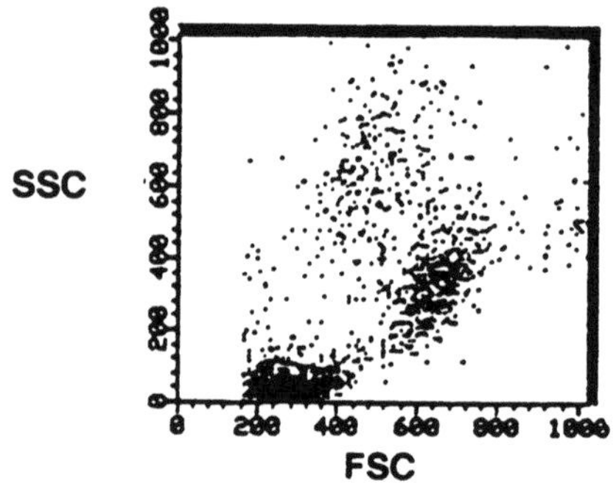

Fig. 1. Light scatter profile of the bone marrow aspirate from a patient with newly diagnosed AML FAB M3. The figure depicts three cell populations: The population with the lowest forward (FSC) and side scatter signals (SSC) are normal lymphocytes. The population on top with the largest SSC signals and an intermediate FSC signals are normal neutrophils, while the population with the largest FSC signals (channels 600–800) represent the leukemic cells poulation. They are located in the area of normal promyelocytes

et al. 1991a). The example in Fig. 1 was cytologically diagnosed as AML FAB M3. Three cell populations are distinguished: The population with the lowest forward (FSC, corresponding to size) and side scatter signals (SSC, corresponding to granularity) are normal lymphocytes. The population on top with the largest SSC signals and an intermediate FSC signal correspond to normal neutrophils, while the population with the largest FSC signals (channels 600–800) and intermediate SSC signals represent the leukemic cell population. They are located in the area of normal promyelocytes. Further analysis of the immunophenotype was performed inside an electronic gate of the leukemic cell population.

Monoclonal Antibodies

Monoclonal antibodies against the T-cell antigens CD3, CD4, and CD8 served as individual, internal controls of setup of gates and for compensation. The leukemic samples frequently displayed more than one subpopulation, based on light scatter and/or staining with combinations of monoclonal antibodies. This has been described previously (Terstappen et al. 1991b; Wörmann et al., submitted a). Samples or subpopulations were called positive for the respective antigen if ≥5% leukemic cells expressed the antigen. Leukemic cells were identified by light scatter plus expression of at least one myeloid antigen. Quadrants were set based on autofluorescence and staining of the isotype controls. Results of antibody staining are listed according to incidence of positive samples, in descending order.

CD45. CD45 was expressed on all samples included in this study. The expression was usually high and rather homogeneous. Two further patients with rapidly progressive pancytopenia were also initially included in this study and had their bone marrow cells phenotyped under the clinical diagnosis of acute leukemia. One of them had a significant population of large CD45-negative cells with intermediate light scatter. The histologic diagnosis was malignant melanoma. The second patient had a dominant population of small cells, slightly larger than the normal lymphocytes, with low SSC signals. The final histologic diagnosis was small cell lung cancer with extensive bone marrow metastasis.

HLA-DR. HLA-DR was present on the leukemic samples of all but eight patients. Five of these were cytologically classified as FAB M3. While this has been previously described, two patients with microscopically characteristic acute promyelocytic leukemia expressed HLA-DR on the leukemic blasts. One of them had two subpopulations of leukemic blasts, one with and one without expression of HLA-DR. This patient also had a coagulation disorder and died of intracerebral bleeding. Cytogenetic analysis did not reveal a 15;17 translocation, neither did the Southern analysis show the characteristic gene rearrangement (de Thé et al. 1990). Figure 2 shows an example of heterogeneous expression of HLA-DR. Within the population of CD13-positive cells, HLA-DR is coexpressed on the majority of cells, but a distinct, minor subpopulation of CD13-positive/HLA-DR negative cells can be distinguished.

CD33. CD33 was present on at least one subpopulation in 89 of the 100 patients. The expression was very heterogeneous. It differed even between the subpopulations from one patient. We previously described a patient with two CD33-positive subpopulations of AML blasts. In relapse, the aspirate was dominated by CD33-negative myeloid cells (Könemann et al. 1991). The lack of a myeloid-lineage-associated antigen as a marker of leukemic cells is more vulnerable to technical errors than other patterns. It should only be used if normal myeloid cells with expression of CD13 are present in the same sample. The examples in Figs. 3 and 4 show a homogeneous population of CD33-positive leukemic cells, one with (Fig. 3) and one without (Fig. 4A) aberrant coexpression of the lymphoid-lineage-associated marker CD7.

CD13. CD13 was a reliable marker of myeloid leukemic cells and was missing in only 13 patients. If present, expression was moderate to intense. In the vast majority of cases, it was coexpressed with CD33. We observed only two patients with lack of CD13 and CD33 on at least one subpopulation.

CD14. Expression was tested on all samples. A total of 125 subpopulations were distinguished, of which 88 were positive with the monoclonal antibody.

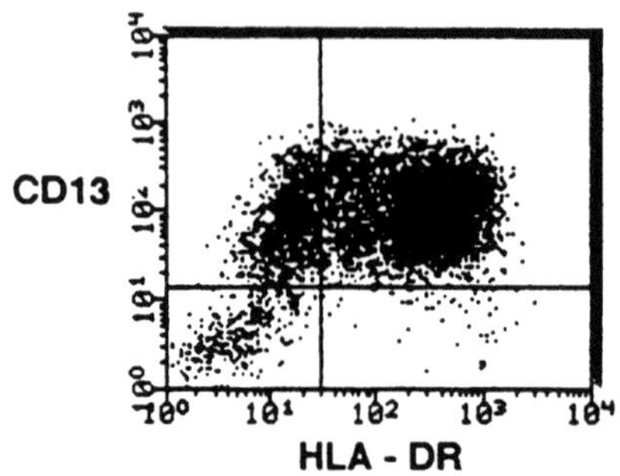

Fig. 2. Coexpression of HLA-DR and CD13. While all cells express CD13, the expression of HLA-DR divides the leukemic cell population into two subpopulation. The majority of cells express HLA-DR strongly, but a minor population of HLA-DR-negative/CD13-positive cells is visible in the upper left quadrant

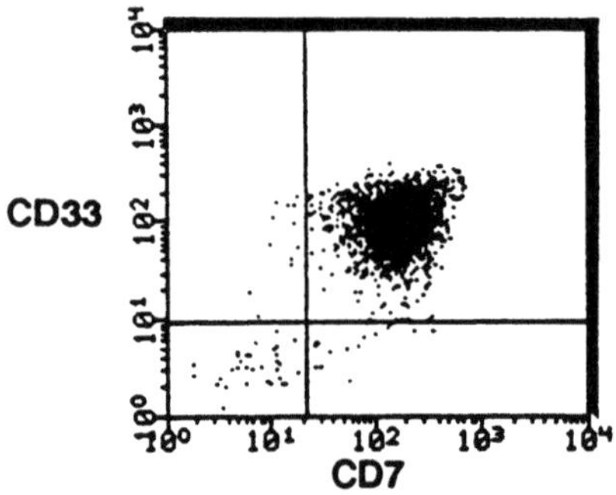

Fig. 3. Coexpression of CD33 and CD7 on the bone marrow aspirate of a patient with newly diagnosed AML. Cells are homogeneously positive for both antigens

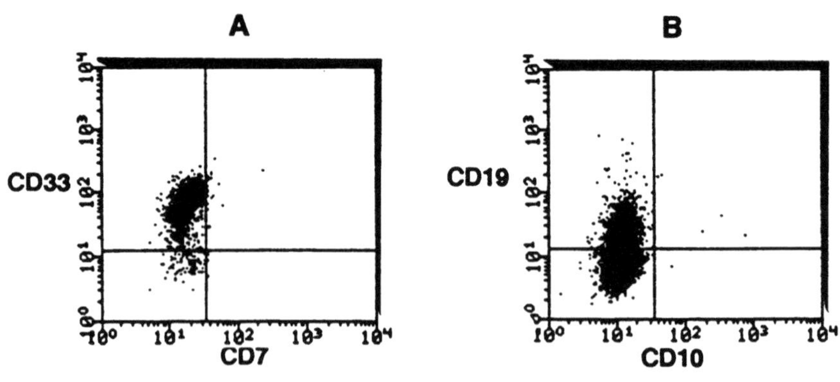

Fig. 4A,B. Expression of CD19 on myeloid leukemic cells. **A** shows the homogeneous staining of CD33 and the negativity for CD7. The expression of CD19 is weakly positive, while CD10 is not expressed on the leukemic cells. The leukemic cells also expressed CD13 (not shown)

Nine of them had a very high expression of CD14, about one log unit more intense than any monocytic cell in normal bone marrow or peripheral blood.

CD34/CD38. The combination of CD34 and CD38 was chosen because of the analogy between leukemic cell antigen presentation and the maturation of normal hematopoietic progenitors (Terstappen et al. 1991c). It also allows the identification of leukemic cells based on the aberrant overexpression of CD34, which is observed in about 15% of cases (Terstappen et al. 1991b). In addition, the distinction of less and more mature leukemic cells may be of prognostic significance (Terstappen et al. 1992). Examples are shown in Fig. 5. They reflect the heterogeneity of CD34/CD38 coexpression. While some leukemic samples are homogeneous, with all blasts clustering at one stage of differentiation, others show heterogeneity ranging from very immature, stem-like cells to more mature progenitor cells (Fig. 5B,D). CD34 expression was observed in 81 samples, and CD38 was present on at least one subpopulation in all AML aspirates. The example in Fig. 5 was chosen to outline further insights into leukemia cell biology that can be gained from multiparameter flow cytometry. Five subpopulations can be distinguished: $CD34^{++}/CD38^{-}$ (1 in Fig. 5B,D), $CD34^{++}/CD38^{+}$ (2 in Fig. 5B,D), $CD34^{+}/CD38^{++}$ (3 in Fig. 5B,D), $CD34^{-}/CD38^{+}$ (4 in Fig. 5B,D), and $CD34^{-}/CD38^{-}$ cells (5 in Fig. 5B,D). Normal hematopoietic progenitor cell differentiation proceeds from the stage of $CD34^{+}/CD38^{-}$ to $CD34^{-}/CD38^{++}$ cells. Gating on the cells with the lowest FSC and SSC signals (Fig. 5C, overlapping with the normal lymphocytes) reveals that the population with the most immature immunophenotype is located in this area (Fig. 5D).

CD5 FITC. CD5 expression was observed on 52 leukemic cell samples. Expression was weak in 60% of the positive subpopulations. It was clearly distinct from the homogeneously high expression of CD5 on T cells and lower than in the majority of CD5-positive B cells in B chronic lymphocytic leukemia (Freedman et al. 1987).

CD7 FITC. CD7 was found on myeloid cells in 38 of the 100 AML samples. The expression was heterogeneous. A homogeneously strong expression, as shown in Fig. 3, was exceptional. As with CD5 and CD2 (monoclonal antibody not included in this study), the staining was weak in the majority of samples (61%). The $CD7^{+}$ T cells was clearly distinguishable based on the homogeneously strong expression of the antigen.

CD19 PE. CD19 expression on myeloid leukemic cells was tested on only 40 samples and found in eight. Expression was weak in six cases and homogeneously strong in two. One example is given in Fig. 4. The leukemic cells were characterized by expression of CD33 (Fig. 4 A) and a weak expression of CD19 (Fig. 4 B), overlapping with the negative control.

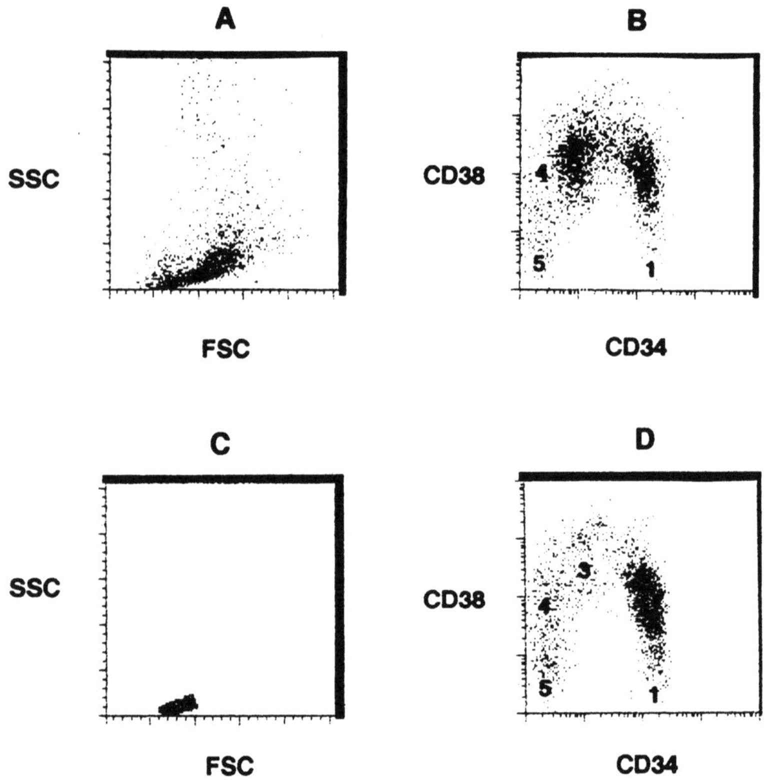

Fig. 5A–D. Coexpression of CD34 and CD38 on myeloid leukemic blasts. Five subpopulations can be distinguished: $CD34^{++}/CD38^{-}$ (1 in **B**, **D**), $CD34^{++}/CD38^{+}$ (2 in **B**, **D**), $CD34^{+}/CD38^{++}$ (3 in **B**, **D**), $CD34^{-}/CD38^{+}$ (4 in **B**, **D**) and $CD34^{-}/CD38^{-}$ cells (5 in **B**, **D**). By gating on the cells with the lowest FSC and SSC signals (overlapping with the normal lymphocytes), the brightly CD34-expressing cells can be distinguished (**D**)

CD10. CD10 was tested on only 37 patients and found on four samples. Expression was weak, and clearly distinct from the homogeneously intensive staining in B-lineage ALL.

Discussion

Therapy results in acute myeloid leukemia in adults have improved in the last decade, but they are not satisfactory. While only 10%–15% of de novo AML patients are initially chemotherapy-resistant and do not reach a complete remission (CR), two-thirds of CR patients will relapse within 2 years. Discussions of new treatment strategies focus on intensity of postremission therapy with or without bone marrow transplantation. A method for distinction of patients with favorable and unfavorable diagnosis would be helpful in designing risk-adapted postremission therapy. The "gold standard" of light microscopic evaluation of bone marrow smears does not provide adequate sensitivity for detection of residual leukemic cells, but no other method has gained wide acceptance. Several authors have proposed the use of monoclonal antibodies for distinction of normal and leukemic myeloid progenitors (Delwel et al. 1988; Terstappen and Loken 1988; Campana et al. 1990). Aberrant expression of surface antigens can be detected using fluorescence-conjugated monoclonal antibodies against differentiation-associated antigens of the myeloid lineage, and/or myeloid- and lymphoid-lineage-associated antigens (Terstappen et al. 1991b). Sensitivity is increased with optimized optical equipment, selection of antibodies with high affinity, and direct conjugation of fluorescence dyes. In a first study, we had used 17 different monoclonal antibodies. Leukemic cells were detectable in 80 of 81 samples. If the method is to gain wide acceptance, a balance must be found between optimal resolution for distinction of leukemic and normal cells and an economically feasible panel of monoclonal antibodies. In the present study, we have restricted the panel to 11 antibodies, based on the previous experiences, plus CD3, CD4, and CD8 as internal standards for the setup of the instrument. This individual standard is a prerequisite for a constant and stable positioning of subpopulations in follow-up analyses. Even in samples with maximal malignant cell infiltration, residual normal T cells were always detected. The first combination of monoclonal antibodies included CD45 and CD14 and was mainly used for distinction of metastatic bone marrow infiltration from nonhematopoietic malignancies. It also served in positioning electronic gates for subpopulations of leukemic cells. In addition, aberrant overexpression of CD14 can be used for identification of leukemic blasts (Terstappen et al. 1991b). The most informative markers for the myeloid lineage were CD13 and CD33, as expected. Only a minor proportion of leukemic subpopulations were negative for both markers. The addition of CD11c, CD15, and/or CD_w65 might be useful in closing this small gap. CD13 was combined with HLA-DR. Inhomogeneous expression of the MHC class II antigens revealed multiple subpopulations in a significant number of samples. It was also most informative in the HLA-DR-negative AML FAB M3. The combination of antibodies against CD10 and CD19 was designed for subclassification of B-lineage ALL. In the context of AML, it served for the detection of aberrant expression of B-lineage-associated antigens. This combination could optimally be complemented with a third monoclonal, e.g., against HLA-DR, or against a myeloid-lineage-associated antigen, e.g., CD_w65. This would provide another useful tool for direct visualization of aberrant antigen expression. The most frequent aberrant antigen expression was the presence of lymphoid-lineage-associated markers on myeloid cells, e.g., CD5, CD7, and CD19. Using these patterns of aberrant antigen expression for follow-up studies, we have recently shown the presence of persistent cells with the leukemic phenotype in AML patients in CR (Wörmann et al., submitted b).

Since the vast majority of AML samples can be safely diagnosed and classified by light microscopy, a major role for immunophenotyping arises in the potential of leukemia monitoring. A prerequisite is the more widespread knowledge of multiparameter analysis. The currently available monoclonal antibodies allow the distinction of normal and leukemic myeloid progenitors at diagnosis in the majority of cases. A feasible technical approach to economic use of these reagents could be based on the panel of this study. If no clear distinction can be made between normal and leukemic cells, it must supplemented with further monoclonal antibodies against differentiation- and non-myeloid-lineage – associated antigens, e.g., CD2, CD11c, CD15, CD16, CD20, and CD_w65. The technical prerequisites have thus been provided for identification of leukemic cells blasts. The method will be most useful for detection of small numbers of leukemic cells in AML patients in CR, in purged bone marrow prior to autologous bone marrow transplantation, and in myelodysplastic syndrome.

References

Argyle JC, Benjamin DR, Lampkin B, Hammond D (1989) Acute nonlymphocytic leukemias of childhood. Inter-observer variability and problems in the use of the FAB classification. Cancer 63:295–301

Ball ED, Lawrence D, Malnar M, Ciminelli N, Mayer R, Wurster-Hill D, Davey FR, Bloomfield CD (1990) Correlation of CD34 and multi-drug resistance P170 with FAB and cytogenetics but not prognosis in acute myeloid leukemia (AML). Blood 76 [Suppl 1]: 252 a (abstr 999)

Bennett JM, Catovsky D, Daniel M-T, Flandrin G, Galton DAG, Gralnick HR, Sultan C (1976) Proposals for the classification of acute leukemias. A report of the French-American-British Cooperative Group. Br J Haematol 33:451–458

Campana D, Coustan-Smith E, Janossy G (1990) The immunologic detection of minimal residual disease in acute leukemia. Blood 76:163–171

Castaigne S, Chomienne C, Daniel MT, Ballerini P, Berger R, Fenaux P, Degos L (1990) All-trans retinoic acid as a differentiation therapy for acute promyelocytic leukemia: I. Clinical results. Blood 76:1704–1709

de Thé H, Chomienne C, Lanotte M, Degos L, Dejean A (1990) The t(15;17) translocation of acute promyelocytic leukaemia fuses the retinoic receptor alpha gene of a novel transcribed locus. Nature 347:558–561

Delwel R, van Gurp R, Bot F, Touw I, Löwenberg B (1988) Phenotyping of acute myelocytic leukemia (AML) progenitors: an approach for tracing minimal numbers of AML cells among normal bone marrow. Leukemia 2:814–819

Foon KA, Gale RP, Todd RF III (1986) Recent advances in the immunologic classification of leukemia. Semin Hematol 23:257–283

Freedman AS, Boyd AW, Bieber FR, Daley J, Rosen K, Horowitz JC, Levy DN, Nadler LM (1987) Normal cellular counterparts of B cell chronic lymphocytic leukemia. Blood 70:418–425

Geller RB, Zahurak M, Hurwitz CA, Burke PJ (1990) Prognostic importance of immunophenotyping in adults with acute myelocytic leukemia: the significance of the stem cell glycoprotein CD34 (My10). Br J Haematol 76:340–347

Greaves MF, Janossy G, Peto J, Kay H (1981) Immunologically defined subclasses of acute lymphobalstic leukaemia in children: their relationship to presentation fetaures and prognosis. Br J Haematol 48:179–197

Ito Y, Tanimoto M, Kumazawa T, Okumura M, Morishima Y, Ohno R, Saito H (1989) Increased p-glycoprotein expression and multidrug resistant gene (MDR 1) amplification in fresh acute leukemia cells – sequential analysis of 15 cases at initial presentation and relapsed stage. Cancer 63:1534–1538

Könemann S, Zurlutter K, Safford M, Schreiber K, Büchner T, Hiddemann W, Wörmann B, Terstappen LWMM (1991) Flow cytometric characterization of therapy resistant leukemic subpopulations in relapse. Ann Hematol 62:A15

Ludwig WD, Seibt-Jung H, Teichmann JV, Komischke B, Gatzke A, Gassner G, Odenwald E, Hofmann J, Riehm H (1989) Clinicopathological features and prognostic implications of immunophenotypic subgroups in childhood ALL: experience of the BFM-ALL study 83. In: Neth R, Gallo RC, Greaves MF, Gaedicke G, Gohla S, Mannweiler K, Ritter J (eds) Modern trends in human leukemia VIII. Springer, Berlin Heidelberg New York, pp 51–57 (Haematology and blood transfusion, vol 32)

MIC Classification (1988) Morphologic, immunologic and cytogenetic (MIC) working classification of the acute myeloid leukaemias. Br J Haematol 68:487–494

Neame PB, Soamboonsrup P, Browman GP, Meyer RM, Benger A, Wilson WE, Walker IR, Saeed N, McBride JA (1986) Classifying acute leukemia by immunophenotyping: a combined FAB-immunologic classification of AML. Blood 68:1355–1362

Sato H, Gottesman MM, Goldstein LJ, Pastan I, Block AM, Sandberg AA, Preisler HD (1990) Expression of the multidrug resistance gene in myeloid leukemias. Leuk Res 14:11–15

Sperling C, Ludwig WD, Seibt–Jung H, Haase D, Becher R, Gassmann W, Schmidt C, Böttcher S, Sauerland C, Gramatzki M, Fonatsch C, Hiddemann W, Löffler H, Büchner T, Thiel E (1991) Immunphänotyp akuter myeloischer Leukämien (AML): Korrelation mit Morphologie, Zytogenetik und Ansprechen auf die Therapie. Onkologie 14 [Suppl 2]: 158 (abstr 454)

Terstappen LWMM, Loken MR (1988) Multidimensional flow cytometric characterization of normal and leukemic cells in acute non-lymphocytic leukemia. Blood 72 [Suppl 1]: 131:230a

Terstappen LWMM, Safford M, Könemann S, Loken MR, Zurlutter K, Büchner T, Hiddemann W, Wörmann B (1991a) Flow cytometric characterization of acute myeloid leukemia: I. Light scattering. Leukemia 5:315–321

Terstappen LWMM, Safford M, Könemann S, Loken MR, Zurlutter K, Büchner T, Hiddemann W, Wörmann B (1991b) Flow cytometric characterization of acute myeloid leukemia: II. Phenotypic heterogeneity at diagnosis. Leukemia 5:757–767

Terstappen LWMM, Huang S, Safford M, Lansdorp PM, Loken MR (1991c) Sequential generations of hematopoietic colonies derived from single non lineage committed progenitor cells. Blood 77:1218–1227

Terstappen LWMM, Safford M, Unterhalt M, Könemann S, Zurlutter K, Piechotka K, Drescher M, Aul C, Büchner T, Hiddemann W, Wörmann B (1992) Flow cytometric characterization of acute myeloid leukemia: IV. Comparison to the differentiation pathway of normal hematopoietic progenitor cells. Leukemia (in press)

Tucker J, Dorey E, Gregory WM, Simpson AP, Amess JA, Lister TA, Horton MA (1990) Immunphenotype of blast cells in acute myeloid leukemia may be a useful predictive factor for outcome. Hematol Oncol 8:47–58

Warrell RP, Frankel SR, Miller WH, Scheinberg DA, Itri LM, Hittelman WN, Vyas R, Andreeff M, Tafuri A, Jakubowski A, Gabrilove J, Gordon MS, Dmitrovsky

E (1991) Differentiation therapy of acute promyelocytic leukemia with tretinoin (all-trans-retinoic acid). N Engl J Med 3243:1385–1393
Wörmann B, Könemann S, Safford M, Loken MR, Zurlutter K, Büchner T, Hiddemann W, Terstappen LWMM. Selective elimination of leukemic subpopulations in acute myeloid leukemia through induction chemotherapy (submitted, a)
Wörmann B, Safford M, Könemann S, Zurlutter K, Piechotka K, Schreiber K, Loken MR, Büchner T, Hiddemann W, Terstappen LWWM. Prognostic significance of residual leukemic cells in patients with acute myeloid leukemia in complete remission (submitted, b)

Detection of Residual Leukemic Cells in Adult Acute Lymphoblastic Leukemia by Analysis of Gene Rearrangements and Correlation with Early Relapses

W.U. Knauf[1], A.D. Ho[2], D. Hoelzer[3] and E. Thiel[1]

[1] Department of Hematology, Klinikum Steglitz, Free University of Berlin, W-1000 Berlin 45, Fed. Rep. of Germany
[2] Northeastern Ontario Oncology Programme, Sudbury, Ontario, Canada
[3] Department of Hematology, University of Frankfurt, W-6000 Frankfurt, Fed. Rep. of Germany

Introduction

Improvements in complete remission (CR) rate and long-term survival in adult acute lymphoblastic leukemia (ALL) have been achieved during the past decade by intensive chemotherapy. Today, more than 75% of the patients attain a CR (Hoelzer et al. 1984; Clarkson et al. 1985; Jacobs and Gale 1984). Nevertheless, the recurrence rate remains high. Only about 40% of patients are still alive and in CR after 5 years (Hoelzer et al. 1984; Clarkson et al. 1985; Jacobs and Gale 1984). Half of the relapses occur within the first year after the diagnosis has been established. Using multivariate analysis, patients can be categorized to be at high risk for relapse according the following criteria: high initial cell count, age over 35 years, null cell ALL immunophenotype, no CR after 4 weeks' induction therapy (Hoelzer et al. 1984). Recurrent disease is probably due to residual leukemic cells. Gene rearrangements are used as markers of clonality and thereby monoclonal lymphoid cells can be detected with an high degree of sensitivity (Korsmeyer et al. 1983; Aisenberg and Wilkes 1985; Raghavachar et al. 1986). Even in bone marrow samples considered morphologically to be free from leukemic cells, analysis of gene rearrangements is still able to give evidence of persisting disease (Zehnbauer et al. 1986). In this study, we have applied the analysis of gene rearrangements to detect residual disease in patients considered to be in CR after a standardized induction therapy. The laboratory findings were correlated with the duration of clinical remission and the relapse rate. The aim of the study was to assess the influence of residual disease on the rate of early relapses in ALL.

Recent Results in Cancer Research, Vol. 131

Patients and Methods

Patient Characteristics

Thirty five patients with newly diagnosed ALL were studied. Their median age was 25 years (range 16–62). The diagnosis of ALL was made by cytomorphological examination of peripheral blood smears and of bone marrow smears, including cytochemistry, and immunophenotyping of peripheral leukemic cells using a panel of monoclonal antibodies (as detailed below). Thirty patients were in the high-risk group (high leukemic cell count at diagnosis or null cell ALL immunophenotype) and five patients in the low-risk group (low cell count and T-cell ALL or pre-B-cell ALL phenotype) according to the classification of the German Multicenter Study Group (Hoelzer et al. 1984). All the patients in this study were considered to be in CR after standardized induction therapy. Details of the chemotherapy regimen have been published elsewhere (Hoelzer et al. 1984). Assessment of response was performed at day 28 after initiation of chemotherapy. CR was defined by clinical and cytomorphological criteria (<5% blasts in the bone marrow, no blasts in the peripheral blood, no detectable disease in other organs). Time to relapse (TTR) was defined as the time interval between the initial diagnosis and the detection of recurrent disease.

Immunophenotyping

At initial diagnosis, peripheral leukemic blasts were enriched on a Ficoll gradient (Pharmacia, FRG). The cells were characterized using monoclonal antibodies directed against the following clusters of determination (CD): CD10 (common ALL antigen), CD24 (pan-B marker), CD20 (pre-B/B antigen), CD1 (thymus associated), CD2 (erythrocyte-rosette-forming T cells), CD7 (pan-T marker). VIM2 (myelocyte associated), VIM13 (monocyte associated), HLA-DR, and terminal deoxynucleotidyl transferase (TdT) activity were also determined.

DNA Extraction

Bone marrow samples were collected before and at day 28 after the start of the induction therapy. The cells were harvested in heparinized tubes and the mononuclear cell fraction was enriched on a Ficoll gradient (Pharmacia, FRG). High molecular weight DNA was extracted from the mononuclear cell fraction by incubation with Proteinase K (Boehringer, FRG) and lysis buffer consisted of 0.07 *M* Tris buffer (pH 8.5), 0.025 *M* EDTA (pH 8.1), and 3% sarcosyl. Then, a phenol/chloroform/isoamylalcohol extraction was carried out. DNA was precipitated in 100% ethanol, washed in 70% ethanol, resuspended in Tris/EDTA buffer and stored at 4°C.

Southern Blot Analysis

10 µg DNA was cleaved with the restriction enzymes *Bam*HI and *Eco*RI, respectively, according to the recommendations given by the supplier (Boehringer, FRG). After a run over a 0.7% agarose gel (Seakem, USA) the DNA was transferred onto nitrocellulose filters (Schleicher and Schuell, FRG) as described by Southern (1975). Hybridization with nick-translated (Rigby et al. 1977) gene probes was performed under high-stringency conditions. Thereafter, an autoradiography followed using XR-AS films (Kodak, USA) and an intensifying screen.

Gene Probes

Cloned DNA sequences coding for the joining regions of the human immunoglobulin heavy chain were kindly provided by P. Leder, Harvard Medical School, Boston, USA. We used a *Sau*3A fragment (JH) of 2.5 kilobases (kb) in length, cloned in pBR 233 (Ravetch et al. 1981). A complementary (c)DNA clone carrying sequences for the constant regions of the β-chain of the human T-cell antigen receptor was kindly provided by T.W. Mak, Ontario Cancer Centre, Toronto, Canada. We used a *Pst*I fragment (Tβ) of 0.77 kb in length, cloned in pBR233 (Yanagi et al. 1984).

Results

Sensitivity Studies

Leukemic cells obtained from a patient with a pre-B-common ALL were diluted with buffy coat cells from healthy control persons before DNA was extracted. Southern blot analysis was performed with the radiolabeled JH probe. Gene rearrangements were detectable down to a content of 1.0% leukemic cells. In a T-ALL, gene rearrangements could also be identified down to a content of 1.0% leukemic cells using the Tβ probe.

Immunotyping and Genotyping

The diagnosis of pre-B-ALL was established in 17 patients, B-ALL in three patients and pre-T/T-ALL in 12 patients by immunophenotyping. Null cell ALL was diagnosed in three patients due to the lack of expression of appropriate surface markers. The immunoglobulin heavy chain gene was found to be rearranged in all the pre-B-ALL and B-ALL and in one T-ALL. The β-chain of the T-cell receptor was rearranged in all the pre-T/T-ALL, but also in four pre-B-ALL and one B-ALL. Both the heavy chain gene and the Tβ gene were rearranged in one null cell ALL, whereas the other two null cell ALL had heavy chain rearrangements only. The data on immunotyping and genotyping are summarized in Table 1.

Persisting Gene Rearrangements and Relapse Rate

Gene rearrangements as determined before therapy were detected in five patients: two pre-B-ALL, one B-ALL, and two T-ALL. All these patients belonged to the high-risk group because of their high initial cell counts. Four of the five patients with persisting gene rearrangements (two pre-B-ALL, one B-ALL, one T-ALL) relapsed within a median TTR of 10 weeks (range 8–20 weeks). The fifth patient with persisting gene rearrangements is still in clinical remission after 1½ years of observation. This patient with a pre-B-common ALL showed a persisting heavy chain and Tβ chain rearrangement after induction therapy. He received an intensified consolidation therapy with high-dose cytosine arabinoside and mitoxantrone. No gene rearrangements could be found thereafter.

Six of the patients without detectable gene rearrangements after standardized induction therapy also relapsed. One of them belonged to the low-risk group and the other five to the high-risk group. Median TTR was 30 weeks (range 16–52 weeks). In one high-risk and the one low-risk patient the relapse became manifest only in the central nervous system (CNS) without detectable BM involvement. One of the high-risk patients without persisting gene rearrangements died due to septicemia after allogeneic bone marrow transplantation, but had been in CR for 6 months. The other high-risk patients are in CR within a median observation time of 20 months (range 6–36 months), and four of the low-risk patients are in CR within a median observation time of 52 weeks (range 20–84 weeks).

There was statistical evidence for a significantly higher relapse rate in patients with detectable persistant gene rearrangments (Fisher's exact test, $p = 0.002$). The characteristics of the relapsed patients are summarized in Table 2.

Discussion

This study shows that Southern blot analysis is an efficient method to detect residual disease preceding early relapses in adult patients with ALL who are considered to be in CR by conventional clinical criteria. After standardized induction therapy, the same gene rearrangements were found as at diagnosis in bone marrow cells from five of 35 patients studied, thus indicating residual disease.

Various attempts have been made to detect residual or even "minimal" disease in ALL, which is thought to cause recurrent disease after initial

Table 1. Patient characteristics

Patient	Age (years)	Diagnosis	Risk score	Gene rearrangements at initial diagnosis	
				JH	Tβ
1	22	null cell	high	+	+
2	39	null cell	high	+	–
3	17	null cell	high	+	–
4	20	pre-B	low	+	–
5	16	pre-B	low	+	–
6	18	pre-B	low	+	–
7	37	pre-B	high	+	+
8	25	pre-B	high	+	+
9	48	pre-B	high	+	–
10	34	pre-B	high	+	–
11	17	pre-B	high	+	–
12	37	pre-B	high	+	–
13	20	pre-B	high	+	–
14	24	pre-B	high	+	–
15	22	pre-B	high	+	+
16	25	pre-B	high	+	–
17	19	pre-B	high	+	–
18	42	pre-B	high	+	–
19	33	pre-B	high	+	+
20	25	pre-B	high	+	–
21	37	B	high	+	+
22	37	B	high	+	–
23	24	B	high	+	–
24	62	pre-T	high	–	+
25	34	T	low	–	+
26	19	T	low	–	+
27	28	T	high	–	+
28	49	T	high	–	+
29	27	T	high	–	+
30	24	T	high	–	+
31	27	T	high	–	+
32	18	T	high	–	+
33	25	T	high	–	+
34	43	T	high	+	+
35	22	T	high	–	+

The diagnosis is listed as determined by immunophenotyping; risk score "high" (white blood cell count, WBC, >30 000 at first diagnosis or null cell ALL) or "low" (WBC <30 000 at first diagnosis and T-ALL or pre-B-ALL) follows the guidelines of the German Multicenter Study Group (Hoelzer et al. 1984); gene rearrangements were detected using gene probes for the immunoglobulin heavy chain and the β-chain of the T-cell antigen receptor (see "Patients and methods")

Table 2. Characteristics of relapsed patients

Diagnosis	Sex	Age (years)	Residual disease	Site of relapse	TTR (weeks)
B-ALL	m	24	JH rearr.	BM, testes	8
Pre-B-ALL	m	20	JH rearr.	BM	12
Pre-B-ALL	m	33	JH rearr.	BM, CNS	20
T-ALL	f	28	Tβ rearr.	BM	8
Null cell ALL	m	22	not detectable	BM	26
B-ALL	f	37	not detectable	BM	52
Pre-B-ALL	m	26	not detectable	BM	16
T-ALL	m	18	not detectable	BM	30
T-ALL	f	24	not detectable	CNS	30
Pre-B-ALL	f	18	not detectable	CNS	45

successful treatment. Examination of surface markers and karyotypes of cultured BM cells have been shown to identify small amounts of residual leukemic blasts (Estrov et al. 1986). But colony growth in vitro might be inconsistent and subject to a variety of appropriate growth factors. Moreover, under the conditions of culturing, the karyotype of the cells may change and can no longer serve as tumor marker. Thus, culture assay systems are highly variable from laboratory to laboratory and it may be difficult to achieve reproducible results.

Gene rearrangements have been used as markers of lineage and clonality in ALL (Korsmeyer et al. 1983; Aisenberg and Wilkes 1985; Raghavachar et al. 1986) and other human lymphoid neoplasms (Aisenberg et al. 1985; Arnold et al. 1983; Cleary et al. 1984). Here, monoclonal lymphoid cells are detected with high sensitivity (Hu et al. 1985). Therefore, gene rearrangements may be sensitive indicators of residual disease in ALL (Wright et al. 1987). In our studies, the sensitivity of the Southern blot analysis was 1.0%, which is within the range reported by other authors (Zehnbauer et al. 1986; Cleary et al. 1984; Minden and Mak 1986).

In this report, five of 35 patients with ALL considered to be in CR were found to have persisting gene rearrangements. A few studies have been reported on the detection of residual disease by analysis of gene rearrangements and the relationship to recurrent disease (Zehnbauer et al. 1986; Bregni et al. 1989) in ALL. However, the patients in these studies did not receive standardized therapy (Zehnbauer et al. 1986), nor were BM specimens taken at standardized time points in the course of treatment (Bregni et al. 1989). The patients in our study were treated with standardized induction therapy and all BM specimens were taken at the time of first assessment of response, i.e., after 4 weeks.

In order to increase the sensitivity, Bregni et al. (1989) selected out lymphoid BM cells using monoclonal antibodies and magnetic beads. They detected residual disease in four of their 11 patients. Without lymphoid cell separation, Zehnbauer et al. (1986) identified residual disease in remission BM specimens in three of seven patients. Whether enrichment of lymphoid cells by immune selection increases the sensitivity for identification of persisting leukemic cells and whether this increase could indeed be of clinical significance has not yet been clarified.

With respect to the sensitivity of Southern blot analysis in detecting monoclonally growing lymphoid cells at a level of 1%, the question arises whether one should use the term "minimal" or only "residual" disease. A sensitivity of 1% is within the sensitivity of conventional cytomorphology, even though the clonality of immature lymphoid cells thereby remains undetermined. Furthermore, a content of lymphoblasts of 1% in a representative BM sample reflects a total mass of leukemic cells representing somewhat "bulky" disease rather than "minimal" residual leukemia.

A new approach to optimize sensitivity and to detect really "minimal" residual disease in ALL may be the use of polymerase chain reaction (PCR) techniques. PCR is reported to detect residual lymphoma cells 3 log units fewer than Southern blotting (Lee et al. 1987). In the case of a consistent chromosomal translocation such as the Philadelphia chromosome, PCR would seem to be the method of first choice (Lee et al. 1988). In order to identify persisting lymphoid blasts which are characterized only by individual clonal gene rearrangements, PCR might not be applicable in a large series of patients because DNA sequencing and synthesis of individual oligomeric primers are needed. The use of consensus sequences of the δ chain of the T cell receptor (TcR) has been described to overcome that particular problem (Hansen-Hagge et al. 1989) but the method will be unsuccessful in about 25% of non-T-ALLs which lack rearrangements of the Tδ chain. A wide application of PCR techniques in ALLs without a consistent chromosomal aberration may be also hampered by the tendency to clonal evolution which leads to altered rearranged gene segments (Wright et al. 1987; Bird et al. 1988). The recently described fingerprinting technique (Deane and Norton 1991) may contribute to solving the problems of sensitivity and specificity. It is reported to identify monoclonal lymphoid cells with a sensitivity of 0.1% and is independent from clonal evolution during the course of the disease. Its usefulness, however, in the detection of minimal residual disease in ALL has to be further determined.

Our data suggest that the detection of residual disease by analysis of gene rearrangements correlates with an high early relapse rate. As two patients relapsed in the CNS without BM involvement, it might be of interest to examine spinal fluid specimens as well. The fact that residual disease was found only in patients of the high-risk group is further evidence that these patients are at a greater risk for recurrent disease. Analysis of gene rearrangements at the time of assessment of the response to primary therapy might therefore be of prognostic value. Because "bulky" rather than "minimal" disease can be detected in patients in clinical CR, analysis of gene rearrangements might contribute to redefine remission criteria in ALL.

References

Aisenberg AC, Wilkes BM (1985) The phenotype and genotype of T-cell and Non-T, Non-B acute lymphoblastic leukemia. Blood 66:1215–1218

Aisenberg AC, Krontiris TG, Mak TW, Wilkes BM (1985) Rearrangement of the gene for the beta chain of the T-cell receptor in T-cell chronic lymphocytic leukemia and related disorders. N Engl J Med 313:538–542

Arnold A, Cossman J, Bakhshi A, Jaffe ES, Waldmann TA, Korsmeyer SJ (1983) Immunoglobulin gene rearrangements as unique clonal markers in human lymphoid neoplasms. N Engl J Med 309:1593–1599

Bird J, Galili N, Link M, Stites D, Sklar J (1988) Continuing rearrangement but absence of somatic hypermutation in immunoglobulin genes of human B cell precursor leukemia. J Exp Med 168:229–245

Bregni M, Siena S, Neri A, Bassan R, Barbui T, Delia D, Bonnadonna G, DallaFavera R, Gianni AM (1989) Minimal residual disease in acute lymphoblastic leukemia detected by immune selection and gene rearrangement analysis. J Clin Oncol 7:338–343

Clarkson B, Ellis S, Little C, Gee T, Arlin Z, Mertelsmann R, Andreef M, Kempin A, Koziner B, Chaganti R, Jhanwar S, McKenzie S, Cirrincione C, Gaynor J (1985) Acute lymphoblastic leukemia in adults. Semin Oncol 12:160–179

Cleary ML, Chao J, Warnke R, Sklar J (1984) Immunoglobulin gene rearrangement as diagnostic criterion of B-cell lymphoma. Proc Natl Acad Sci USA 81:539–597

Deane M, Norton JD (1991) Immunoglobulin gene "fingerprinting": an approach to analysis of B lymphoid clonality in lymphoproliferative disorders. Br J Haematol 77:274–281

Estrov Z, Grunberger T, Dube ID, Wang YP, Freedman MH (1986) Detection of residual acute lymphoblastic leukemia cells in cultures of bone marrow obtained during remission. N Engl J Med 315:538–542

Hansen-Hagge TE, Yokota S, Bartram CR (1989) Detection of minimal residual disease in acute lymphoblastic leukemia by in vitro amplification of rearranged T-cell receptor delta chain sequences. Blood 74:1762–1767

Hoelzer D, Thiel E, Löffler H, Bodenstein H, Plaumann L, Büchner T, Urbanitz D, Koch P, Heimpel H, Engelhardt R, Müller U, Wendt EC, Sodomann H, Rühl H, Herrmann F, Kaboth W, Dietzfelbinger H, Pralle H, Lunscken C, Hellriegel KP, Spors S, Nowrousian RM, Fischer J, Fülle H, Mitrou PS, Pfreundschuh M, Görg C, Emmerich B, Queisser W, Meyer P, Labedzki L, Essers U, König H, Mainzer K, Herrmann R, Messerer D, Zwingers T (1984) Intensified therapy in acute lymphoblastic and acute undifferentiated leukemia in adults. Blood 64:38–47

Hu E, Thompson J, Horning S, Trela M, Lowder J, Levy R, Sklar J (1985) Detection of B-cell lymphoma in peripheral blood by DNA hybridization. Lancet II:1092–1095

Jacobs AD, Gale RP (1984) Recent advances in the biology and treatment of acute lymphoblastic leukemia in adults. N Engl J Med 311:1219–1231

Korsmeyer SJ, Arnold A, Bakhshi A, Ravetch JV, Siebenlist U, Hieter PA, Sharrow SO, LeBien TW, Kersey JH, Poplack DG, Leder P, Waldmann TA (1983) Immunoglobulin gene rearrangement and cell surface antigen expression in acute lymphocytic leukemias of T cell and B cell precursor origins. J Clin Invest 71:301–313

Lee MS, Chang KS, Cabanillas F, Freireich EJ, Trujillo JM, Stass SA (1987) Detection of minimal residual cells carrying the t(14;18) by DNA sequence amplification. Science 237:175–178

Lee MS, Chang KS, Freireich EJ, Kantarijan HM, Talpaz M, Trujillo JM, Stass SA (1988) Detection of minimal residual bcr/abl transcripts by a modified polymerase chain reaction. Blood 72:893–897

Minden MD, Mak TW (1986) The structure of the T cell antigen receptor in normal and malignant T cells. Blood 68:327–336
Raghavachar A, Bartram CR, Ganser A, Heil G, Kleihauer E, Kubanek B (1986) Acute undifferentiated leukemia: Implications for cellular origin and clonality suggested by analysis of surface markers and immunoglobulin gene rearrangement. Blood 68:658–662
Ravetch JV, Siebenlist U, Korsmeyer SJ, Waldmann T, Leder P (1981) The structure of the immunoglobulin mu locus: characterization of embryonic and rearranged J and D genes. Cell 27:583–591
Rigby DJ, Dieckman M, Rhodes C, Berg P (1977) Labeling deoxyribonucleic acid to high specific activity in-vitro by nick translation with DNA polymerase I. J Mol Biol 113:237–251
Southern EM (1975) Detection of specific sequences among DNA fragments separated by gel electrophoresis. J Mol Biol 98:1860–1861
Wright PP, Poplack DG, Bakhshi A, Reaman DG, Cole D, Jensen JP, Korsmeyer SJ (1987) Gene rearrangements as markers of clonal variation and minimal residual disease in acute lymphoblastic leukemia. J Clin Oncol 5:735–741
Yanagi Y, Yoshikai Y, Legget K, Clark SP, Aleksander I, Mak TW (1984) A human T cell-specific cDNA clone encodes a protein having extensive homology to immunoglobulin chains. Nature 308:145–149
Zehnbauer BA, Pardoll DM, Burke PJ, Graham ML, Vogelstein B (1986) Immunoglobulin gene rearrangements in remission bone marrow specimens from patients with acute lymphoblastic leukemia. Blood 67:835–838

Interleukin-2-Based Immunotherapy in the Management of Minimal Residual Disease in Acute Leukemia Patients

R. Foa[1,2], G. Meloni[3], A. Guarini[1], M. Vignetti[3], D. Marchis[1], S. Tosti[3], A. Gillio Tos[1], F. Mandelli[3], and F. Gavosto[1]

[1] Dipartimento di Scienze Biomediche e Oncologia Umana, Sezione di Clinica Medica, University of Turin, Via Genova 3, 10126 Turin, Italy
[2] Centro CNR "Immunogenetica e Istocompatibilità", University of Turin, 10126 Turin, Italy
[3] Dipartimento di Biopatologia Umana, Sezione di Ematologia, University of Rome, Via Benevento 6, 00161 Rome, Italy

Background

Following extensive preclinical studies both in vitro and in vivo in experimental models (Grimm et al. 1982; Lafraniere and Rosenberg 1985), the possibility of exploiting interleukin-2 (IL-2), with or without ex vivo activated lymphokine activated killer (LAK) cells, as an immunotherapeutic tool in the treatment of solid tumor patients has over the last 5–6 years become a new and promising reality in the management of cancer (Rosenberg et al. 1985, 1987; West et al. 1987). More recently, the feasibility of extending such an approach to the treatment of acute leukemia patients has been investigated, first preclinically in vitro and thereafter in vivo. The necessity for new therapeutic strategies originates from a number of clinical and biological considerations. The first and more relevant clinical consideration is that despite achieving ever-increasing incidences of complete remissions (CR) following induction chemotherapy, in the great majority of adult acute leukemias this is unfortunately short-lived, indicating that the neoplastic clone has not been eradicated by treatment. Only a minority of adults with acute leukemias in fact survive long. This confirms that the definition of CR, which is still mainly based on morphological criteria, is operational and that the tools for defining a true remission are, thus, largely inadequate. On biological grounds, it is well known that some patients may live for a variable period of time with a detectable proportion of steady-state blasts even in the absence of chemotherapy. This implies that some host defense mechanism is capable of controlling the disease and of impeding its rapid expansion. The evidence that small proportions of blasts may remain silent is further confirmed by the knowledge that individual cases may relapse several years after entering a clinicohematological remission, suggesting that the clone had never been completely eradicated and that it had remained in a dormant state. The likelihood that the immune system plays a primary role in controlling disease progression is given support by the evidence that the natural killer (NK) cell

Recent Results in Cancer Research, Vol. 131

activity is often defective in acute leukemia patients at presentation (Lotzova et al. 1983) and that the monitoring of the NK function may provide an early indicator of relapse (Pizzolo et al. 1988).

Preclinical Findings in Acute Leukemia

The preclinical data determined first in vitro and thereafter in vivo in immunosuppressed nude mice have demonstrated that acute leukemia blasts may be killed by LAK precursors and that normal LAK effectors, as well as recombinant IL-2 alone, may block the growth in nude mice of human leukemic blasts (Oshimi et al. 1986; Adler et al. 1988; Fierro et al. 1988; Lista et al. 1989). In addition, studies in vitro have shown that only in a minority of acute leukemias can IL-2 induce a proliferative signal on the neoplastic clone (Foa et al. 1990a). Most often IL-2 is ineffective or reduces the degree of proliferation of the blasts. This has been further substantiated by experiments carried out in vivo in immunosuppressed nude mice, which have shown that IL-2 alone is capable of blocking the growth of human leukemic cell lines and of primary leukemic blasts (Foa et al. 1990a). These data represented the requisite preclinical observations which have allowed the in vivo use of IL-2-based immunotherapeutic protocols to be used in the management of acute leukemia patients.

Here we shall review the results obtained so far by our group, which, in collaboration with the Chair of Hematology in Rome, started to treat acute leukemia patients with recombinant IL-2 over 4½ years ago, as well as some of the biological modifications induced by such treatment. The experience of other European and American groups will also be discussed.

Clinical Results

The protocol employed by our group involves administering IL-2 alone by continuous intravenous infusion and using a daily escalating protocol. Up to December 1990, Glaxo Imb material was used; thereafter, Cetus IL-2 has been employed. The induction protocol consists of repeated 5-day cycles of IL-2 followed by 2–3 days off. In the presence of detectable disease, the goal is to administer, according to toxicity, four courses of IL-2 in a row. Two cycles are scheduled for patients in apparent CR. If the patients obtain a remission or an objective response, the clinicohematological picture is "maintained" with monthly 5-day courses of a lower dose of IL-2 given on an out-patient basis.

Treated patients are monitored closely on hematological, morphological, and biological grounds at both bone marrow and peripheral blood levels.

The early patients treated, who necessarily had to be relapsed and resistant to chemotherapy, allowed us to demonstrate that IL-2 could be administered to acute leukemias and that the dose-escalating scheme produced acceptable side effects, allowing high doses of IL-2 (up to 18×10^6 units Cetus IL-2/m^2 daily) to be administered.

On clinicohematological grounds, IL-2 alone appears in our experience of little value in patients with an elevated marrow blastosis (Foa et al. 1991a). On the other hand, unexpected responses have been observed in individual patients who, after the unsuccessful administration of IL-2 alone, were put back on the same chemotherapeutic agents to which they were previously resistant (Foa et al. 1991a). These findings point to a potential synergistic action between IL-2 and cytotoxic drugs. This possibility has been more recently confirmed in vitro by our group, which found that in a proportion of acute myeloid leukemia cases capable of growing blastic colonies in semisolid media, preincubation of the blasts with IL-2 made them more susceptible to the cytolytic action of cytosine arabinoside (personal data).

The overall scenario appeared quite different when patients with more limited disease were enrolled. In our experience, in fact, CR may be obtained with IL-2 alone in patients who display a relatively small proportion (5%–30%) of chemoresistant residual bone marrow blasts (Foa et al. 1990b, 1991a). These remissions may be long-lived. One acute myeloid leukemia patient has achieved his fourth CR with IL-2 alone and remains in remission more than 4 years later.

Taken together, these data strongly indicate that should immunotherapy with IL-2/LAK cells play a role in the management of acute leukemia, this is likely to occur in patients with limited or minimal residual disease. While this latter aspect will be dealt with later (see "Future perspectives"), another most relevant area of application is that of immunotherapy as a booster after an autologous bone marrow transplant. Several lines of thought make this approach of conceptual promise: (1) It is widely accepted that an antileukemic role of the host, probably via the immune system, against the neoplastic clone would be a desirable effect. (2) Cytotoxic cells may be relevant in such a context. (3) After an autologous bone marrow transplant cytotoxic progenitors can be found in the peripheral blood (Reittie et al. 1989). Based on these considerations, IL-2 has been given to acute leukemia patients after a bone marrow autograft in an attempt to stimulate or activate the immune system. The results so far obtained indicate that this approach is feasible in terms of toxicity and of doses of IL-2 administered. This holds true for adults (Blaise et al. 1990; Higuchi et al. 1991), and in our experience also for children (Meloni et al. 1992). The biological considerations linked with this treatment modality and the best possible approach in the context of this particular setting will be discussed below.

Clinical, Hematological, and Biological Modifications

As in solid tumor patients treated with IL2/LAK cells, also in acute leukemia the administration of IL-2 is followed by marked clinical, hematological, and biological modifications (Foa et al. 1991a,b). Side effects have been observed in all patients, but they appear to be better controlled with the daily dose-escalating protocol. No patient had to be transferred to an emergency care unit and all were managed in a conventional ward. Complications were similar to those described in other categories of patients treated with IL-2. Biochemical alterations reversed rapidly after stopping IL-2 administration.

Clinically, in most patients the infusion of IL-2 is followed by a more or less evident hepatosplenomegaly. Hematologically, during the administration a marked neutrophilia is observed together with an increase in eosinophils. After stopping IL-2, there is an evident leukocytosis and lymphocytosis with an increase in large granular lymphocytes and a persistent eosinophilia. A moderate anemia and, frequently, a marked thrombocytopenia most often occur. The latter may be severe and require supportive treatment. In addition to a possible sequestration mechanism (Paciucci et al. 1990), in vitro studies have shown that LAK effectors from the patients may profoundly hamper the in vitro growth of autologous bone marrow megakaryocytic progenitor cells and that this effect is contributed by tumor necrosis factor α (Guarini et al. 1991). It is, therefore, likely that an inhibitory action exerted by IL-2-activated LAK cells directly in the marrow of the IL-2-treated patients plays an important contributory role in the pathogenesis of the thrombocytopenia.

Several marked immunological modifications are linked to treatment with IL-2 (Foa et al. 1991b). These include an overall increase in circulating $CD3^+$ and $CD8^+$ lymphocytes, the expression of the IL-2 receptor α chain (Tac/CD25 antigen), an enhancement of NK and LAK functions in blood and marrow lymphocytes, and the generation of endogenous LAK effectors. Of relevance, these endogenous LAK cells can also be found in the marrow of the treated patients. Furthermore, the administration of IL-2 is followed by increased serum levels of tumor necrosis factor α and interferon-γ (in preparation).

The same biological follow-up has been applied to patients who underwent treatment with IL-2 following an autologous bone marrow transplantation. Interestingly, and in agreement with the suggestion that in these patients there may be an amplification of the cytotoxic compartment, the infusion of IL-2 was followed by a very marked activation of endogenous LAK cells, to values greater than those observed in patients treated with IL-2 but who had not undergone an autologous bone marrow transplant (Meloni et al. 1992).

Future Perspectives

The analysis of the data so far accumulated on the use of IL-2 in the management of acute leukemia patients allows some conclusions. It seems convincingly established that this innovative approach may be extended to this category of patients, both in terms of toxicity and of possible clinical responses. The likelihood that IL-2 may induce a proliferative signal on the leukemic clone, a potentially worrying issue, also appears to be a relatively limited risk. This is further confirmed by recent data by our group which indicate that human leukemic cells transduced with the IL-2 gene do not modify their proliferation pattern (in preparation). On clinical grounds, IL-2 alone has proven in our experience of little value for patients with a marked marrow blastosis. This may be due to the fact that few effectors are potentially "inducible" because admixed with the largely blastic population, and that the daily escalating protocol employed probably allows therapeutic doses of IL-2 to be reached when the clone is further expanded. Furthermore, recent biological data have shown that the blasts of patients at diagnosis and, to a further extent, at the time of relapse are in the great majority of cases resistant to autologous LAK effectors, while being susceptible to normal allogeneic LAK cells (Foa et al. 1991c). Thus, if the potential therapeutic effect of IL-2-based immunotherapy is contributed by LAK effectors generated in vivo, the latter may be ineffective against the autologous clone in patients with active disease. Should an immunotherapeutic strategy be considered for such advanced disease patients, it is conceivable that this should not be based on IL-2 alone, but rather that it should take into account combination protocols with IL-2 and chemotherapy or, possibly, with LAK cells generated ex vivo.

In view of the results so far obtained, it appears that patients with limited or minimal disease are the best target of these new therapeutic modalities. This is based on the clinicohematological evidence that CR may be induced in patients with a limited proportion of residual blasts by repeated courses of IL-2 alone. These findings are confirmed by the demonstration that in patients in CR LAK effectors may regain their capacity to lyse autologous blasts (Foa et al. 1991c).

On the basis of these findings, the ongoing studies are mainly devoted to confirming in larger series of patients with limited and chemoresistant disease the potential antileukemic effect of IL-2. Furthermore, they strenghthen the necessity for carrying out pilot and randomized studies with IL-2 administered to acute leukemia patients in first and second CR. These studies, which are currently underway, should conclusively clarify if and to what extent IL-2 may be valuable in the management of acute leukemia.

Particular attention is being devoted to the role of IL-2 given after an autologous bone marrow transplant in an attempt to combine the potentially most eradicating chemotherapeutic approach with a biological boosting of the immune system of the host to further control or eradicate minimal residual disease. The preliminary studies so far carried out have shown the feasibility of such an approach both in adults and in children and opened the way to randomized studies. The problem of the best time to start IL-2 administration and of the doses to be employed is a relevant and difficult issue in the context of the autografted patients. IL-2 shortly after grafting – theoretically preferable, particularly in acute lymphoblastic leukemia in view of the high rate of early posttransplant relapses – needs to be administered at low doses in order to limit the toxicities, particularly on the megakaryocytic compartment. One may argue that these low doses may be of limited therapeutic validity. Higher doses of IL-2 have so far been given at approximately day 80 after grafting. The value of these different approaches, as well as the addition of exogenous LAK cells will probably be clarified by the currently ongoing studies.

A particularly important aspect is that concerning the relevance of pre- and post-treatment biological studies. Though it has been clearly shown that in acute leukemia the administration of IL-2 is followed by a marked amplification of the immune system, we have so far failed to show a correlation between biological data and clinical response (Foa et al. 1991b). Most likely, this is largely due to the fact that the triggering of the LAK compartment has been investigated against allogeneic targets. Studies aimed at assessing the generation of specific LAK effectors directed against the autologous leukemic population will be a potentially more accurate marker of response. In this respect, the demonstration that blasts from acute leukemia patients at diagnosis and at relapse are often resistant to autologous LAK effectors, while autologous killing is frequently restored at the time of remission, suggests that this approach may help to identify patients potentially responsive to IL-2-based protocols.

In conclusion, the data so far accumulated indicate that IL-2/LAK cells appear to have an antileukemic effect, and clinical responses have been documented, particularly in patients with limited disease. These findings, coupled to the biological information obtained, justify the currently ongoing attempts to clarify in larger series of acute leukemia patients and in randomized trials the real impact IL-2/LAK immunotherapy, and the search for possible response-predictive factors.

Acknowledgments. This work was supported by Istituto Superiore di Sanità, Rome (Italy–USA Program on "Therapy of Neoplasias") and by CNR, Special Project "Applicazioni Cliniche della Ricerca Oncologica", Rome, Italy. A.G.T was in receipt of a fellowship from the Associazione Italiana per la Ricerca sul Cancro (AIRC), Milan, Italy.

References

Adler A, Chervenick PA, Whiteside TL, Lotzova E, Herberman RB (1988) Interleukin 2 induction of lymphokine-activated killer (LAK) activity in the peripheral blood and bone marrow of acute leukemia patients: I. Feasibility of LAK generation in adult patients with active disease and in remission. Blood 71:709–716

Blaise D, Olive D, Stoppa AM, Viens P, Pourreau C, Lopez M, Attal M, Jasmin C, Monges G, Mawas C, Mannoni P, Palmer P, Franks C, Philip T, Maraninchi D (1990) Hematologic and immunologic effects of the systemic administration of

recombinant interleukin-2 after autologous bone marrow transplantation. Blood 76:1092–1097
Fierro MT, Xin-Sheng L, Lusso P, Bonferroni M, Matera L, Cesano A, Lista P, Arione R, Forni G, Foa R (1988) In vitro and in vivo susceptibility of human leukemic cells to lymphokine activated killer activity. Leukemia 2:50–54
Foa R, Caretto P, Fierro MT, Bonferroni M, Cardona S, Guarini A, Lista P, Pegoraro L, Mandelli F, Forni G, Gavosto F (1990a) Interleukin 2 does not promote the in vitro and in vivo proliferation and growth of human acute leukaemia cells of myeloid and lymphoid origin. Br J Haematol 75:34–40
Foa R, Fierro MT, Tosti S, Meloni G, Gavosto F, Mandelli F (1990b) Induction and persistence of complete remission in a resistant acute myeloid leukemia patient after treatment with recombinant Interleukin 2. Leuk Lymph 1:113–117
Foa R, Meloni G, Tosti S, Novarino A, Fenu S, Gavosto F, Mandelli A (1991a) Treatment of acute myeloid leukaemia patients with recombinant interleukin 2: a pilot study. Br J Haematol 77:491–496
Foa R, Guarini A, Gillio Tos A, Cardona S, Fierro MT, Meloni G, Tosti S, Mandelli F, Gavosto F (1991b) Peripheral blood and bone marrow immunophenotypic and functional modifications induced in acute leukemia patients treated with Interleukin 2: evidence of in vivo lymphokine activated killer cell generation. Cancer Res 51:964–968
Foa R, Fierro MT, Cesano A, Guarini A, Bonferroni M, Raspadori D, Miniero R, Lauria F, Gavosto F (1991c) Defective lymphokine-activated killer cell generation and activity in acute leukemia patients with active disease. Blood 78:1041–1046
Grimm EA, Mazumder A, Zhang HZ, Rosenberg SA (1982) Lymphokine activated killer cell phenomenon. Lysis of natural killer-resistant fresh solid tumor cells by interleukin 2-activated autologous human peripheral blood lymphocytes. J Exp Med 155:1823–1841
Guarini A, Sanavio F, Novarino A, Gillio Tos A, Aglietta M, Foa R (1991) Thrombocytopenia in acute leukaemia patients treated with IL2: cytolytic effect of LAK cells on megakaryocytic progenitors. Br J Haematol 79:451–456
Higuchi CM, Thompson JA, Petersen FB, Buckner CD, Fefer A (1991) Toxixity and immunomodulatory effects of interleukin-2 after autologous bone marrow transplantation for hematologic malignancies. Blood 77:2561–2568
Lafraniere R, Rosenberg SA (1985) Successful immunotherapy of murine experimental hepatic metastases with lymphokine activated killer cells and recombinant interleukin-2. Cancer Res 45:3735–3741
Lista P, Fierro MT, Xin-Sheng L, Bonferroni M, Brizzi MF, Porcu PL, Pegoraro L, Foa R (1989) Lymphokine-activated killer (LAK) cells inhibit the clonogenic growth of human leukemic stem cells. Eur J Haematol 42:425–430
Lotzova E, Savary CA, Keating MJ (1983) Leukemia diseased patients exhibit multiple defects in natural killer cell lytic machinery. Exp Hematol 10:83–95
Meloni G, Foa R, Tosti S, Vignetti M, Mancini F, Guarini A, Marchis D, Gavosto F, Mandelli F (1992) Autologous bone marrow transplantation followed by interleukin-2 in children with advanced leukemia: a pilot study. Leukemia 6:780–785
Oshimi K, Oshimi Y, Akutsu M, Takei Y, Saito H, Okada M, Mizoguchi H (1986) Cytotoxicity of interleukin 2 activated lymphocytes for leukemia and lymphoma cells. Blood 68:938–948
Paciucci PA, Mandeli J, Oleksowicz L, Ameglio F, Holland JF (1990) Thrombocytopenia during immunotherapy with interleukin-2 by constant infusion. Am J Med 89:309–312
Pizzolo G, Trentin L, Vinante F, Agostini C, Zambello R, Masciarelli M, Feruglio C, Dazzi F, Todeschini G, Chilosi M, Veneri D, Zanotti R, Benedetti F, Perona G, Semenzato G (1988) Natural killer cell function and lymphoid subpopulations

in acute non-lymphoblastic leukaemia in complete remission. Br J Cancer 58: 368–372

Reittie JE, Gottlieb D, Heslop HE, Leger O, Drexler HG, Hazlehurst G, Hoffbrand AV, Prentice G, Brenner K (1989) Endogenously generated activated killer cells circulate after autologous and allogeneic marrow transplantation but not after chemotherapy. Blood 73:1351–1358

Rosenberg SA, Lotze MT, Muul LM, Leitman S, Chang AE, Ettinghausen SE, Matory YL, Skibber JM, Shiloni E, Vetto JT, Seipp CA, Simpson C, Reichert CM (1985) Observations on the systemic administration of autologous lymphokine activated killer cells and recombinant interleukin-2 to patients with metastatic cancer. N Engl J Med 313:1485–1492

Rosenberg SA, Lotze MT, Muul LM, Chang AE, Avis EP, Leitman S, Linehan WM, Robertson CN, Lee RE, Rubin JT, Seipp CA, Simpson CG, White DE (1987) A progress report on the treatment of 157 patients with advanced cancer using lymphokine activated killer cells and interleukin-2 or high dose interleukin-2 alone. N Engl J Med 316:889–897

West WH, Tauer KW, Yannelli JR, Marshall GD, Orr DW, Thurman GB, Oldham RK (1987) Constant-infusion recombinant interleukin-2 in adoptive immunotherapy of advanced cancer. N Engl J Med 316:898–905

Preclinical Studies of T-Cell-Mediated Immune Responses Against Autologous Tumor Cells in Patients with Acute Leukemia

M. Notter, W.-D. Ludwig, and E. Thiel

Department of Hematology and Oncology, Free University of Berlin, Hindenburgdamm 30, W-1000 Berlin 45, Fed. Rep. of Germany

Immunotherapy in Acute Leukemia: Rationale, Concepts, and Problems

Risk-adapted therapy in patients with acute leukemia has significantly improved prognosis. As a result of relapsing disease and increasing resistance to chemotherapy, however, long-term survival in nontransplanted patients does not exceed 30% (Büchner et al. 1985). Clearly, new therapeutic approaches are needed.

At present, the best cure rates are achieved in patients eligible for allogeneic bone marrow transplantation. The relapse-free survival advantage in this population, which is partially lost following depletion of T lymphocytes from the marrow graft, demonstrates that T lymphocytes may exert antileukemic activity which is associated with clinical benefit. This observation of an immune cell-mediated "graft-versus-leukemia reaction" in conjunction with the availability of recombinant cytokines for clinical use and with the low tumor burden present in stages of minimal residual disease provides a rationale for immunotherapeutic strategies in the treatment of leukemia.

Interleukin-2 (IL-2), the central T and NK cell-stimulating cytokine, was used in pilot and phase I trials to stimulate antileukemic activity of host lymphocytes in the postremission phase or following bone marrow transplantation (Gottlieb et al. 1989; Foa et al. 1991a,b). In these early trials IL-2 had no impact on relapse-free survival. Several problems, however, associated with administration of IL-2 in this setting became obvious. At present no in vitro assay or clinical predictor is available that allows one to identify patients likely to respond to IL-2. Optimal timing and dosing schedules are unknown. Systemic administration of high doses of IL-2 is associated with significant toxicity (Lotze et al. 1985). Counterregulatory mechanisms are activated when IL-2 alone is used in vivo. These include factors known to suppress immune responses such as interleukin-10 (Vieira et al. 1991) and soluble LFA-3 (Meuer, personal communication). Tumor progression may also lead to the selection of nonimmunogenic tumor cells or of malignant

Recent Results in Cancer Research, Vol. 131

clones that stimulate suppressor cells, as has been shown for Burkitt's lymphoma (Gregory et al. 1988) and malignant melanoma (Mukherji et al. 1987), respectively. IL-2 administered in this scenario might tip the balance in favor of antileukemic immunosuppression rather than elimination of residual malignant cells. The issue is furthermore complicated by the observation that IL-2 therapy can obviously select for relapsing nonlymphocytic leukemic cells with de novo expression of both the p75 and p55 subunits of the IL-2 receptor (Rosolen et al. 1989; Macdonald et al. 1991). The functional significance of this finding, however, is still under debate (Foa et al. 1990).

At this point, it becomes obvious that the knowledge base available as of yet is insufficient to allow for selective immunointervention with a predicted antileukemic outcome. More efficient and less toxic modalities of generating cytotoxic lymphocytes to eliminate residual leukemia have to be established. Combinations of cytokines may be more efficient than single agents in this regard.

How can we arrive at meaningful strategies, however? On a purely empirical basis, testing numerous permutations of the ever-growing number of cytokines is simply not feasible. Rather, we propose that immunotherapeutic strategies should be rationally developed on the basis of understanding tumor–host relationships on a cellular and molecular level. In vitro test systems are required that provide answers to the key questions: (1) What is the potency and specificity of cytotoxic immune cells activated in vitro against autologous tumor cells of leukemia patients? (2) What cell surface molecules and which cytokines are involved in the host–tumor interaction? This information will prove instrumental in designing controlled interventions to augment the specificity and efficiency of the host antileukemia response. In the following, an in vitro test system is described developed along these guidelines, and results of two applications are presented.

Method of Studying Cytotoxic Lymphocyte-Mediated Effector Mechanisms Against Autologous Leukemic Cells (Table 1)

To establish an autologous test system in vitro, fresh leukemic cells from bone marrow or peripheral blood isolated at primary diagnosis or relapse are cryopreserved in large numbers. From each patient, a nonmalignant reference cell line is prepared by transforming autologous B lymphocytes or T cells with Epstein-Barr virus (EBV) or phytohemagglutinin (PHA), respectively. Effector T lymphocytes are isolated at various time points in the patient's clinical course. T cells are activated by various modes. In mixed lymphocyte tumor cultures (MLTC) effector cells are cocultured with autologous tumor cells in the presence of low doses of IL-2 (25 U/ml), followed by cloning of responding cells by limiting dilution. Long-term cultivation in high doses of IL-2 (1000 U/ml) results in expansion of effector cells consisting

Table 1. Outline of methods used to study cell-mediated immune responses against autologous tumor cells of patients with acute leukemia

Autologous test system
- Leukemia cells at diagnosis and relapse
- Effector lymphocytes in remission
- Nonmalignant reference cells: EBV transformation, PHA stimulation

In vitro activation of T cells
- Mixed-lymphocyte tumor culture: cloning of T cells
- Interleukin-2
- Anti-CD3 monoclonal antibody in effector phase

Characterization of effector cells
- Cell-mediated cytotoxicity (chromium release)
- Proliferation
- Immunophenotyping

of more than 80% of T cells. We have extensively studied anti-CD3 monoclonal antibodies present during the effector phase because they have been reported to increase antileukemic cytotoxicity (Lotzova et al. 1987). Activated T cells are characterized in the chromium-release assay by repeatedly testing their cytotoxic potential against autologous leukemic cells and nonmalignant reference cells in addition to known cultured leukemic cell lines such as K562, representing the classic NK-sensitive target. We believe HLA class II-positive autologous nonmalignant cells represent an essential reference target, because activation of autoreactive T cells directed against HLA class II molecules by a so-called "autologous mixed lymphocyte response" is a well-described phenomenon (Takeuchi et al. 1987) that needs to be distinguished from true antileukemic cytotoxicity. Effector cells are also characterized in terms of their proliferative potential and of their immunophenotype. Applications of this system will now be described in the investigation of T cell-mediated antileukemic cytotoxicity for time-sequential analysis in a single patient and for screening a series of 15 consecutive patients with acute leukemia.

Sequential Analysis of Lymphocyte-Mediated Autologous Antileukemic Cytotoxicity

Figure 1 shows T and NK cell-mediated cytotoxicity against autologous leukemia cells, EBV-transformed B cells (EBV-B), and K562 tested at various time points during the clinical course of a 22-year old patient with acute myeloid leukemia (AML) M4 of the eosinophilic subtype. This patient readily achieved complete remission (CR) following three cycles of chemotherapy. Exactly 1 year after the primary diagnosis had been made, he suffered an early relapse of his disease including central nervous system (CNS) involvement. Relapsed AML was refractory to salvage chemotherapy,

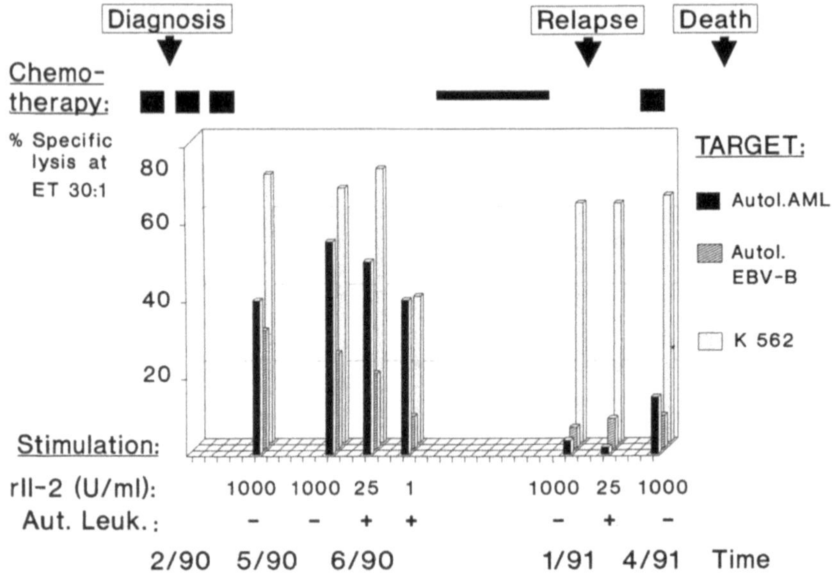

Fig. 1. Sequential activated T cell-mediated antileukemic cytotoxicity of a patient with AML M4 of the eosinophilic subtype. Peripheral blood lymphocytes were activated by long-term culture for 7–40 days in the presence of high doses of IL-2, or by cocultivation with autologous leukemic cell in the presence of the indicated lower amounts of IL-2, as described (Notter et al. 1990). Effector cells were tested at weekly intervals by the standard 4-h chromium-release assay against the indicated target cells. Peak cytotoxic responses are shown

resulting in a rapid fatal outcome. T cells collected at various points in time were activated by long-term culture for 7–40 days in the presence of high doses of IL-2 (1000 U/ml) or by MLTC with lower doses of IL-2. Effector cells were tested in weekly intervals and peak responses are shown.

NK-like activity as measured against K562 was uniformly high during remission and relapse and was considered an internal control to assure comparable activation conditions. After recovery from the aplastic phase following consolidation chemotherapy, we detected a fairly high level of cytotoxicity against both autologous leukemic cells and EBV-B cells (40% and 31% specific lysis, respectively, at effector: target (ET) ratio of 30:1). This increased even further when the patient was out 1 month further into CR (55% and 25% specific lysis). Surprisingly, at this point in time, doses of IL-2 as low as 25 U/ml and even 1 U/ml were sufficient to very efficiently activate cytotoxic T cells against autologous fresh leukemic cells. With decreasing IL-2 amounts, specificity against malignant cells increased, demonstrated by 40% versus 8% specific lysis (ET ratio 30:1) of autologous tumor and EBV-B cells, respectively, which was mediated by T cells activated by MLTC in the presence of IL-2 1 U/ml. In contrast, T cells activated in an identical fashion could either not or only minimally be induced to cytotoxicity against autologous tumor cells during relapse.

Based on this case report, the following conclusions can be drawn: (1) NK-like cytotoxicity of activated T cells clearly does not correlate with killing of fresh autologous leukemic cells, although opposite reports exist in the literature (Oshimi et al. 1986). (2) Potency and specificity of autologous antileukemic cytotoxicity vary during the clinical course of an individual patient. (3) This system allows detection of prominent cytotoxicity, being selectively directed against autologous malignant cells during CR. This finding supports the hypothesis that one ultimately established time point for initiation of adjuvant immunotherapy in AML will be shortly following achievement of first clinical remission. Although we will never know, it is tempting to speculate on what would have happened to the patient's clinical course if he had received IL-2 at a time when his host antileukemic cytotoxicity was being measured by this test system.

Cross-sectional Analysis of Lymphocyte-Mediated Autologous Antileukemic Cytotoxicity

Figure 2 shows screening results of a series of 15 consecutive nonselected patients (12 with AML, 3 with acute lymphoblastic leukemia, ALL). Activated T lymphocytes were generated from remission peripheral blood lymphocytes by culture in IL-2 (1000 U/ml) for 7–35 days. Again, maximum cytotoxic responses against autologous leukemic and EBV-B cells of weekly repeated measurements are presented. In general, three patterns of cytotoxicity are apparent. In some cases, as exemplified by patients 1–3 and 7–10, activated T cells are selectively cytotoxic for autologous leukemic cells. T cells of patients 4, 5, 11, and 12 have similar cytotoxic activities against both malignant and EBV-B cells. In ALL patients and in AML patient 6, an overall small cytotoxic response against autologous leukemic cells or EBV-B cells was detected. The basis for the observed heterogeneity of cytotoxicity patterns remains unclear. It may be due to different degrees of immunogenicity of malignant cells, to differential expression of adhesion molecules, to different cytokine secretion profiles of tumor and of immune effector cells, or to different genetic idiotypic repertoires of the effector cell populations. It may also be merely a reflection of time-related variation of antileukemic cytotoxicity in an individual patient, as was described above. These hypotheses are the subjects of ongoing studies and await further clarification.

In contrast to the heterogeneous specificity patterns of activated patient T cells, a rather uniform picture emerges when the same screening assay is performed in the presence of anti-CD3 monoclonal antibody (MAb). In all AML patients studied, addition of, in this case, OKT3 MAb enhanced antileukemic cytotoxicity 1.5- to 9.3-fold. Cytotoxicity against autologous EBV-B cells was not affected or even reduced. The minimal cytotoxic

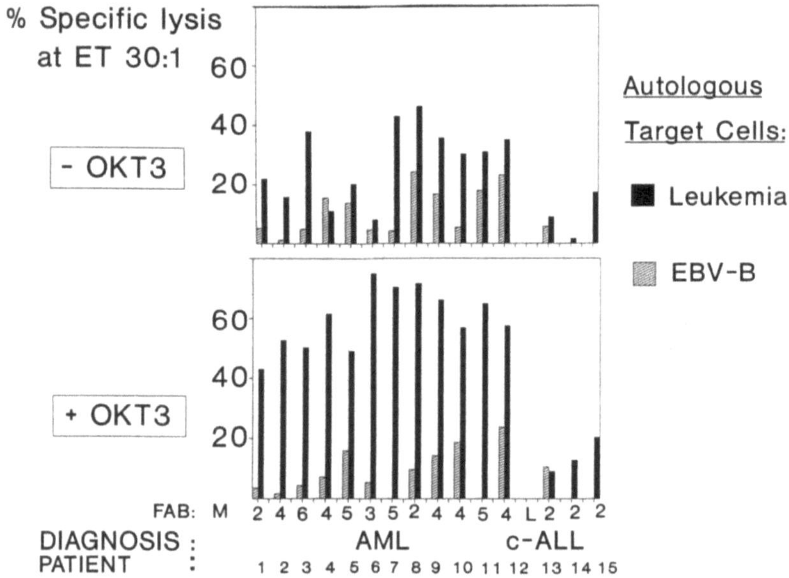

Fig. 2. Cytotoxicity against autologous leukemic cells and autologous nonmalignant B cells of 15 patients with acute leukemia. Remission peripheral blood lymphocytes were activated by culture in the presence of IL-2 (1000 U/ml) for 7–35 days and tested at weekly intervals for cytotoxicity by a standard 4-h chromium-release assay in the presence or absence of OKT3 (80 ng/ml) during the effector phase. Diagnoses including FAB subtypes are indicated. Each pair of *bars* represents the results of an individual patient. Only test results with a spontaneous chromium release of less than 30% were included in the analysis

activity against the three lymphatic leukemic cell samples studied was unaltered or only marginally increased. Since addition of anti-CD3 MAbs increased efficiency and specificity of effector cells against autologous nonlymphocytic leukemic cells, the mechanisms underlying this phenomenon were investigated. Several lines of evidence indicate that high-affinity Fc receptors for immunoglobulin G on AML blasts are the predominant target cell ligands for OKT3-coated effector T lymphocytes. We found that expression of this molecule on malignant and non-malignant cells is rather restricted to monocytic and myeloid cells and that it is inducible by interferons, resulting in increased sensitivity for autologous T cells targeted by anti-CD3 MAbs (manuscripts in preparation).

Summary and Perspectives

Treatment of AML in adults by chemotherapy alone is not curative in the majority of patients. The observation of a graft-versus-leukemia reaction following allogeneic bone marrow transplantation suggests that recombinant cytokines might be a new treatment modality. Several clinical studies using IL-2 have been reported. However, none has yet proved superior to conventional therapy. These failures may be a result of the host–tumor relationship being insufficiently understood with regard to the cell surface molecules involved and cytokines produced by both tumor and immune cells. In this context, a test system was described here revealing heterogeneous patterns of cytotoxicity against autologous tumor and nonmalignant cells in patients with acute leukemia. In individual patients, marked temporal variation in antileukemic activity mediated predominantly by activated T lymphocytes is detected. In addition, cell surface molecules and their modulation by interferons involved in the interaction between myeloid tumor cells and T lymphocytes targeted with anti-CD3 monoclonal antibodies were identified on the basis of this system. This information is crucial for designing rational treatment strategies. The investigation of tumor–host cell interactions at a cellular and molecular level provides essential criteria to define indications for immunotherapeutic interventions in patients with acute leukemia. We feel that attempts at using immunologic means to eliminate residual leukemic cells, although a promising approach, should at present be preceded by preclinical evaluation of the type described. At least in this phase, therapy should be guided by immunologic testing in the laboratory on an individualized basis. Clinical trials conducted along these guidelines in the future will have to demonstrate whether in vitro findings will translate into therapeutic benefit in vivo.

Acknowledgement. Part of this work was supported by a grant from the Deutsche Krebshilfe (W10/90/No 1).

References

Büchner T, Urbanitz D, Hiddemann W, Rühl H, Ludwig WD, Fischer J, Aul HC, Vaupel HA, Kuse R, Zeile G, Nowrousian MR, König HJ, Walter M, Wendt FC, Sodomann H, Hossfeld DK, von Paleske A, Löffler H, Gassmann W, Hellriegel KP, Fülle HH, Lunschken C, Emmerich B, Pralle H, Pees HW, Pfreundschuh M, Bartels H, Koeppen KM, Schwerdtfeger R, Donhuijsen-Ant R, Mainzer K, Bonfert B, Köppler H, Zurborn KH, Ranft K, Thiel E, Heinecke A (1985) Intensified induction and consolidation with or without maintenance chemotherapy for acute myeloid leukemia (AML). J Clin Oncol 3:9–17

Foa R, Caretto P, Fierro MT, Bonferroni M, Cardona S, Guarinio A, Lista P, Pegoraro L, Mandelli F, Forni G, Gavosto F (1990) Interleukin 2 does not promote the in vitro and in vivo proliferation and growth of human acute leukemia cells of myeloid and lymphoid origin. Br J Haematol 75:34–40

Foa R, Guarini A, Tos AG, Cardona S, Fierro MT, Meloni G, Tosti S, Mandelli F, Gavosto F (1991a) Peripheral blood and bone marrow immunophenotypic and functional modifications induced in acute leukemia patients treated with interleukin 2: evidence of in vivo lymphokine activated killer cell generation. Cancer Res 51:964–968

Foa R, Meloni G, Tosti S, Novarino A, Fenu S, Gavosto F, Mandelli F (1991b) Treatment of acute leukaemia patients with recombinant interleukin 2: a pilot study. Br J Haematol 77:491–496

Gottlieb DJ, Prentice HG, Heslop HE, Bello-Fernandez C, Bianchi AC, Galazka AR, Brenner MK (1989) Effects of recombinant interleukin-2 administration on cytotoxic function following high-dose radiochemotherapy for hematological malignancy. Blood 74:2335–2342

Gregory CD, Murray RJ, Edwards CF, Rickinson AB (1988) Downregulation of cell adhesion molecules LFA-3 and ICAM-1 in Epstein-Barr virus-positive Burkitt's lymphoma underlies tumor cell escape from virus-specific T cell surveillance. J Exp Med 167:1811–1824

Lotze MT, Matory YL, Ettinghausen SE, Rayner AA, Sharrow SO, Seipp CAY, Custer MC, Rosenberg SA (1985) In vivo administration of purified human Interleukin-2. J Immunol 4:2865–2875

Lotzova E, Savary CA, Herberman RB, McCredie KB, Keating MJ, Freireich EJ (1987) Augmentation of antileukemia lytic activity by OKT3 monoclonal antibody: Synergism of OKT3 and Interleukin-2. Nat Immun Cell Growth Regul 6:219–223

MacDonald D, Jiang YZ, Swirsky D, Vulliamy T, Morilla R, Bungey J, Barrett AJ (1991) Acute myeloid leukemia relapsing following interleukin-2 treatment expresses the alpha chain of the interleukin-2 receptor. Br J Haematol 77:43–49

Mukherji B, Guha A, Loomis R, Ergin MT (1987) Cell-mediated amplification and downregulation of cytotoxic immune response against autologous human cancer. J Immunol 138:1987–1991

Notter M, Schirrmacher V (1990) Tumor-specific T-cell clones recognize different protein determinants of autologous human malignant melanoma cells. Int J Cancer 45:834–841

Oshimi K, Oshimi Y, Akutsu M, Takei Y, Saito H, Okada M, Mizogouchi H (1986) Cytotoxicity of Interleukin 2-activated lymphocytes for leukemia and lymphoma cells. Blood 68:938–948

Rosolen A, Nakanishi M, Poplack DG, Cole D, Quinones R, Reaman G, Cotelingam JD, Trepel JB, Sausville E, Marti GE, Jaffe E, Neckers LM, Colamonici OR (1989) Expression of interleukin-2 receptor beta subunit in haematopoietic malignancies. Blood 73:1968–1972

Takeuchi T, Rudd CE, Schlossmann SF, Morimoto C (1987) Induction of suppression following autologous mixed lymphocyte reaction; role of a novel 2H4 antigen. Eur J Immunol 17:97–103

Vieira P, De Waal-Malefyt R, Dang MN, Johnson KE, Kastelen R, Fiorentino DF, DeVries JE, Roncarolo MG, Mosmann TR, Moore KW (1991) Isolation and expression of human cytokine synthesis inhibitory factor cDNA clones: Homology to Epstein-Barr virus open reading frame BCRFI. Proc Natl Acad Sci USA 88:1172–1176

Susceptibility of Human Leukemia Cells to Allogeneic and Autologous Lymphokine-Activated Killer Cells and Its Augmentation by Exposure of Leukemia Target Cells to Cytotoxic Drugs In Vitro and In Vivo

J.V. Teichmann, W.-D. Ludwig, and E. Thiel

Department of Hematology and Oncology, Universitätsklinikum Steglitz, Free University of Berlin, Hindenburgdamm 30, W-1000 Berlin 45, Fed. Rep. of Germany

Introduction

Interleukin-2- (IL-2-)activated cytotoxic effector cells, known as lymphokine-activated killer (LAK) cells, lyse a wide variety of fresh solid tumor cells (Grimm et al. 1982; Itoh et al. 1986) as well as fresh noncultured leukemia cells (Oshimi et al. 1986; Lotzová et al. 1987; Fierro et al. 1988; Teichmann et al. 1989) in a fashion not restricted by the major histocompatibility complex (MHC). LAK cell cytotoxicity is predominantly mediated by $CD3^-/CD56^+$ activated natural killer (NK) cells and only to a small degree by MHC-unrestricted $CD3^+/CD56^+$ T cells (Phillips and Lanier 1986; Herberman et al. 1987; Tilden et al. 1987; Saito et al. 1988). Human leukemia cells possess a distinct LAK cell susceptibility which varies considerably in different subtypes of leukemia (Teichmann et al. 1992). Maximal cytolysis by activated effector cells is desirable for therapy. The current study therefore aimed at investigating whether in vitro exposure of leukemic cells to cytotoxic agents, relevant for leukemia treatment, can augment the susceptibility of fresh noncultured leukemia cells to LAK cell lysis. In addition, we also studied the susceptibility of leukemia cells both before and after exposure to cytotoxic drugs given in vivo during induction chemotherapy.

Material and Methods

Effector Cells. Allogeneic human LAK cells were generated from peripheral blood mononuclear cells (PBMC) of healthy volunteers. Our group of normal PBMC donors was selected for low interindividual variation of their LAK cell function (Teichmann et al. 1992). To induce autologous LAK cells, PBMC were obtained from leukemia patients in complete remission (CR) for 3–9 months. All of these patients were under maintenance therapy

Recent Results in Cancer Research, Vol. 131

according to the regimen of the AML Cooperative Group in the Federal Republic of Germany (Buechner et al. 1990). Blood samples from patients were drawn after regeneration of the peripheral blood count right before the next course of chemotherapy. PBMC isolated from heparinized venous blood were cultured with recombinant IL-2 1000 U/ml for 6 days. The assays with allogeneic LAK cells were performed with two or three different LAK cell donors. The highest cytotoxicity value achieved was used for the analyses.

Target Cells. Fresh leukemic cells were obtained from bone marrow or peripheral blood of untreated patients by Ficoll-Hypaque gradient centrifugation. For some experiments leukemia cells were collected on different days of induction therapy according to the TAD-9 regimen right before injection of the drugs scheduled for the given day. The leukemic cells were cryopreserved until use in the cytotoxicity assays. Phenotypic characterization of leukemia samples was performed by standard indirect immunofluorescence assays using monoclonal antibodies as described elsewhere (Ludwig et al. 1988; Thiel et al. 1989). Normal bone-marrow cells were obtained from patients who had marrow aspiration for nonmalignant diseases. The K562 and Daudi cell lines maintained as continuous cultures served as standard target cells.

Drug Treatment of Target Cells. Leukemia target cells were suspended in culture medium and incubated with cytosine arabinoside (Ara-C) or daunorubicin (DNR) for 18 h. After incubation, the cells were washed twice, and their viability was assessed. The viability of drug-exposed cells was between 85% and 95%.

Cytotoxicity Assays. Cytotoxicity was determined in a standard 4-h chromium-51-release assay at four different effector-to-target (ET) ratios. The results were expressed as a percentage of specific chromium release or as lytic units (LU). LU were calculated by exponential regression analysis according to the method of Pross et al. (1981). One LU was defined as the number of effector cells/10^7 required to lyse 20% of the target cells. The statistical analysis was performed using Student's *t* test.

Results

Standardization and Definition of Susceptibility. Allogeneic LAK cells were used to examine fresh leukemia cells for susceptibility to LAK cell cytotoxicity and to analyze the differential sensitivity of the various leukemia subgroups. In separate studies, we determined the LAK cell cytotoxicity of PBMC from 18 healthy volunteers and selected a group of 15 normal donors with very low interindividual variation of LAK cell cytotoxicity (Teichmann

Table 1. Susceptibility of normal bone-marrow cells to allogeneic LAK cells

	Cytotoxicity[a]				
	Specific chromium release (%)				LU/10[7]
	100:1	50:1	25:1	12.5:1	
Mean[b]	5.48	3.85	2.63	1.54	2.38
SD[c]	±3.64	±2.82	±2.09	±1.70	±1.73
99% confidence interval (upper limit)	14.85	11.12	8.01	5.91	6.86

Effector cells were induced from PBMC of normal donors incubated with recombinant IL-2 10^3 U/ml for 6 days. Target cells were normal bone-marrow cells obtained from 52 donors, as described in "Material and Methods."

[a] Cytotoxicity is given as percentage specific chromium release and as lytic units ($LU/10^7$).

[b] Mean of 52 independent experiments.

[c] Standard deviation.

et al. 1992). The "susceptibility" of a given leukemia sample was defined on the basis of chromium release from normal bone-marrow cells achieved by LAK cells from the allogeneic donor group. We analyzed chromium releases in 52 normal bone-marrow samples and found that the mean release from normal bone marrow (ET of 50:1) was 3.8 ± 2.8% (Table 1). The upper limit of the 99% confidence interval was used as the threshold value for defining "susceptibility" of leukemia cells to the lytic activity of LAK cells. By definition, all leukemia samples with a specific chromium release >11.12% at an ET of 50:1 are considered susceptible to LAK cell lysis.

Susceptibility of Leukemic Cells to Allogeneic Lymphokine-Activated Killer Cells. The study with 252 samples of different leukemia subtypes from untreated leukemia patients using allogeneic LAK cells showed that 155 of 252 leukemias (62%) are susceptible (mean chromium release 28.8 ± 13.5%) and 97 of 252 (38%) resistant (mean chromium release 5.2 ± 3.2%) to LAK-cell-mediated cytolysis (Table 2). A differential analysis of leukemia subgroups revealed a considerably higher frequency of susceptible samples from acute leukemias or chronic myelogenous leukemia in blast crisis (65%) than from chronic leukemias (39%) (Fig. 1). Within the group of acute leukemias, no significant differences could be detected between acute myeloid leukemia (AML) and acute lymphoblastic leukemia (ALL). Considering the different FAB subgroups of AML, we observed a susceptibility of 66% for the subgroups M1 and M2 and of 57% for M4, while a considerably higher freqency (88%) was found for M5 leukemias. The M3 and M6 subgroups could not be evaluated because of the limited number of

Table 2. Susceptibility of leukemic cells to allogeneic LAK cells

Target cells	Total no. of samples	Cytotoxicity (% specific Cr release, ET 50:1)			
		n (pos)[a]	% ± SD	*n* (neg)[b]	% ± SD
AML	102	69 (68)[c]	28.5 ± 13.4	33 (32)[c]	5.2 ± 3.2
M1/M2	68	45 (66)	28.1 ± 13.2	23 (34)	4.6 ± 3.3
M3	2	0	–	2 (100)	4.5 ± 0.7
M4	14	8 (57)	31.1 ± 14.2	6 (43)	6.8 ± 2.4
M5	16	14 (88)	25.1 ± 10.2	2 (12)	7.5 ± 4.9
M6	2	2 (100)	49.5 ± 24.7	0	–
CML-BC	13	12 (92)	34.6 ± 16.3	1 (8)	8.0
CML in chronic phase	9	2 (22)	22.5 ± 10.6	7 (78)	6.0 ± 2.9
ALL	99	59 (60)	29.2 ± 13.4	40 (40)	5.2 ± 3.3
0-ALL	10	4 (40)	35.0 ± 10.1	6 (60)	6.5 ± 3.0
c-ALL	62	45 (73)	29.6 ± 14.8	17 (27)	5.1 ± 3.2
B-ALL	2	1 (50)	63.0	1 (50)	0.0
T-ALL	25	9 (36)	20.7 ± 7.7	16 (64)	5.3 ± 3.4
B-CLL	13	6 (46)	16.2 ± 5.2	7 (54)	7.7 ± 2.9
LP-IC	4	3 (75)	42.3 ± 11.7	1 (25)	1.0
B-PLL	6	3 (50)	26.7 ± 4.5	3 (50)	6.0 ± 2.8
T-PLL	2	0	–	2 (100)	4.5 ± 6.3
HCL	4	1 (25)	14.0	3 (75)	5.7 ± 1.5
Total	252	155 (62)	28.8 ± 13.5	97 (38)	5.2 ± 3.2

Effector cells were induced from PBMC of normal donors incubated with recombinant IL-2 10^3 U/ml for 6 days. Cytotoxicity against different fresh noncultured leukemia cells was tested in a 4-h chromium release assay at four effector-to-target (ET) ratios. The results are given as percentage specific chromium release at an ET of 50:1. The values represent the mean ± standard deviation (SD) of independent experiments.
AML, acute myeloid leukemia; M1–M6, subtypes according to the FAB classification; CML-BC, chronic myelogenous leukemia in blast crisis; ALL, acute lymphoblastic leukemia; 0-ALL, null ALL; c-ALL, common ALL; B-ALL, ALL of B-cell type; T-ALL, ALL of T-cell type; B-CLL, B-cell chronic lymphocytic leukemia; LP-IC, lymphoplasmocytic immunocytoma; B-PLL, prolymphocytic leukemia of B-cell type; T-PLL, prolymphocytic leukemia of T-cell type; HCL, hairy cell leukemia.
[a] Number of samples susceptible to LAK cells (specific chromium release >11.12%).
[b] Number of samples not susceptible to LAK cells (specific chromium release ≤11.12%).
[c] Numbers in parentheses give percentage of total samples tested.

samples examined. Almost all samples of chronic myelogenous leukemia in blast crisis (CML-BC) proved to be susceptible to LAK cell lysis (12 of 13 samples, 92%). Comparison of the different immunologic subtypes of ALL revealed exceptionally high susceptibility (73%) for common ALLs, whereas T-cell ALLs and null ALLs seemed to be mostly resistant to LAK-cell-mediated lysis (Table 2, Fig. 1).

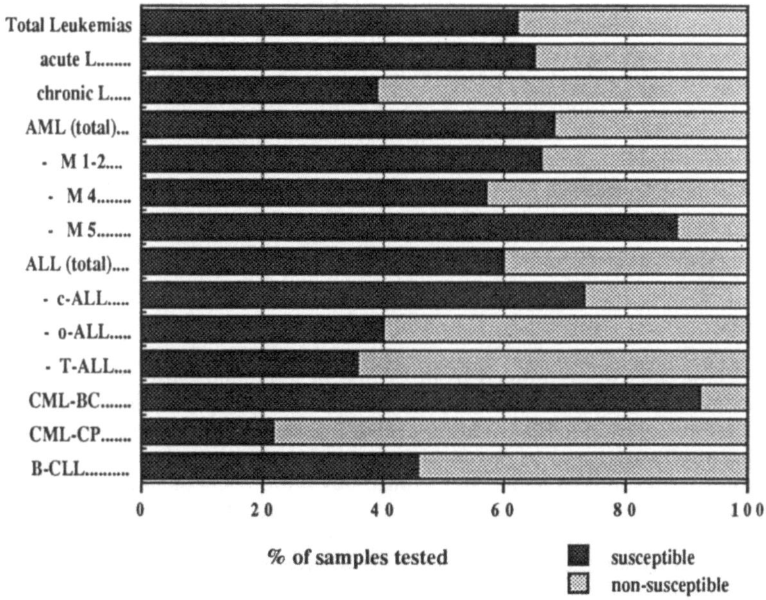

Fig. 1. Susceptibility of leukemia cells to allogeneic LAK cells. Effector cells were induced from PBMC of normal donors incubated with recombinant IL-2 10^3 U/ml for 6 days. Cytotoxicity against noncultured leukemia cells was tested in a 4-h chromium release assay. The relation is depicted between susceptible and nonsusceptible samples of the major leukemia subgroups. *acute L*, AML, ALL, and CML-BC; *chronic L*, CML-CP, B-CLL, LP-IC, B-PLL, T-PLL, HCL; for abbreviations, see footnote to Table 2

Susceptibility of Leukemic Cells to Autologous Lymphokine-Activated Killer Cells. In 40 acute leukemia patients (24 AML, 16 ALL), LAK cell activity against autologous leukemia cells isolated before treatment was examined during CR. Leukemia cells were found to be susceptible to the autologous LAK cells in 63% of the patients (75% AML, 44% ALL), whereas 37% developed no significant cytotoxicity against their autologous leukemic cells (Table 3). The cytotoxicity level achieved in terms of specific chromium release was 23.5% ± 11.0% for susceptible versus 3.9 ± 3.6% for resistant leukemias.

LAK cell activity of leukemia patients against their autologous leukemic cells can in many cases only be examined after CR is reached. Therefore, with a view to therapeutic considerations, we tried to determine whether the results of allogeneic tests allow a prediction of the results with autologous leukemia targets. Our analysis revealed that 20 of 25 samples (80%) were susceptible not only to allogeneic but also to autologous LAK cells, and 11 of 15 samples (73%) were resistant not only to allogeneic but also to autologous LAK cells (Table 4). Thus in 70%–80% of the samples a correct

Table 3. LAK cell cytotoxicity of patients with acute leukemia in complete remission (CR) against their autologous leukemia cells

Target cells	Total no. of samples	Cytotoxicity (% specific Cr release ET 50:1)			
		n (pos)[a]	% ± SD	*n* (neg)[b]	% ± SD
AML	24	18 (75)[c]	22.1 ± 9.3	6 (25)[c]	4.8 ± 3.6
ALL	16	7 (44)	27.1 ± 14.6	9 (56)	3.3 ± 3.7
c-ALL	9	5 (56)	32.2 ± 14.4	4 (44)	4.5 ± 4.4
T-ALL	7	2 (29)	14.5 ± 2.1	5 (71)	2.4 ± 3.3
Total	40	25 (63)	23.5 ± 11.0	15 (37)	3.9 ± 3.6

Effector cells were induced from PBMC of leukemia patients in CR incubated with recombinant IL-2 10^3 U/ml for 6 days. Cytotoxicity against their autologous leukemia cells was tested in a 4-h chromium release assay at four effector-to-target (ET) ratios. The results are given as percentage specific chromium release at an ET of 50:1. The values represent the mean ± standard deviation (SD) of independent experiments. AML, acute myeloid leukemia; ALL, acute lymphoblastic leukemia; c-ALL, common ALL; T-ALL, ALL of T-cell type.

[a] Number of samples susceptible to autologous LAK cells (specific chromium release >11.12%).

[b] Number of samples not susceptible to autologous LAK cells (specific chromium release ≤11.12%).

[c] Numbers in parentheses give percentage of total samples tested.

Table 4. Susceptibility of leukemia cells to allogeneic LAK cells compared with their susceptibility to autologous LAK cells from patients in complete remission

Effector cells	Number of samples				
	Susceptible (Cr release >11.12%) (+)		Nonsusceptible (Cr release ≤11.12%) (−)		Total
Allogeneic	25		15		40
	(+)	(−)	(+)	(−)	
Autologous	20	5	4	11	40
Predictive values	80%			73%	

The susceptibility of leukemia cells to LAK cells was tested in 40 patients with allogeneic and autologous effector cells; for details see "Material and Methods" and legends to Tables 2 and 3. The results of both test methods were compared.

prediction is possible of whether patients will develop relevant LAK-cell cytotoxicity to their autologous leukemia cells.

Augmentation of the Susceptibility of Leukemia Target Cells to LAK Cell Lysis by Exposure to Cytotoxic Drugs In Vitro. As demonstrated in Table 2,

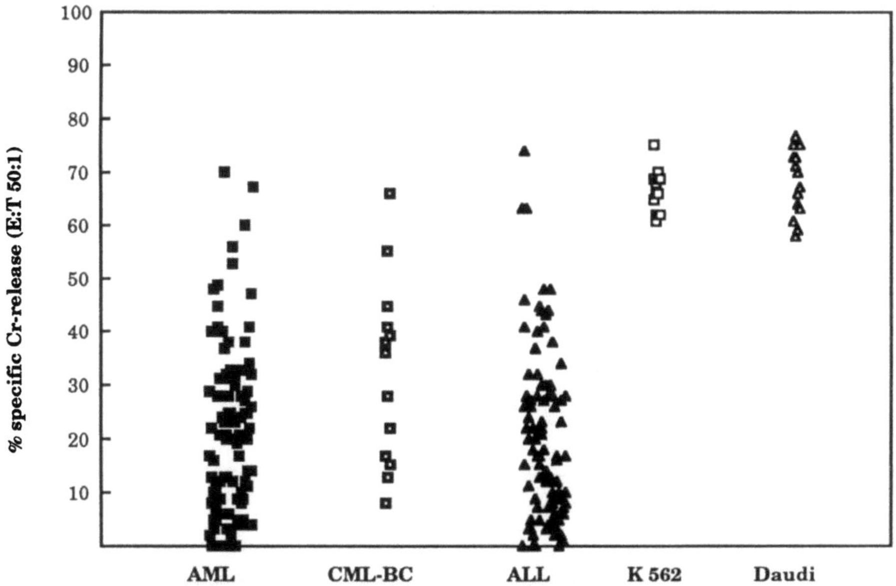

Fig. 2. Susceptibility of leukemic cells to allogeneic LAK cells. Fresh noncultured leukemia cells were compared to the K562 and Daudi cell lines. Effector cells were induced by incubating PBMC of normal donors with recombinant IL-2 10^3 U/ml for 6 days. Cytotoxicity was tested in a 4-h chromium release assay at four effector-to-target (ET) ratios. The results are given as percentage specific chromium release at an ET ratio of 50:1 (fresh leukemia cells) or 25:1 (K562, Daudi). *AML*, acute myeloid leukemia (n = 102); *CML-BC*, chronic myelogenous leukemia in blast crisis (n = 13); *ALL*, acute lymphoblastic leukemia (n = 99); K562 (n = 15); Daudi (n = 15)

the mean specific chromium release of fresh noncultured leukemic cells is about 30%. A survey of the individual cytotoxicity data (Fig. 2) revealed that chromium release of fresh noncultured leukemias varied considerably and only few leukemis reached a cytolysis comparable to that of cell lines. However, maximal cytolysis is desirable for therapy. Therefore the augmentation of susceptibility by treating leukemia cells with cytotoxic drugs was investigated.

Leukemia target cells were exposed to Ara-C and DNR in vitro for 18 h prior to the cytotoxicity assays. Incubation with Ara-C significantly augments the susceptibility of leukemia targets to LAK cell cytolysis (Fig. 3). It is remarkable that exposure of LAK-cell-resistant leukemia samples to Ara-C rendered them susceptible to the lytic action of LAK cells (Fig. 3b,e,f). These effects could not be observed with DNR which we studied in parallel (data not shown).

Augmentation of the Susceptibility of Leukemia Target Cells to LAK-Cell Lysis by Exposure to Cytotoxic Drugs In Vivo. In the light of the results

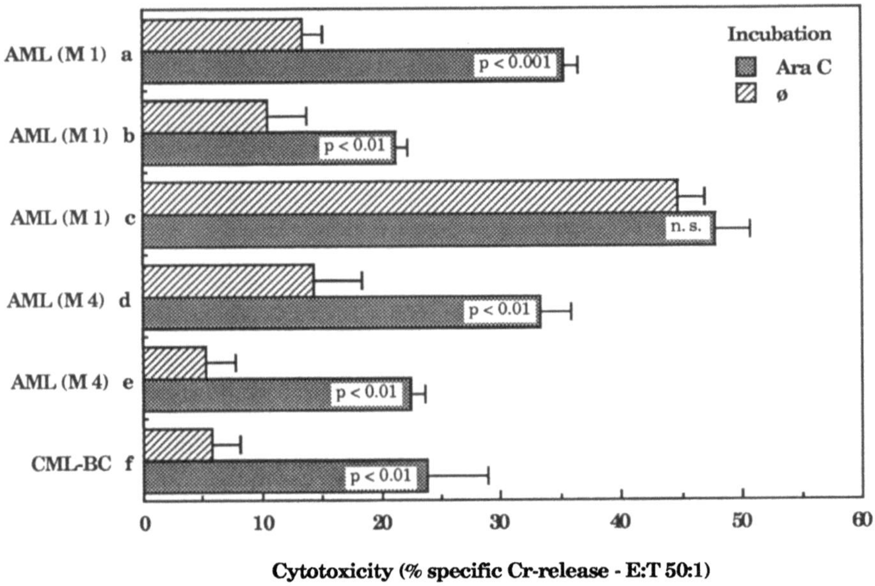

Fig. 3. Augmentation of the susceptibility of leukemia cells to LAK cell lysis by incubation with cytotoxic drugs. Effector cells were induced from PBMC of normal donors incubated with recombinant IL-2 10^3 U/ml for 6 days. The leukemia target cells were incubated without (Ø) or with Ara-C (5 µg/ml) 18 h prior to the cytotoxicity assay. The chromium release assays were performed at effector-to-target ratios of 100:1, 50:1, 25:1, and 12.5:1. The results are given as mean percentage specific chromium release ± standard deviation. *AML*, acute myeloid leukemia; *M1, M4*, subtypes of AML according to the FAB classification; *CML-BC*, chronic myelogenous leukemia in blast crisis; *n.s.*, not significant

obtained in vitro it was of utmost interest to examine whether the susceptibility of leukemia cells to LAK cell lysis would be augmented by in vivo exposure to cytotoxic drugs during induction therapy. Leukemia cells from AML patients were therefore collected during the first days of induction therapy, isolated, and cryopreserved. The cytotoxicity assays with the leukemia cells collected on different days were performed in parallel. It was observed that almost all series tested displayed a significant increase in the LAK cell susceptibility of leukemia cells during induction chemotherapy (Fig. 4 shows representative experiments).

Similar results could be observed with autologous LAK cells from a patient with AML in CR. As demonstrated in Fig. 5, the susceptibility of leukemia cells to autologous LAK cells was also significantly augmented during induction therapy with cytotoxic drugs.

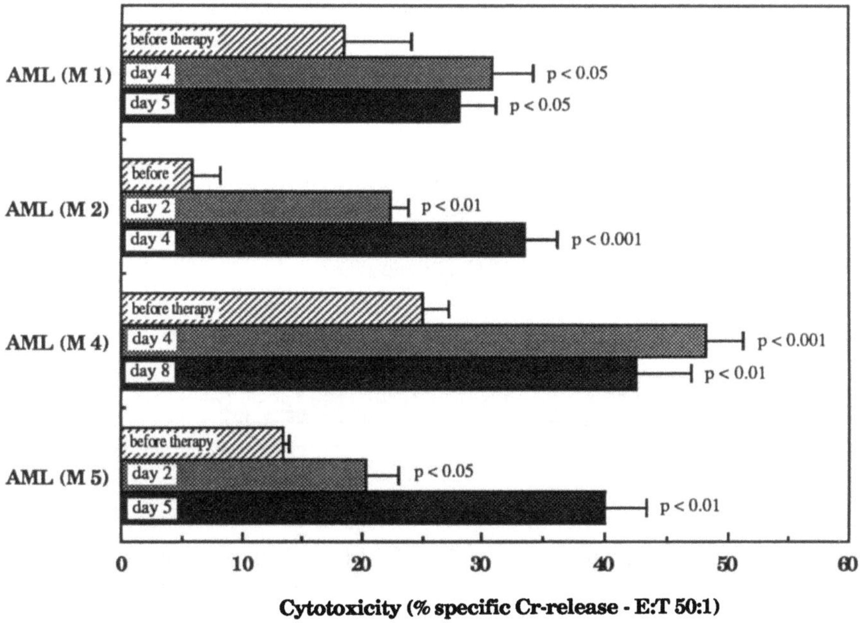

Fig. 4. Augmentation of the susceptibility of leukemia cells to LAK cell lysis by in vivo exposure of the target cells to cytotoxic drugs during induction chemotherapy according to the TAD-9 protocol. Effector cells were induced from PBMC of normal donors incubated with recombinant IL-2 10^3 U/ml for 6 days. The leukemia target cells were collected from patients with AML before therapy and on the specified days of therapy and cryopreserved until use. Susceptibility of the different target cell fractions to LAK cell lysis was tested in parallel. The chromium release assays were performed at effector-to-target ratios of 100:1, 50:1, 25:1, and 12.5:1. The results are given as mean percentage specific chromium release ± standard deviation. *AML*, acute myeloid leukemia; *M1–M5*, subtypes of AML according to the FAB classification. Significant differences between the susceptibility of the leukemia cells before therapy and on the given day of therapy. TAD-9 protocol: days 1 and 2, ara-C 100 mg/m^2 per 24 hours as continuous infusion; days 3–5, DNR 60 mg/m^2; days 3–8, ara-C 100 mg/m^2 per 12 hours as short-term infusion; days 3–9, thioguanine 100 mg/m^2 per 12 hours

Discussion

Systemic administration of IL-2 alone or combined with adoptive cellular immunotherapy using ex-vivo-generated LAK cells are known to be promising approaches in cancer therapy. There have been numerous clinical reports on solid tumors (Rosenberg et al. 1987; West et al. 1987; Fisher et al. 1988; Gambacorti-Passerini et al. 1988; Mitchell et al. 1988; Sosman et al. 1988; Dutcher et al. 1989), but there is still insufficient information available on the clinical significance of IL-2 and LAK cells in connection with human leukemia. As this type of immunotherapy is associated with

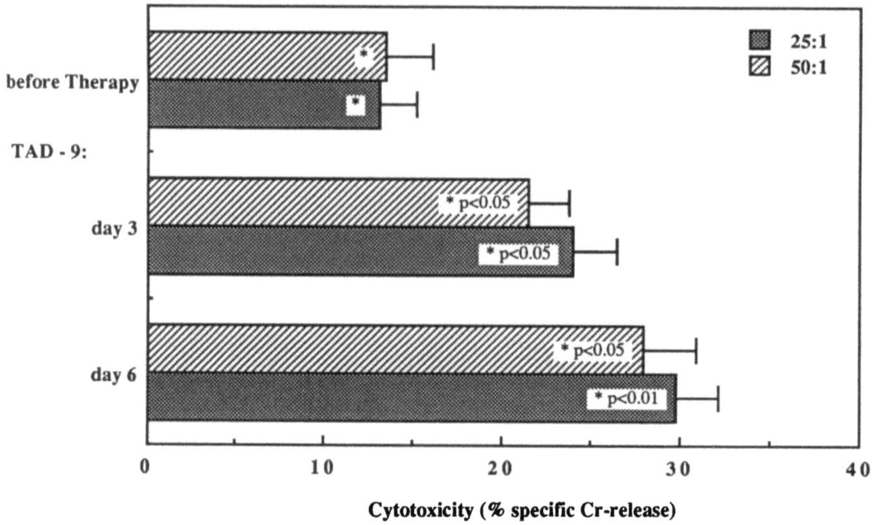

Fig. 5. Augmentation of the susceptibility of AML cells to autologous LAK cells by in vivo exposure of the target cells to cytotoxic drugs during induction chemotherapy according to the TAD-9 protocol. Autologous effector cells were induced from PBMC of a patient with AML during CR incubated with recombinant IL-2 10^3 U/ml for 6 dyas. The leukemia target cells were collected from the patient before therapy and on the specified days of therapy and cryopreserved until use. Susceptibility of the different target cell fractions to LAK cell lysis was tested in parallel. The chromium release assay was performed at effector-to-target ratios of 100:1, 50:1, 25:1, and 12.5:1. Depicted are the mean percentage specifc chromium release ± standard deviation at an ET ratio of 50:1 and 25:1.
* Significant differences between the susceptibility of leukemia cells before therapy and on day 3 and 6 of therapy. TAD-9 protocol: days 1 and 2, ara-C 100 mg/m^2 per 24 hours as continuous infusion; days 3–5, DNR 60 mg/m^2; days 3–8 ara-C 100 mg/m^2 per 12 hours as short-term infusion; days 3–9 thioguanine, 100 mg/m^2 per 12 hours.

considerable toxicity, criteria should be found for determining which patients it may benefit. This study therefore aimed at investigating the differential susceptibility of leukemia subtypes towards lytic effects of allogeneic and autologous LAK cells.

The degree of cytotoxicity achieved in the interaction between effector and target cells depends not only on the cytotoxic activity of the effector cells but also on the target-cell's distinctive features, which are still not known in detail. Expression of intercellular adhesion molecules by the tumor cells may play a role in this connection (Rothlein et al. 1986; Billaud et al. 1987; Marlin and Springer 1987; Boyed et al. 1988, 1989). There is no generally accepted definition of the "susceptibility" of a given target cell sample to cytotoxic effector cells; some authors arbitrarily define a certain percentage of chromium release as their threshold value for susceptible/

nonsusceptible, e.g., 6% or 10% (Rayner et al. 1985; Itoh et al. 1986; Panayotides et al. 1988; Allavena et al. 1989; van der Harst et al. 1989), while others seem to regard all specific chromium release >0% as relevant (Oshimi et al. 1986; Fierro et al. 1988). Since LAK cells are known to exert little or no cytotoxic influence on normal nonmalignant cells (Oshimi et al. 1986; Sondel et al. 1986; Djeu and Blanchard 1988; Agah et al. 1989), their cytolytic effect on normal bone-marrow cells seems to be appropriate for defining LAK cell "susceptibility" of leukemic cells. A clinically relevant comparison can thus be made to determine whether malignant hemopoietic cells are more susceptible to LAK cell cytolysis than normal bone-marrow cells. The "susceptibility" of a given leukemia sample was defined on the basis of the chromium release achieved by allogeneic LAK cells from 52 samples of normal bone-marrow cells (Table 1). The upper limit of the 99% confidence interval was used as threshold value for defining "susceptibility" of leukemia cells to the lytic activity of LAK cells. All leukemia samples with chromium releases >11.12% (ET 50:1) are considered susceptible to LAK cell cytolysis.

In the current study, investigating the susceptibility of 252 samples of different leukemias from untreated patients, we observed that 62% of the leukemias are susceptible and 38% resistant to LAK cell lysis (Table 2). The mean cytotoxicity in terms of the specific chromium release (ET 50:1) was 28.8 ± 13.5% for susceptible versus 5.2 ± 3.2% for resistant samples. These results are in contrast to reports indicating susceptibility of most leukemias to LAK cell cytolysis (Oshimi et al. 1986; Fierro et al. 1988). The discrepancies may be due to differences in the numbers of leukemias examined and the definition of "susceptibility" applied, as already discussed. There have been no studies with sufficient leukemia samples for analysis of the differential susceptibility of leukemia subgroups. Our study makes it possible to analyze certain different subgroups. The frequency of susceptible samples is considerably higher (65%) from acute leukemias or CML-BC than from chronic leukemias (39%), as demonstrated in Fig. 1. This may be connected with the stage of differentiation, as ALL in the primitive stages were shown to be more susceptible than those in mature differentiation stages (Oshimi et al. 1986). Within the group of acute leukemias, no significant differences could be observed between AML and ALL. Analysis of AML according to the different FAB subgroups revealed that the frequency of susceptible samples was average for M1/M2 and M4 leukemias (66% and 57%) but considerably higher for M5 (88%). Samples from CML-BC were extraordinarily often susceptible to LAK cell lysis (92%). When considering the different immunologic subtypes of ALL, we observed a 73% susceptibility of common ALLs to LAK-cell-mediated lysis, whereas T-cell ALLs and null ALLs seem to be mainly resistant (Table 2, Fig. 1). The finding of differential susceptibilities in various leukemia subtypes is particularly relevant for therapeutic considerations and may help to define patients who can benefit from immunologic therapy modalities.

The most important question is whether acute leukemia patients in CR are able to develop significant cytotoxic activity against their autologous leukemia cells. As demonstrated in Table 3, the leukemia cells of 63% of the patients (AML 75%, ALL 44%) were found to be susceptible to autologous LAK cells. In other words, these patients developed considerable LAK cell activity against their autologous leukemia cells during CR. As cytotoxicity assays with autologous effector cells from leukemia patients are difficult to perform during active disease, we tried to determine whether the results of the allogeneic and autologous tests are related. The analysis of our data revealed that examinations with allogeneic LAK cells can correctly predict the development of autologous LAK cell activity in 70%–80%of cases (Table 4). These observations are interesting, particularly in determining which patients may benefit from immunologic therapy modalities and in scheduling immunotherapy.

In this study it was observed that the LAK cell susceptibility of fresh noncultured leukemia cells varies considerably and that cytolysis is substantially lower for fresh leukemias than for leukemia cell lines (Fig. 2). For therapy, maximal cytolysis by activated effector cells would be desirable. Studies designed to improve susceptibility of fresh leukemia target cells to cytolytic effector cells are therefore essential. As previous studies have suggested that some anticancer agents increase tumor-cell sensitivity to NK cells, cytotoxic T cells, or macrophages (Kunkel and Welsh 1981; Ziegler-Heitbrock et al. 1983; Colotta et al. 1984; Uchida and Klein 1985; Leroux et al. 1986; Lichtenstein and Pende 1986; Nagarkatti et al. 1988), our investigations attempted to determine whether cytotoxic drugs used in leukemia treatment augment the susceptibility of human leukemia cells to LAK cells. The results showed that incubating leukemia cells from AML or CML-BC with Ara-C significantly increases their susceptibility to LAK cell cytolysis (Fig. 3). It is noteworthy that this augmentation by Ara-C renders some resistant leukemias susceptible to the lytic LAK cell effect. However, incubating leukemia cells with DNR prior to the cytotoxicity test does not augment their susceptibility to LAK cells.

Our observation that leukemia cell susceptibility to LAK cells is augmented by in vitro incubation of the target cells with cytotoxic agents led us to study whether it would also increase during induction therapy with cytotoxic drugs used in the TAD-9 protocol. The results demonstrate significantly increased susceptibility of AML cells in most samples tested (Fig. 4). Moreover, pretreatment insensitive leukemia cells became susceptible to LAK-cell-mediated cytolysis during chemotherapy. However, which of the drugs applied (Ara-C, DNR, thioguanine) is in fact responsible for augmenting the susceptibility of leukemic cells cannot be determined. These observations could be reproduced in one patient using autologous LAK cells generated during CR. The leukemic cells of this patient became significantly more susceptible to autologous LAK cells during induction therapy than before treatment (Fig. 5). These findings are of interest in relation to the clinical application of IL-2 or IL-2 induced LAK cells, particularly if cytotoxic agents are combined with immunotherapeutic approaches during maintenance therapy in order to eliminate residual leukemia cells. In this respect, important findings from murine models have shown that a combination of chemotherapy with adoptive immunotherapy or in vivo IL-2 application eliminates some disseminated tumors more effectively than either chemotherapy or immunotherapy alone (Ades et al. 1987; Salup et al. 1987). Further studies in a murine system indicate that the synergistic effect of the two treatment modalities consists in a reduction of the tumor load by chemotherapy, an augmentation of tumor cell susceptibility to cell-mediated cytotoxicity, and a reduction of suppressor cell activity by chemotherapy (Papa et al. 1988).

In conclusion, we have shown that human leukemia cells have a distinct susceptibility to LAK-cell-mediated cytolysis. Cytotoxic drugs, relevant for leukemia treatment, augment leukemia cell susceptibility to LAK cells in vitro, and, more importantly, exposure of leukemia cells to anticancer agents in vivo during induction chemotherapy also increases their sensitivity to the lytic effect of LAK cells. These observations are encouraging for the possibility of combining chemotherapy with immunotherapeutic approaches. As the clinical response to immunotherapy is probably related to the tumor burden, such combined modalities will be most effective in situations when the leukemia mass is small, for example in minimal residual disease (MRD). Patients with acute leukemia in CR seem to be the most suitable candidates for chemoimmunotherapy. Combining conventional maintenance chemotherapy with IL-2/LAK cell therapy or IL-2 alone may help to eliminate MRD in an attempt to prevent relapses and possibly augment the cure rate of leukemia. Future clinical trials will have to clarify their potential value and determine the best schedules of these therapeutic approaches.

Acknowledgements. These studies were supported by grant W 19/87/Te 1 from the Deutsche Krebshilfe e.V./Mildred Scheel Stiftung für Krebsforschung, Bonn, FRG. The authors wish to thank the Glaxo Institute for Molecular Biology, Geneva, Switzerland, for the generous gift of recombinant IL-2 and the participants of the ALL/AUL-BMFT trials and ALL-BFM trials for fruitful cooperation. The skillful technical assistance of Mrs. G. Bochert and Mrs. A. Maass and the valuable help of J. Weirowski, Ph.D., in preparing the manuscript are gratefully acknowledged.

References

Ades EW, McKemie III CR, Wright S, Peacocke N, Pantazis C, Lockhart III WL (1987) Chemotherapy subsequent to recombinant interleukin-2 immunotherapy: protocol for enhanced tumoricidal activity. Nat Immun Cell Growth Regul 6:260–268

Agah R, Malloy B, Kerner M, Mazumder A (1989) Generation and characterization of IL-2-activated bone marrow cells as a potent graft vs tumor effector in transplantation. J Immunol 143:3093–3099
Allavena P, Damia G, Colombo T, Maggioni D, D'Incalci M, Mantovani A (1989) Lymphokine-activated killer (LAK) and monocyte-mediated cytotoxicity on tumor cell lines resistant to antitumor agents. Cell Immunol 120:250–258
Billaud M, Calender A, Seigneurin JM, Lenoir GM (1987) LFA-1, LFA-3, and ICAM-1 expression in Burkitt's lymphoma. Lancet II:1327–1328
Boyed AW, Wawryk SO, Burns GF, Fecondo JV (1988) Intercellular adhesion molecule-1 (ICAM-1) has a central role in cell-cell contact mediated immune mechanisms. Proc Natl Acad Sci USA 85:3095–3099
Boyed AW, Dunn SM, Fecondo JV, Culvenor JG, Duehrsen U, Burns GF, Wawryk SO (1989) Regulation of expression of a human intercellular adhesion molecule (ICAM-1) during lymphohematopoietic differentiation. Blood 73:1896–1903
Buechner T, Hiddemann W, Maschmeyer G, Ludwig WD, Loeffler H, Nowrousian M, Aul C, Heinecke A (1990) How to improve therapy for adult acute myeloid leukemia: studies of the AML Cooperative Group in the Federal Republic of Germany. J Cancer Res Clin Oncol 116:97–99
Colotta F, Peri G, Villa A, Mantovani A (1984) Rapid killing of actinomycin D-treated tumor cells by human mononuclear cells. J Immunol 132:936–944
Djeu JY, Blanchard DK (1988) Lysis of human monocytes by lymphokine-activated killer cells. Cell Immunol 111:55–65
Dutcher JP, Creekmore S, Weiss GR, Margolin K, Markowitz AB, Roper M, Parkinson D, Ciobanu N, Fisher RI, Boldt DH, Doroshow JH, Rayner AA, Hawkins M, Atkins M (1989) A phase II study of interleukin-2 and lymphokine-activated killer cells in patients with metastatic malignant melanoma. J Clin Oncol 7:477–485
Fierro MT, Liao XS, Lusso P, Bonferroni M, Matera L, Cesano A, Lista P, Arione R, Forni G, Foa R (1988) In vitro and in vivo susceptibility of human leukemic cells to lymphokine activated killer activity. Leukemia 2:50–54
Fisher RI, Coltman CA, Doroshow JH, Rayner AA, Hawkins MJ, Mier JW, Wiernik P, McMannis JD, Weiss GR, Margolin KA, Gemlo BT, Hoth DF, Parkinson DR, Paietta E (1988) Metastatic renal cancer treated with interleukin-2 and lymphokine-activated killer cells. Ann Intern Med 108:518–523
Gambacorti-Passerini C, Radrizzani M, Marolda R, Belli F, Sciorelli G, Galazka AR, Schindler JD, Cascinelli N, Parmiani G (1988) In vivo activation of lymphocytes in melanoma patients receiving escalating doses of recombinant interleukin-2. Int J Cancer 41:700–706
Grimm EA, Mazumder A, Zhang HZ, Rosenberg SA (1982) Lymphokine-activated killer cell phenomenon. Lysis of natural killer-resistant fresh solid tumor cells by interleukin 2-activated autologous human peripheral blood lymphocytes. J Exp Med 155:1823–1841
Herberman RB, Hiserodt JC, Vujanovic N, Balch CM, Lotzová E, Bolhuis R, Golub S, Lanier LL, Phillips JH, Riccardi C, Ritz J, Santoni A, Schmidt RE, Uchida A (1987) Lymphokine-activated killer cell activity. Characteristics of effector cells and their progenitors in blood and spleen. Immunol Today 8:178–181
Itoh K, Tilden AB, Balch CM (1986) Lysis of human solid tumor cells by lymphokine-activated natural killer cells. J Immunol 136:3910–3915
Kunkel LA, Welsh RM (1981) Metabolic inhibitors render "resistant" target cells sensitive to natural killer cell-mediated lysis. Int J Cancer 27:73–79
Leroux JY, Mercier G, Oth D (1986) Enhancement of murine lymphoma cell lysability by CTL and by LAK cells after treatments with mitomycin C and with adriamycin. Int J Immunopharmacol 8:369–375

Lichtenstein A, Pende KD (1986) Enhancement of natural killer cytotoxicity by cis-diammine-dichloroplatinum (II) in vivo and in vitro. Cancer Res 46:639–644
Lotzová E, Savary CA, Herberman RB (1987) Induction of NK cell activity against fresh human leukemia in culture with interleukin 2. J Immunol 138:2718–2727
Ludwig WD, Bartram CR, Ritter J, Raghavachar A, Hiddemann W, Heil G, Harbott J, Seibt-Jung H, Teichmann JV, Riehm H (1988) Ambiguous phenotypes and genotypes in 16 children with acute leukemia as characterized by multi-parameter analysis. Blood 71:1518–1528
Marlin SD, Springer TA (1987) Purified intercellular adhesion molecule-1 (ICAM-1) is a ligand for lymphocyte function-associated antigen-1 (LFA-1). Cell 51:813–819
Mitchell MS, Kempf RA, Harel W, Shau H, Boswell WD, Lind S, Bradley EC (1988) Effectiveness and tolerability of low-dose cyclophosphamide and low-dose intravenous interleukin-2 in disseminated melanoma. J Clin Oncol 6:409–424
Nagarkatti M, Nagarkatti PS, Kaplan AM (1988) Differential effects of BCNU on T cell, macrophage, natural killer and lymphokine-activated killer cell activities in mice bearing a syngeneic tumor. Caner Immunol Immunother 27:38–46
Oshimi K, Oshimi Y, Akutsu M, Takei Y, Saito H, Okada M, Mizoguchi H (1986) Cytotoxicity of interleukin-2-activated lymphocytes for leukemia and lymphoma cells. Blood 68:938–948
Panayotides P, Porwit A, Sjögren AM, Wasserman J, Reizenstein P (1988) Resistance of some leukemic blasts to lysis by lymphokine activated killer (LAK) cells. Eur J Haematol 40:362–367
Papa MZ, Yang JC, Vetto JT, Shiloni E, Eisenthal A, Rosenberg SA (1988) Combined effects of chemotherapy and interleukin-2 in the therapy of mice with advanced pulmonary tumors. Cancer Res 48:122–129
Phillips JH, Lanier LL (1986) Dissection of the lymphokine-activated killer phenomenon. Relative contribution of peripheral blood natural killer cells and T lymphocytes to cytolysis. J Exp Med 164:814–825
Pross HF, Baines MG, Rubin P, Shragge P, Patterson MS (1981) Spontaneous human lymphocyte-mediated cytotoxicity against tumor target cells. IX. The quantitation of natural killer cell activity. J Clin Immunol 1:51–63
Rayner AA, Grimm EA, Lotze MT, Chu EW, Rosenberg SA (1985) Lymphokine-activated killer (LAK) cells. Analysis of factors relevant to the immunotherapy of human cancer. Cancer 55:1327–1333
Rosenberg SA, Lotze MT, Muul LM, Chang AE, Avis FP, Leitman S, Linehan WM, Robertson CN, Lee RE, Rubin JT, Seipp CA, Simpson C, White DE (1987) A progress report on the treatment of 157 patients with advanced cancer using lymphokine-activated killer cells and interleukin-2 or high-dose interleukin-2 alone. N Engl J Med 316:889–897
Rothlein R, Dustin ML, Marlin SD, Springer TA (1986) A human intercellular adhesion molecule (ICAM-1) distinct from LFA-1. J Immunol 137:1270–1274
Saito H, Oshimi K, Oshimi Y, Mizoguchi H (1988) Characterization of interleukin 2-expanded human peripheral blood lymphocytes: Not only NKH-1^+ NK cells but also NKH-1^+ and NKH-1^- T cells are LAK effectors. Cell Immunol 117:253–263
Salup RR, Back TC, Wiltrout RH (1987) Successful treatment of advanced murine renal cell cancer by bicompartmental adoptive chemoimmunotherapy. J Immunol 138:641–647
Sondel PM, Hank JA, Kohler PC, Chen BP, Minkoff DZ, Molenda JA (1986) Destruction of autologous human lymphocytes by interleukin-2-activated cytotoxic cells. J Immunol 137:502–511
Sosman JA, Kohler PC, Hank J, Moor KH, Bechhofer R, Storer B, Sondel PM (1988) Repetitive weekly cycles of recombinant human interleukin-2: responses of renal carcinoma with acceptable toxicity. J Natl Cancer Inst 80:60–63

Teichmann JV, Ludwig WD, Seibt-Jung H, Thiel E (1989) Induction of lymphokine-activated killer (LAK) cells against human leukemia cells in vitro. Blut 59:21–24
Teichmann JV, Ludwig W-D, Thiel E (1992) Susceptibility of human leukemia to allogeneic and autologous lymphokine-activated killer cells in an analysis of 252 samples. Nat Immun 11:117–132
Thiel E, Kranz BR, Raghavachar A, Bartram CR, Löffler H, Messerer D, Ganser A, Ludwig WD, Büchner T, Hoelzer D (1989) Prethymic phenotype and genotype of pre-T (CD $7^+/ER^-$) – cell leukemia and its clinical significance within adult acute lymphoblastic leukemia. Blood 73:1247–1258
Tilden AB, Itoh K, Balch CM (1987) Human lymphokine-activated killer (LAK) cells: identification of two types of effector cells. J Immunol 138:1068–1073
Uchida A, Klein E (1985) Natural cytotoxicity of human blood monocytes and natural killer cells and their cytotoxic factors: discriminating effects of actinomycin D. Int J Cancer 35:691–699
van der Harst D, Brand A, van Luxemburg-Heys SAP, Kooy-Winkelaar EMC, van Rood JJ (1989) Lymphokine-activated killer cell functions in patients with leukemic B-lympho-proliferative diseases. Blood 74:2464–2470
West WH, Tauer KW, Yannelli JR, Marshall GD, Orr DW, Thurman GB, Oldham RK (1987) Constant infusion of recombinant interleukin-2 in adoptive immunotherapy of advanced cancer. N Engl J Med 316:898–905
Ziegler-Heitbrock HWL, Erhardt J, Riethmüller G (1983) Treatment of fresh human leukaemia cells with actinomycin D enhances their lysability by natural killer cells. Br J Cancer 48:507–514

V. Immunophenotypic and Molecular Genetic Characterization of Acute Lymphoblastic Leukemia: Biological and Clinical Implications

Regulation of Protooncogenes and Cytokine Genes in Acute Lymphoblastic Leukemia

H. Tesch[1], M. Jücker[1], H. Abts, R. Laumann[1], W.-D. Ludwig[2] and I. Pahl[1]

[1] Medizinische Klinik I, Universität Köln, W-5000 Cologne, Fed. Rep. of Germany
[2] Department of Hematology and Oncology, Universitaätsklinikum Steglitz, Free University of Berlin, W-1000 Berlin 45, Fed. Rep. of Germany

Introduction

It is assumed that both inherited and environmental factors may be responsible for the induction of a leukemia by various mechanisms. These events include mutations, insertional events, translocations, defects of DNA repair mechanisms, and immune suppression. Also, lymphotropic viruses of the herpesvirus group such as Epstein-Barr virus (EBV) and retroviruses like human T-lymphotropic virus type I (HTLV-I) are candidates in leukemogenesis. The genes which are the targets of these events include cellular oncogenes, tumor suppressor genes, and cytokine and cytokine receptor genes.

Oncogenes have been implicated in the generation and/or maintenance of neoplastic cells (Weinberg 1989). Their cellular counterparts, protooncogenes, were shown to be involved in the regulation of growth and differentiation in normal cells. The genes were originally described in acute transforming retroviruses. Later studies revealed that the genes were transduced from cellular sequences called cellular oncogenes or protooncogenes, which are highly conserved genes during evolution. Another group of oncogenes have been detected by transfection experiments into nonmalignant fibroblast cell lines. Today, more than 60 cellular oncogenes have been described and the list is still expanding.

Finally, it has been suggested that genes which are not expressed in the tumor cells but are present in nontransformed cells, the so-called tumor suppressor genes or antioncogenes, may also play a role in leukemogenesis (Weinberg 1989). Additional cellular genes may be responsible for the deregulated growth and differentiation of the malignant cells. These genes include cytokine and cytokine receptor genes, which are involved in proliferation and differentiation of the normal counterparts of the leukemic cells.

We would like to discuss here some of the evidence and some hypotheses about how these genes are involved in the biology of acute lymphoblastic leukemia (ALL).

Chromosomal Translocations

More than 15 consistently occurring chromosomal translocations have been identified in ALL. The chromosomal aberrations include a number of translocations which involve both protooncogenes and antigen receptor genes. The translocations can be divided into two categories (Table 1).

In the first type the translocation leads to the juxtaposition of an oncogene and one of the genes which encode for the antigen receptors on B or T cells. The best-studied type of this translocation is the Ig/*myc* translocation in Burkitt's lymphoma (BL) (Leder et al. 1983). Other examples of such translocations involve the *bcl2* gene in follicular lymphomas (Tsujimoto et al. 1984), *lyl1*, which codes for a DNA binding protein and is joined with T-cell receptor β (TCRβ) genes in the t(7;19) translocation in T-ALL, *ttg*, which also codes for a DNA binding protein and is translocated into the TCRδ locus in the t(11;14) translocation in certain T-ALL (McGuire et al. 1989), and the IL-3 lymphokine gene (in the t(5;14) translocation the J_H gene is joined with the promoter region of the IL-3 gene in opposite transcriptional orientations in a B-lineage ALL).

The second class of translocations leads to the formation of a fusion gene and to a chimeric protein which expresses an altered function not present in the original gene. The best-studied translocation of this type which is also very frequent in ALL is the t(9;22) translocation which leads to the formation

Table 1. Translocations in human leukemia

Type	Genes involved	Product	Examples
I	Antigen receptor gene + cellular oncogene	Deregulation of oncogene	Ig/c-*myc* Ig/*bcl2* Ig/*bcl1* TCRβ/*lyl1* TCRδ/*ttg1* J_H/IL-3
II	Cellular oncogene + cellular gene	Chimeric protein	*bcr*/c-*abl* *prl1*/*E2a*

Table 2. Model of the development of Burkitt's lymphoma and B-ALL

Step 1	Step 2	Step 3
Suppression of helper T cells: malaria (Africa), HIV-1	Oligoclonal B cell activation: IL-6	Monoclonal B cell tumor: translocation Ig/c-*myc*

of the Philadelphia chromosome. Similar translocations occur in chronic myeloid leukemia (CML). However, whereas in CML the translocation result in an 8.5-kilobase (kb) messenger (m)RNA and a 210-kDa protein, in ALL a 7-kb transcript results in a 190-kDa fusion protein. In CML most of the breakpoints are clustered in the major breakpoint region in the body of the *bcr* gene, but are widely dispersed over 100 kb of the c-*abl* gene. Using the polymerase chain reaction method it is possible to detect the fusion transcripts with a high sensitivity and to differentiate clearly between the CML blast crisis and the Ph^+ ALL. Maurer and colleagues showed that 77/179 adults with ALL carried *bcr*/*abl* transcripts, which were restricted to B-precursor leukemias. There was a correlation between the presence of these transcripts and poor overall survival and remission duration (Maurer et al. 1991). In children with ALL 6% of primary and 17% of recurrent leukemias carried the translocation.

Also in this second group is the t(1;19) translocation which occurs in pre-B ALL. The translocation leads to the formation of a 85-kDa fusion protein. The genes joined in this translocation are the *E2a* gene, which codes for enhancer binding transcription factors E12 and E47. In the translocation the DNA binding domain of *E2a* is replaced by the putative DNA binding domain of the second gene, called *prl-1* for pre-B cell leukemia, which contains a homeodomain. The *E2a* gene was found to be rearranged in 10/10 ALL with the t(1;19) translocation (Nourse et al. 1990).

The 8;14 translocation is implicated in B-cell ALL. This translocation is also found together with the variant translocations 2;8 and 8;22 in all BL cases and in a high number of patients with acquired immune deficiency syndrome (AIDS). However, it is not clear how the translocations lead to the transformation. A current model is shown in Table 2.

One assumes that several steps are involved in the tumor. The first event may be in African-type BL immunosuppression – it is known that the African type of BL is associated with malaria – which leads to suppression of T cells. In AIDS patients the suppression of T cells is caused most likely by the human immunodeficiency virus (HIV) itself, which infects and eliminates CD4-positive T cells. The next step could be the polyclonal proliferation of B cells, which can be detected in large proportion of AIDS patients. This polyclonal proliferation could be induced by viral or by cellular factors. A candidate gene possibly involved is the IL-6 gene, since high IL-6 serum levels are found in HIV-infected patients during the later stages. In the third step, the translocation event, involving the Ig and the c-*myc* gene, occurs; this affects one clone, and this clone is positively selected and carries the malignant phenotype. Whether this scenario is really true is not known at present. There is, however, good evidence that the translocation event is necessary but not sufficient for the generation of the tumor. This evidence comes from experiments in transgenic mice where several authors have shown that the deregulated c-*myc* gene alone, when expressed in all B cells, leads only rarely to B cell tumors, and so additional events must have occurred.

Activation of Protein Kinase Genes

We were especially interested in such additional events and therefore looked for genes which might cooperate with c-*myc*. In a series of BL cell lines with the 8;14 translocation northern blot analyses were performed. Hybridization with a c-*fes*-specific probe revealed the expression of a short mRNA of 1.0 kb, whereas the mature c-*fes* transcripts of myeloid and monocytic cells are 3.0 kb in size. These short transcripts were found in 6/12 BL lines. Southern blot, pulsed field gel electrophoresis, and cytogenetic experiments did not show any difference from normal cells in the c-*fes* locus, thus it is unlikely that the transcripts are due to translocation or insertional events (M. Jücker et al., submitted for publication).

To further characterize the structure of the truncated c-*fes* transcripts we isolated in cooperation with W. van de Ven, Leuven, (isolated) complementary (c)DNA clones from a Hodgkin cell line. There is no point mutation present in the sequence. S1 experiments revealed that the truncated transcripts start within exon 16 and encode a part but not the entire kinase domain. We could also demonstrate a DNAse I hypersensitive site 5′ in exon 16 in the cells which express the short transcripts, indicating the presence of a cryptic promoter (M. Jücker et al., submitted for publication). When a cDNA clone was translated in vitro a 17-kDa c-*fes*-specific protein could be identified which encompasses the phosphotransfer motif and the tyrosine which serves as a phosphoacceptor site during auto-phosphorylation. Since the 17-kDa c-*fes* protein lacks the ATP binding site which is required for full kinase activity it is unlikely that a functional protein kinase is encoded by the truncated c-*fes* trancript (M. Jücker et al., submitted for publication). At present we are investigating the function of the protein in more detail. In ALL we have not so far detected these transcripts. Northern blots, however, show expression of the mature 3.0-kb transcript in some ALL (data not shown).

Expression of the normal c-*fes* transcripts was detected in some common ALL, pre-B ALL, and progenitor ALL. This is in contrast with results from other groups and we are currently performing single cell analyses to rule out contamination by monocytic cells. In normal cells expression of c-*fes* is restricted to monocytes and cannot be detected in lymphoid cells.

A large group of protooncogenes encode protein tyrosine kinases. Within this group, *lck* and c-*fgr* seem to be involved in growth and/or differentiation of lymphocytes. Both c-*fgr* and *lck* belong to the *src* gene family, which shows a conserved intron–exon structure and varies only in the N-terminal exons of c-*fgr*, *lck*, and c-*src*; these genes have thus probably evolved from an ancestral gene by exon shuffling. In normal tissues, *lck* and c-*fgr* show a distinct pattern of expression. The *lck* gene encodes a 56-kDa protein and is normally expressed exclusively in cells of lymphoid lineage, predominantly in T lymphocytes. The c-*fgr* gene encodes a 58-kDa protein ($p58^{c\text{-}fgr}$) and is expressed in mature peripheral blood monocytes and granulocytes and in alveolar and splenic macrophages.

Investigation of *lck* expression in the ALL cells by northern analysis revealed in all cases a single 2.2-kb *lck*-specific mRNA species, as expected in most T-ALL but also in some common ALL and B-ALL. In addition, we have seen expression of *lck* in most BL and chronic lymphocytic leukemia (CLL) cells (Jücker et al. 1991a; Abts et al. 1991). Although the number of T cells in the leukemic cell population is drastically reduced, at least some of the *lck* mRNA detected could be due to contaminating T cells. To test this hypothesis the CD3-positive T cells were depleted by magnetic sorting in two cases with CLL. Although the amount of T cells was reduced to 1%, no corresponding decrease of *lck* mRNA was observed, suggesting that *lck* mRNA was indeed produced by the malignant B cells.

c-*fgr* mRNA was not detected in ALL, except in one case with B-ALL. However, in all 21 cases with CLL significant amounts of c-*fgr* mRNA were detected. In normal B cells no c-*fgr* or *lck* mRNA could be detected (Tesch et al. 1989). Both *lck* and c-*fgr* belong to the of nonreceptor-type tyrosine kinases since they lack transmembrane or ligand-binding domains. These kinases are most likely involved in signal transduction and must therefore interact with other membrane proteins. The recent observation that the gene product of *lck* ($p56^{lck}$) is capable of forming complexes with the CD4 and CD8 antigens in T lymphocytes is the first demonstrated example of such an interaction (Veilette et al. 1989). Thus, in MHC-mediated stimulation of T cells with antigen the *lck* kinase could phosphorylate molecules of the CD3 complex and thus lead to signal transduction. This demonstrates that nonreceptor tyrosine kinases are involved in the growth control of normal T cells and maybe also of malignant B and T lymphocytes.

Tumor Suppressor Genes

Alterations within the coding sequence of the p53 tumor suppressor genes are among the most frequent genetic changes that have been observed in human cancer. Current data indicate that half or more of adult cancers of the lung, breast, colon, prostate, esophagus, and skin contain p53 mutations. The nuclear phosphoprotein p53 was initially classified as the product of an oncogene; however, more recent evidence has suggested that p53 is a tumor suppressor or anti-oncogene: First, p53 binds to DNA tumor virus proteins, including SV40 T and adenovirus Elb proteins. Secondly, compared to nontumor tissues there is a frequent loss of heterozygosity at the p53 locus in human tumors and the second allele is almost always mutated. Thirdly, the wild-type p53 protein expresses growth suppressive activity in various tumor systems. Mutations within the conserved regions of the p53 coding sequence induce conformational changes which extend the half-life of the mutated protein, which is then detectable in the tumor cells.

We have stained fresh ALL cells with p53-specific monoclonal antibodies and can detect high levels of expression. By contrast, in some cases with AML no p53 protein was detected, whereas the cells expressed the antigen Ki67, which is a good marker for proliferating cells. In northern blot analyses p53 mRNA was present in most but not all ALL cells. In four cases of common ALL and one case of 0-ALL there was no message for the gene.

The p53 gene is highly conserved in evolution and five domains have 90% sequence homology between humans and rodents. The majority of the mutations occur in the conserved domains in exons 5–8, with some hotspots where the mutations are very frequent. Some of these mutational hotspots are associated with certain malignancies and are indicative of a carcinogen or a tumor type. We have analyzed the mutations in 10 cases of AML but could not detect any mutations in the highly conserved regions. Interestingly, two such mutations were found in a T-ALL cell line (R. Laumann and H. Tesch, manuscript in preparation).

The retinoblastoma susceptibility gene *Rb* located in the chromosome 13q14 region was the prototype of the class of tumor suppressor genes. Inactivation of the *Rb* gene has been demonstrated not only in human retinoblastoma but also in some cases with osteogenic and other sarcomas, small cell lung cancers, gliomas, breast cancers, etc. Chen et al. analyzed by Southern blotting 52 cases with ALL and found deletion of part of the *Rb* gene in one case with pre-B ALL and a t(14;16) translocation (Chen et al. 1990). The cells lacked the 110-kDa Rb protein. Another case was described by Hansen and coworkers (Hansen et al. 1990). The putative function of the Rb protein is the regulation of the transition from G_1 to S phase of the cell cycle. Diaz and coworkers observed a frequent homozygous or hemizygous deletions of interferon-α and interferon-β_1 genes on chromosome 9p (18/62 cases, 29%) and speculated that a suppressor gene may be present at this locus (Diaz et al. 1990).

Cytokine and Cytokine Receptor Genes

Another group of genes deregulated in ALL are genes which code for cytokine or cytokine receptors. The malignant cells of the acute T cell leukemia which is endemic in Japan and the Caribbean islands, and some other parts, are associated with the HTLV-I retrovirus. The leukemic cells express constitutively the light chain p55 of the interleukin-2 (IL-2) receptor. The expression is regulated by viral transactivation factors. Also, in some other cases with T-ALL expression of IL-2 receptors and also of IL-2 had been reported, suggesting a stimulation via autocrine or paracrine mechanisms. We analyzed whether IL-2 and IL-2 receptors are expressed in other cases of ALL.

Expression of IL-2 was detected in rare cases of T-ALL, in some B-ALL, and in most pre-B ALL. mRNA for the IL-2 receptor light chain could not be detected in any case. In a few cases, IL-6-specific mRNA was found, but IL-6 receptor mRNA was only detected in one case. IL-6 and IL-6 receptors are involved in plasmocytomas and it has been suggested that the tumor cells may be stimulated by autocrine or paracrine pathways. We have recently found both IL-6 and IL-6 receptor mRNA and protein in Hodgkin and Reed-Sternberg cells (Jücker et al. 1991b). IL-1 mRNA was also detected in some cases with common ALL. Currently, we are investigating additional lymphokines in the ALL cells and attempting to correlate the data with clinical and immunological markers.

An experiment relating to the regulation of lymphokine expression in tumor cells has recently been carried out by S. Kochanek in W. Doerfler's group. They asked the question whether cells at various stages of differentiation or tumor cells exhibit changes in their profiles of DNA-methylation. The genomic sequencing technique worked out by Church and Guilbert allows the methylation state of individual cytidine residues in the DNA to be assessed.

For the tumor necrosis factor β (TNF-β) gene a decrease in DNA methylation has been observed in several examples of acute or chronic myeloid leukemias in comparison to normal human granulocytes or monocytes, which show almost complete methylation between nucleotides 700 and 900. In human T and B cells, the main producers of TNF-β, all 5′CG3′ sequences are unmethylated in this region, and the same is true for three cases of CLL and two cases of non-Hodgkin lymphoma (Kochanek et al. 1991). Also, human leukemias and lymphomas frequently show hypo-methylation in the TNF-α and TNF-β genes, and it will be interesting to investigate to what extent this finding relates to alterations in the differentiation and expression programs of these tumor cells.

Altogether, there is evidence that in most cases of ALL genetic changes of cellular genes lead to deregulated growth and differentiation. The genes affected and deregulated include protooncogenes, cytokine and cytokine receptor genes, and tumor suppressor genes. Although the whole cascade of the transforming events is not understood yet, analysis of these aberrations will allow us to distinguish certain molecular forms of ALL which have distinct clinical features. The correlation of genetic abnormalities with clinical parameters will lead to the identification of prognostic markers and thus to new treatment strategies for high risk patients. Finally, with powerful molecular techniques such as the polymerase chain reaction, residual disease can be more accurately identified. Follow-up studies will tell whether positive cases with residual tumor cells are clinically relevant and should be treated early after detection.

Acknowledgement. This work was supported by the Bundesministerium für Forschung und Technologie (BMFT) and the Deutsche Forschungsgemeinschaft.

References

Abts H, Jücker M, Diehl V, Tesch H (1991) Human chronic lymphocytic leukemia cells regularly express lck and c-fgr mRNAs. Leuk Res 15:987–997

Chen YC, Chen PJ, Yeh SH, Tien HF, Wang CH, Tang JL, Hong (1990) RL Deletion of the human retinoblastoma gene in primary leukemias. Blood 76: 2060–2064

Diaz MO, Rubin CM, Harden A, Ziemin S, Larson RA, Le Beau MM, Rowley JD (1990) Deletions of interferon genes in acute lymphoblastic leukemia. N Engl J Med 322:77–82

Hansen MF, Morgan R, Sandberg A, Cavenee (1990) WK Structural alteratilon at the putative retinoblastoma locus in some human leukemias and preleukemia. Cancer Genet. Cytogenet 49:15–23

Ince C, Blick M, Pathak S, Vadhan-Raj S, Selvanagam P, Gutterman JU, Cabanillas F (1988) Bcl-1 gene rearrangements in B cell lymphoma. Leukemia 2:343

Jücker M, Abts H, Eick D, Lenoir G, Tesch H (1991a) Overexpression of lck in Burkitt's lymphoma cells lines. Leukemia 5:528–530

Jücker M, Abts H, Li W, Schindler R, Merz H, Günther A, von Kalle C, Schaadt M, Diamantstein T, Feller AC, Krueger GRF, Diehl V, Blankenstein T, Tesch H (1991b) Expression of interleukin-6 and interleukin-6 receptor in Hodgkin's disease. Blood 77:2413–2418

Kawano M, Hirano T, Matsuda T, Taga T, Horii Y, Ewato K, Asaoku H, Tang B, Tanabe O, Tanaka H, Kuramoto A, Kishimoto T (1988) Autocrine generation and requirement of BSF-2/IL-6 for human multiple myelomas. Nature 332:83

Kochanek S, Radbruch A, Tesch H, Renz D, Doerfler W (1991), DNA methylation profiles in subpopulations of white blood cells and in leukemias in the human genes for tumor necrosis factor alpha and beta. Proc Natl Acad Sci USA 88: 5759–5763

Leder P, Battey J, Lenoir G, Moulding C, Murphy W, Potter H, Stewart T, Taub R (1983) Translocations among antibody genes in human cancer. Science 222: 765–771

Maurer J, Janssen JWG, Thiel E, Denderen J, Ludwig WD, Aydemir Ü, Heinze B, Fonatsch C, Harbott J, Reiter A, Riehm H, Hoelzer D, Bartram C (1991) Detection of chimeric BCR-ABL genes in acute lymphoblastic leukaemia by the polymerase chain reaction. Lancet 337:1055–1058

McGuire EA, Hockett RD, Pollock KM, Bartholdi MF, O'Brien SJ, Korsmeyer SJ (1989) The t(11;14)(p15;q11) in a T-cell acute lymphoblastic leukemia cell line activates multiple transcripts, including Ttg-1, a gene encoding a potential zinc finger protein. Mol Cell Biol 9:2124–2132

Nourse J, Mellentin JD, Galili N, Wilkinson J, Stanbridge E, Smith SD, Clearly ML (1990) Chromosomal translocation t(1;19) results in synthesis of a homeobox fusion mRNA that codes for a potential chimeric transcription factor. Cell 60: 535–545

Tesch H, Abts H, Jücker M, Mays K, Lenoir G, Diehl V (1989) Expression of c-fgr in EBV positive and negative B cell tumors. Leukemia 3:897–898

Tsujimoto Y, Finger LR, Yunis J, Nowell PC, Croce CM (1984) Cloning of the chromosomal breakpoint of neoplastic B cells with the t(14;18) chromosome translocation. Science 226:1097

Veilette A, Bookman MA, Horak EM, Samelson LE, Bolen JB (1989) Signal transduction through the CD4 receptor involves the activation of the internal membrane tyrosine-protein kinase p56lck. Nature 338:257–259

Weinberg RA (1989) Oncogenes, antioncogenes and the molecular basis of multistep carcinogenesis. Cancer Res 49:3713–3721

Cellular Drug Sensitivity of Immunophenotypic Subgroups of Childhood Acute Lymphoblastic Leukemia

R. Pieters[1], G.J.L. Kaspers[1], E.R. van Wering[2], D.R. Huismans[1], A.H. Loonen[1], K. Hählen[2,3], and A.J.P. Veerman[1,2]

[1] Free University Hospital, Department of Pediatrics, 1081 HV Amsterdam, The Netherlands
[2] Dutch Childhood Leukemia Study Group, The Hague, The Netherlands
[3] Sophia's Children's Hospital, Subdivision Haemato-Oncology, Erasmus University, Rotterdam, The Netherlands

Introduction

The immunophenotype is one of the prognostic factors in children with acute lymphoblastic leukemia (ALL) (Crist et al. 1984, 1985, 1989; Sallan et al. 1980; Greaves et al. 1981; Pui et al. 1986). B-cell ALL (B-ALL) cases have the worst prognosis and patients with B-cell precursor ALL the most favorable prognosis. Precursor B-ALL can be subdivided into three groups: pro-B-ALL ($CD10^-$, cytoplasmic μ chain$^-$ [$c\mu^-$]; common ALL (c-ALL) ($CD10^+/c\mu^-$) and pre-B-ALL ($CD10^{+\text{ or }-}/c\mu^+$). The small group of patients whose cells lack the common ALL (c-ALL) antigen characteristic of the earliest stage of B-cell differentiation (pro-B-ALL) show poorer responses by comparison with the c-ALL$^+$ cases. In some studies the pre-B-ALL cases did worse than the cALL cases, but this is probably due to a small subset of patients with a specific chromosomal abnormality on their leukemic cells (Crist et al. 1990). Also, patients with T-cell ALL (T-ALL) have an unfavorable prognosis. Some of these findings are still controversial because in some studies the immunophenotype is related to other clinical and biological features like white blood cell (WBC) count and organomegaly. Also, when effective treatments are used, the prognostic value of immunophenotype could be diminished (Borowitz 1990; Poplack and Reaman 1988; Miller 1988).

The cell-biological basis for the associations between immunophenotype and treatment outcome is not understood. It has been shown that immunophenotype is correlated with karyotype, but this itself does not elucidate the relationship with prognosis (Pui et al. 1988). It is often suggested that differences in phenotype and karyotype reflect differences in drug resistance, but no studies have been performed to support this hypothesis. Recently, we adapted the MTT (3-[4,5-dimethylthiazol-2-yl]-2,5-diphenyltetrazolium bromide) assay for in vitro drug sensitivity testing in ALL patient samples (Pieters et al. 1988, 1989, 1990). This assay shows good correlations between

Recent Results in Cancer Research, Vol. 131

in vitro results and clinical response to chemotherapy (Santini et al. 1989; Sargent and Taylor 1989; Hongo et al. 1990; Veerman and Pieters 1990; Pieters 1991). Recently, we showed that cellular drug resistance determined at initial diagnosis with the MTT assay is related to long-term clinical outcome in childhood ALL (Pieters et al. 1991). We report here the relation of immunophenotype and drug resistance in children with ALL.

Material and Methods

Cells. Bone marrow or peripheral blood cells from 84 children with untreated ALL were used. In 46 cases cells had been cryopreserved in liquid nitrogen at −170°C. Leukemic cells were isolated on a Ficoll-Isopaque gradient (Lymphoprep 1.077 g/ml). The median percentage of malignant cells was 94 (range 66–100) and was not different between the immunological subtypes. Cryopreservation does not alter drug sensitivity (Pieters et al. 1989) and bone marrow and peripheral blood cells did not differ as to drug sensitivity (Kaspers et al. 1991). Immunophenotyping was done in the research laboratory for Pediatric Hemato-Onco-Immunology of the Free University Hospital and in the laboratory of the DCLSG using an indirect peroxidase staining method. The samples of the B-lineage ALL, the B-cell origin of which was confirmed by the expression of CD19 and HLA-DR, were classified into four sequential differentiation stages: pro-B-ALL cells were $CD10^-$, cytoplasmic μ chain$^-$ ($c\mu^-$) and surface immunoglobulin$^-$ (sIg^-); c-ALL cells $CD10^+/c\mu^-/sIg^-$; pre-B-ALL cells $CD10^{+ \text{ or } -}/c\mu^+/sIg^-$; and B-ALL cells $CD10^-/c\mu^-/sIg^+$.

Drug Sensitivity Assay. In vitro drug sensitivity was assessed with the MTT assay as described elsewhere (Pieters et al. 1990). Briefly, 96-well microculture plates contained 100 μl cell suspension with six duplicate concentrations of the following drugs: 6-thioguanine (6-TG), vincristine (VCR), prednisolone (Pred), daunorubicin (DNR), mafosfamide (Maf, an active derivative of cyclophosphamide), cytosine arabinoside (ara-C), mustine HCl (Must), and L-asparaginase (L-Asp). Untreated control cells were set up six fold. After incubation in a humidified incubator in 5% CO_2 for 4 days at 37°C, 10 μl MTT solution was added for 6 h. MTT is reduced to a colored formazan by living but not by dead cells. The formazan crystals were dissolved with 100 μl acid isopropanol. The optical density (OD) was measured with a microplate reader at 540 nm. The OD is linearily related to cell number (Pieters et al. 1988). Leukemic cell survival (LCS) was calculated by the equation:

$$\text{LCS} = (\text{OD treated well/mean OD control wells}) \times 100\%.$$

The LC_{50} is the drug concentration lethal to 50% of the cells.

Statistics. The Mann–Whitney *U* test was used for two-tailed testing at a significance level of 0.05.

Results

Twenty patients had the T-ALL phenotype; seven had pro-B-ALL, 37 c-ALL, 17 pre-B-ALL and three B-ALL. The relationship between immunophenotype and in vitro drug resistance is shown in Fig. 1 and Table 1. Several observations can be made from these data:

- Large variations in sensitivity were detected with overlaps between the different immunological subtypes. In general, c-ALL and pre-B-ALL cells had the lowest median LC_{50} values, i.e., were the most chemosensitive cells. This was especially true for Pred and L-Asp.
- T-ALL cells were significantly more resistant to Pred, DNR, ara-C, Maf and L-Asp than c-ALL and pre-B-ALL cells and more resistant to VCR than pre-B ALL cells. The largest absolute differences were for Pred and L-Asp: The median LC_{50} values in T-ALL were 180 and 12–25 times of those in c-ALL and pre-B-ALL, respectively. In 6/18 (33%) T-ALL cases the LC_{50} for Pred was higher than the maximum concentration tested (250 μg/ml), compared to 2/43 (4%) c-ALL and pre-B-ALL cases. In only 1/18 (6%) T-ALL cases was the LC_{50} lower than the minimum concentration tested (0.1 μg/ml), compared to 16/43 (37%) c-ALL and pre-B-ALL cases.
- Pro-B-ALL cells showed a significant resistance to 6-TG, Pred, and DNR, and a trend to resistance to L-Asp compared to cALL and pre-B-ALL cells. Pro-B-ALL cells were more resistant to Maf than pre-B-ALL cells. In 4/6 (67%) pro-B-ALL cases the LC_{50} for Pred was higher than 250 μg/ml and in no pro-B cases was it lower than 0.1 μg/ml, compared to 2/43 (4%) and 16/43 (37%) c-ALL and pre-B-ALL cases, respectively.
- No differences were found between c-ALL and pre-B-ALL cases, with the exception of the alkylating drugs Maf and Must. Pre-B cells were more sensitive than c-ALL cells to these drugs with a two- to threefold difference in median LC_{50} values.
- All three B-ALL cases were highly resistant to VCR and DNR compared to all other phenotypes. Two out of three B-ALL cases were resistant to Pred. One B-ALL case was also highly resistant to all other drugs tested, while one other was relatively sensitive to these, especially to the alkylating drugs.

Discussion

With most treatment protocols for children with ALL, the immunophenotype has prognostic value. c-ALL and pre-B-ALL cases have the best prognosis, pro-B-ALL and T-ALL a poorer one, and B-ALL the worst (Crist et al. 1984, 1985, 1989; Sallan et al. 1980; Greaves et al. 1981; Pui et al. 1986; Borowitz 1990; Poplack and Reaman 1988; Miller 1988). It is hypothesized that differences in cellular drug sensitivity account for these differences in clinical responsiveness to chemotherapy. The present study reports on differ-

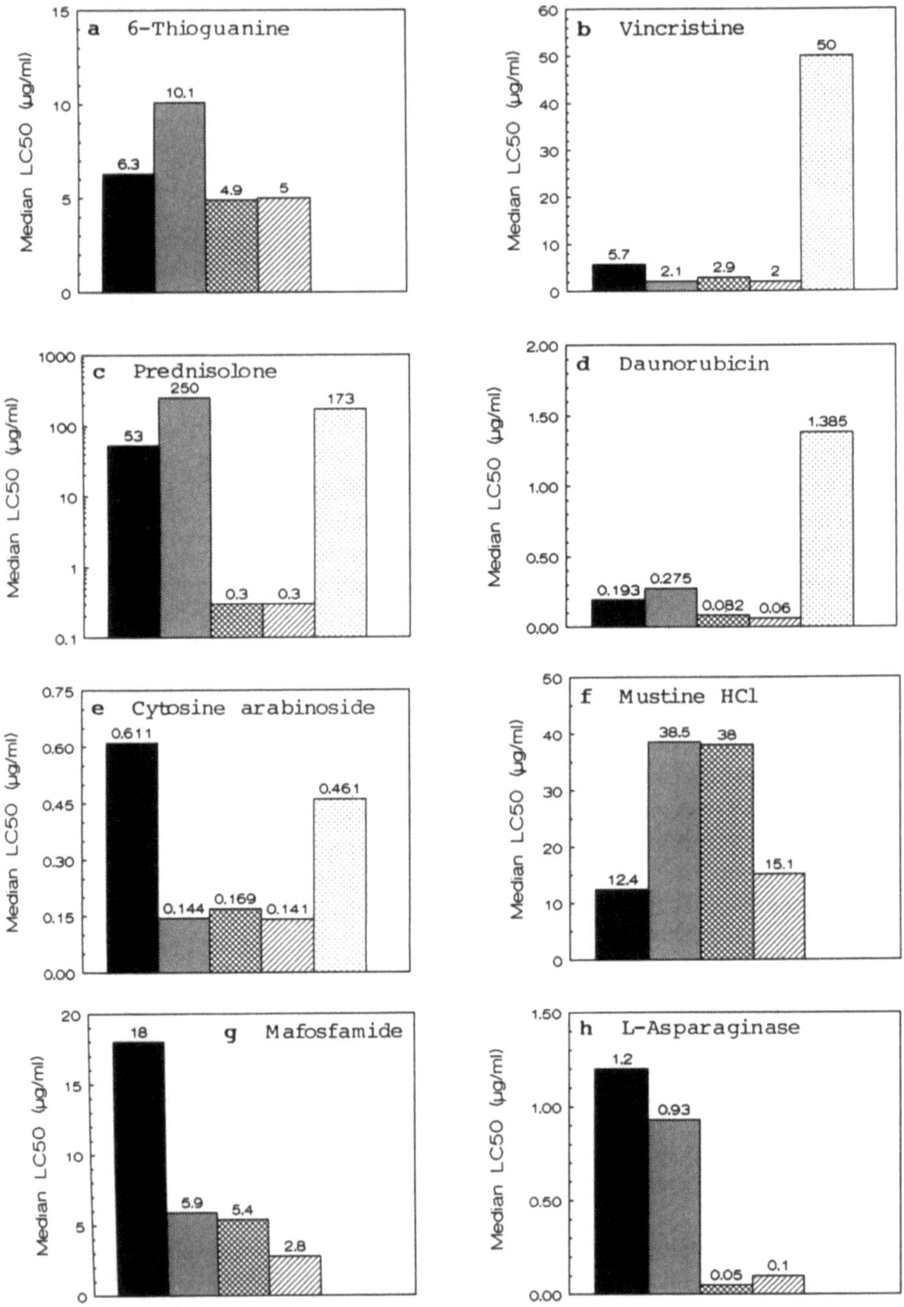

Fig. 1a–h. Relationship between immunophenotype and in vitro drug resistance in childhood ALL. Median LC_{50} values in μg/ml (for L-Asp in IU/ml). ■, T-ALL; ▨, pro-B-ALL; ▩, c-ALL; ▧, pre-B-ALL; ▤, B-ALL

Table 1. Immunophenotype and drug resistance in childhood ALL

Drug	Phenotype	LC_{50}		2-tailed p-values		
		Median	Range	n	c-ALL	Pre-B
6-TG	T-ALL	6.3	1.6–50.0	18	0.074	
	Pro-B	10.1	2.5–17.9	7	0.015	0.057
	c-ALL	4.9	1.6–15.3	30		
	Pre-B	5.0	2.1–14.9	15		
	B		5.3–50.0	2		
VCR	T-ALL	5.7	0.3–50.0	18		0.047
	Pro-B	2.1	0.5–50.0	7		
	c-ALL	2.9	0.3–50.0	28		
	Pre-B	2.0	0.3–36.8	16		
	B	50.0	24.4–50.0	3	0.011	0.010
Pred	T-ALL	53.4	0.1–250.0	18	0.005	0.002
	Pro-B	250.0	1.0–250.0	6	0.006	0.004
	c-ALL	0.3	0.1–250.0	28		
	Pre-B	0.3	0.1–168.2	15		
	B	172.6	0.1–250.0	3		
DNR	T-ALL	0.193	0.023–2.000	18	0.025	0.024
	Pro-B	0.275	0.074–0.863	7	0.026	0.014
	c-ALL	0.082	0.002–0.895	24		
	Pre-B	0.060	0.002–0.378	14		
	B	1.385	0.444–1.470	3	0.009	0.008
Ara-C	T-ALL	0.611	0.018–2.500	14	0.013	0.004
	Pro-B	0.144	0.029–0.986	7		
	c-ALL	0.169	0.002–2.500	26		
	Pre-B	0.141	0.002–0.478	13		
	B	0.461	0.082–2.266	3		
Must	T-ALL	12.4	1.7–60.0	6		
	Pro-B	38.5	4.7–48.5	5		
	c-ALL	38.0	1.1–115.4	18		0.032
	Pre-B	15.1	4.6–34.7	7	0.032	
	B		0.7–214.3	2		
Maf	T-ALL	18.0	3.3–100.0	14	0.048	0.0003
	Pro-B	5.9	1.6–28.0	7		0.035
	c-ALL	5.4	0.5–44.2	22		0.021
	Pre-B	2.8	0.2–15.6	12	0.021	
	B		0.8–38.1	2		
L-Asp	T-ALL	1.20	0.016–10.00	14	0.024	0.022
	Pro-B	0.93	0.020–1.58	7	0.073	0.051
	c-ALL	0.05	0.016–10.00	26		
	Pre-B	0.10	0.016–1.06	12		
	B		0.080–10.00	2		

LC_{50} values in μg/ml (in U/ml for L-Asp). Two-tailed p-values of the comparison of T-ALL, pro-B ALL, and B-ALL with, c-ALL and pre-B ALL, respectively, which were <0.10 are shown.

ences in in vitro drug resistance between the immunophenotypic subgroups of childhood ALL.

In general, c-ALL and pre-B-ALL cells showed a higher chemosensitivity than cells of the other phenotypes. Pre-B-ALL cells were more sensitive to the alkylating agents Maf and Must than c-ALL cells. This suggests that sensitivity to alkylating drugs increases with B-cell maturation. We could not test this hypothesis further because of the low number of B-ALL samples. One B-ALL sample was highly sensitive but the other highly resistant to Maf and Must. Single-agent cyclophosphamide has been curative in some patients with advanced B-cell malignancies (Arseneau et al. 1975).

From the comparison of the T-, pro-B-, and B-ALL cases with the c-ALL and pre-B-ALL cases, the following differences are evident:

- T-ALL cases showed a resistance to Pred, DNR, ara-C, Maf, and L-Asp. T-ALL cells were more VCR resistant than pre-B-ALL cells.
- Pro-B-ALL cases were resistant to 6-TG, Pred, DNR, and L-Asp. Pro-B-ALL cells were more Maf resistant than pre-B-ALL cells.
- The number of B-ALL cases studied was too small to draw general conclusions. All three samples were resistant to VCR and DNR and 2/3 also to Pred. For most other drugs only two samples could be evaluated, one showing a general resistance while cells from the other were relatively chemosensitive, especially to the alkylating agents.

The finding that T- and B-ALL are relatively resistant to Pred correlates well with the fact that the number of glucocorticoid receptors differs among the phenotypes, with a higher density in c-ALL and pre-B-ALL than in T-ALL and B-ALL (Costlow et al. 1982; Quddus et al. 1985; Vogler et al. 1981). Low number of receptors usually imply Pred resistance, but high numbers do not guarantee a response to this drug (Pui et al. 1984; Pui and Costlow 1986; Mastrangelo et al. 1980; Thompson et al. 1985; Thompson and Harmon 1986). Therefore, studies of Pred resistance should incorporate a drug sensitivity assay, e.g., the MTT assay, because this measures cell lysis, which is the endpoint of all mechanisms of resistance, rather than the presence of receptors.

We conclude that the prognostic value of the immunophenotype might at least partly be explained by differences in drug sensitivity. This remains to be confirmed in larger studies. It might then be possible to design more specific treatment protocols for the different risk groups.

Acknowledgements. This study was supported by the Dutch Cancer Society (IKA 87-17 and 89-06). We acknowledge the Dutch Childhood Leukemia Study Group (DCLSG) for their help in performing this study. Board members of the DCLSG are W.A. Kamps, K. Hählen, F.A.E. Nabben, J.A. Rammeloo, G.A.M. de Vaan, P.J. van Dijken, A.J.P. Veerman, R.S. Weening, E.Th. van't Veer-Korthof, A. Postma, I. Risseeuw-Appel, J.P.M.

Bökkerink, M.V.A. Bruin, F.C. de Waal, E.F. van Leeuwen, and M. van Weel-Sipman.

References

Arseneau JC, Canellos GP, Banks PM, Berard CW, Gralnick HR, DeVita VT (1975) American Burkitt's lymphoma: a clinicopathologic study of 30 cases: I. Clinical factors relating to prolonged survival. Am J Med 58:314–321

Borowitz MJ (1990) Immunologic markers in childhood acute lymphoblastic leukemia. Hematol Oncol Clin North Am 4:743–765

Costlow ME, Pui C-H, Dahl GV (1982) Glucocorticoid receptors in childhood acute lymphocytic leukemia. Cancer Res 42:4801–4806

Crist W, Boyett J, Roper M, Pullen J, Metzgar R, van Eys J, Ragab A, Starling K, Vietti T, Cooper M (1984) Pre-B cell leukemia responds poorly to treatment: a Pediatric Oncology Group study. Blood 63:407–414

Crist WM, Grossi CE, Pullen J, Cooper M (1985) Immunologic markers in childhood acute lymphocytic leukemia. Semin Oncol 12:105–121

Crist W, Boyett J, Jackson J, Vietti T, Borowitz M, Chauvenet A, Winick N, Ragab A, Mahoney D, Head D, Iyer R, Wagner H, Pullen J (1989) Prognostic importance of the pre-B-cell immunophenotype and other presenting features in B-lineage childhood acute lymphoblastic leukemia: a Pediatric Oncology Group Study. Blood 74:1252–1259

Crist WM, Carroll AJ, Shuster JJ, Behm FG, Whitehead M, Vietti TJ, Look AT, Mahoney D, Ragab A, Pullen DJ, Land VJ (1990) Poor prognosis of children with pre-B acute lymphoblastic leukemia is associated with the t(1;19)(q23;p13): a Pediatric Oncology Group study. Blood 76:117–122

Greaves MF, Janossy G, Peto J, Kay H (1981) Immunologically defined subclasses of acute lymphoblastic leukemia in children: their relationship to presentation features and prognosis. Br J Haematol 48:179–197

Hongo T, Fujii Y, Igarashi Y (1990) An in vitro chemosensitivity test for the screening of anti-cancer drugs in childhood leukemia. Cancer 65:1263–1272

Kaspers GJL, Pieters R, van Zantwijk CH, de Laat PAJM, de Waal FC, van Wering ER, Veerman AJP (1991) In vitro drug sensitivity of normal peripheral blood lymphocytes and childhood leukaemic cells from bone marrow and peripheral blood. Br J Cancer 64:469–474

Mastrangelo R, Malandrino R, Riccardi R, Longo O, Ranelletti FO, Iacobelli S (1980) Clinical implications of glucocorticoid receptor studies in childhood acute lymphoblastic leukemia. Blood 56:1036–1040

Miller DR (1988) Childhood acute lymphoblastic leukemia: 1. Biological features and their use in predicting outcome of treatment. Am J Pediatr Hematol Oncol 10:163–173

Pieters R (1991) Drug resistance in childhood leukemia. Thesis, Free University, Amsterdam

Pieters R, Huismans DR, Leyva A, Veerman AJP (1988) Adaptation of a rapid automated tetrazolium based (MTT-) assay for chemosensitivity testing in childhood leukemia. Cancer Lett 41:323–332

Pieters R, Huismans DR, Leyva A, Veerman AJP (1989) Comparison of a rapid automated tetrazolium based (MTT-) assay with a dye exclusion assay for chemosensitivity testing in childhood leukemia. Br J Cancer 59:217–220

Pieters R, Loonen AH, Huismans DR, Broekema GJ, Dirven MWJ, Heyenbrok MW, Hählen K, Veerman AJP (1990) In vitro drug sensitivity of cells from

children with leukemia using the MTT assay with improved culture conditions. Blood 76:2327–2336
Pieters R, Huismans DR, Loonen AH, van der Does-van den Berg A, van Wering ER, Hählen K, Veerman AJP (1991) Relation of cellular drug resistance to long-term clinical outcome in childhood acute lymphoblastic leukemia. Lancet 338:399–403
Poplack DG, Reaman G (1988) Acute lymphoblastic leukemia in childhood. Pediatr Clin North Am 35:903–932
Pui C-H, Costlow ME (1986) Sequential studies of lymphoblast glucocorticoid receptor levels at diagnosis and relapse in childhood leukemia: an update. Leuk Res 10:227–229
Pui C-H, Dahl GV, Rivera G, Murphy SB, Costlow ME (1984) The relationship of blast cell glucocorticoid receptor levels to response to single-agent steroid trial and remission response in children with acute lymphoblastic leukemia. Leuk Res 8:579–585
Pui CH, Williams DL, Raimondi SC, Melvin SL, Behm FG, Look AT, Dahl GV, Rivera GK, Kalwinsky DK, Mirro J, Dodge RK, Murphy SB (1986) Unfavorable presenting clinical and laboratory features are associated with calla-negative non-T, non-B lymphoblastic leukemia in children. Leuk Res 10:1287–1292
Pui C-H, Williams DL, Roberson PK, Raimondi SC, Behm FG, Lewis SH, Rivera GK, Kalwinsky DK, Abromowitch M, Crist WM, Murphy SB (1988) Correlation of karyotype and immunophenotype in childhood acute lymphoblastic leukemia. J Clin Oncol 6:56–61
Quddus FF, Leventhal BG, Boyett JM, Pullen DJ, Crist WM, Borowitz MJ (1985) Glucocorticoid receptors in immunological subtypes of childhood acute lymphocytic leukemia: A Pediatric Oncology Group study. Cancer Res 45:6482–6486
Sallan SE, Ritz J, Pesando J, Gelber R, O'Brien C, Hithcock S, Coral F, Schlossman SF (1980) Cell surface antigens: prognostic implications in childhood acute lymphoblastic leukemia. Blood 55:395–402
Santini V, Bernabei PA, Silvestro L, Dal Pozzo O, Bezzini R, Viano I, Gattei V, Saccardi R, Rossi Ferrini P (1989) In vitro chemosensitivity testing of leukemic cells: prediction of response to chemotherapy in patients with acute non-lymphocytic leukemia. Hematol Oncol 7:287–293
Sargent JM, Taylor CG (1989) Appraisal of the MTT assay as a rapid test of chemosensitivity in acute myeloid leukaemia. Br J Cancer 60:206–210
Thompson EB, Harmon JM (1986) Glucocorticoid receptors and glucocorticoid resistance in human leukemia in vivo and in vitro. Adv Exp Med Biol 196:111–127
Thompson EB, Smith JR, Bourgeois S, Harmon JM (1985) Glucocorticoid receptors in human leukemias and related diseases. Klin Wochenschr 63:689–698
Veerman AJP, Pieters R (1990) Drug sensitivity assays in leukemia and lymphoma. Br J Haematol 74:381–384
Vogler LB, Crist WM, Sarrif AM, Pullen J, Bartolucci AA, Falletta JM, Dowell B, Humphrey GB, Blackstock R, van Eys J, Metzgar RS, Cooper MD (1981) An analysis of clinical and laboratory features of acute lymphocytic leukemias with emphasis on 35 children with pre-B leukemia. Blood 58:135–140

Use of Clinical and Laboratory Features to Define Prognostic Subgroups in B-Precursor Acute Lymphoblastic Leukemia: Experience of the Pediatric Oncology Group

M.J. Borowitz[1,8], A.J. Carroll[2,8], J.J. Shuster[3,8], A.T. Look[4,8], F.G. Behm[4,8], D.J. Pullen[5,8], V.J. Land[6,8], P. Steuber[7,8], and W.M. Crist[4,8]

[1] Duke University Medical Center, Durham, NC 27710, USA
[2] University of Alabama at Birmingham, Birmingham, AL, USA
[3] Statistial Office, Pediatric Oncology Group, University of Florida, Gainesville, FL, USA
[4] St. Jude Children's Regional Hospital, Memphis, TN, USA
[5] University of Mississippi Medical Center, Jackson, MS, USA
[6] Washington University, St. Louis, MO, USA
[7] Baylor College of Medicine, Houston, TX, USA
[8] The Pediatric Oncology Group, St. Louis, MO, USA

Introduction

For more than a decade, the Pediatric Oncology Group (POG) has been engaged in a series of studies of acute lymphocytic leukemia in childhood in which advances in therapeutic approaches have been undertaken in conjunction with biologic studies of the properties of leukemic cells. Historically, the POG has assigned children to treatment arms on the basis of clinical and laboratory measurements at the time of diagnosis (Pullen et al. 1983, 1984). In early studies, attention was focused on the immunophenotypic differences among leukemias, and specific treatments were derived for patients with T-cell ALL (T-ALL), B-precursor ALL, and B-cell ALL (B-ALL) (Pullen et al. 1982, 1983; Sullivan et al. 1990). Patients with T-ALL, originally defined by serologic studies first with heteroantisera and later with monoclonal antibodies (Borowitz et al. 1985), have been treated as poor prognosis leukemia irrespective of clinical risk factors. In addition, the small number of patients with surface Ig-positive (sIg^+) B-ALL have been treated in a manner similar to patients with Burkitt's lymphoma (Sullivan et al. 1990). Patients with B-precursor ALL have been assigned to treatment groups on the basis of clinical criteria, including age at diagnosis, leukocyte count, and adenopathy and organomegaly (Pullen et al. 1984; Crist et al. 1990).

Children with pre-B ALL, defined as those with blasts expressing cytoplasmic (cIg) but not surface immunoglobulin (sIg), were shown to have a poorer outcome than those with early pre-B-ALL in two consecutive POG

Recent Results in Cancer Research, Vol. 131

studies (Crist et al. 1984, 1989). Thus, in the most recent study, ALinC 14, patients with pre-B-ALL were not randomized to all of the treatment regimens (Crist et al. 1990a).

More recently, we have expanded our biologic studies, using investigators at several different reference laboratories, to include ploidy analysis by flow cytometry and leukemic cell karyotyping, as well as an expanded investigation into immunophenotype using a large number of monoclonal antibodies. The present report summarizes some of the experience of the POG with these expanded biologic studies, emphasizing how new insights into the complex biology of childhood ALL can be used to refine our approach to therapy.

Materials and Methods

Patients. From February 1986 to November 1990, 2661 patients with newly diagnosed ALL were enrolled in the classification study ALinC 14C. All patients had myeloperoxidase- and nonspecific esterase-negative blasts and were tested with a screening cocktail of monoclonal antibodies including CD7/CD5 and HLA-DR. Patients with DR^+, $CD7/5^-$ ALL were considered to have B-precursor ALL, and samples were sent to the reference laboratory at Duke University for immunophenotypic confirmation and to the St. Jude Children's Research Hospital reference laboratory for cIg and sIg determination. Additional reference laboratory testing is described below.

The results presented include cases of early pre-B-ALL and pre-B-ALL, defined as those lacking the T antigens CD7 or CD5 and also lacking sIg. A total of 1953 samples were satisfactorily tested at the Duke reference laboratory and verified as B-precursor ALL, but different numbers of cases are used in the analyses described depending on which specific laboratory tests were required by the active study at that time.

Immunophenotyping and Flow Cytometry Studies. Heparinized bone marrow was sent by overnight carrier to the Duke reference laboratory where it was stained by the single-color immunofluorescence technique with a panel of monoclonal antibodies and assayed by flow cytometry as previously described (Borowitz et al. 1990). cIg and sIg testing was performed by visual immunofluorescence, as described (Gathings et al. 1977). Pre-B-ALL was defined as $\geq 10\%$ marrow lymphoblasts cIg^+. For ploidy analysis, blasts were stained with propidium iodide and analyzed by flow cytometry, as described previously (Look et al. 1982). Hyperdiploidy was defined as a DNA index (DI) >1.16.

Cytogenetic Analysis. Bone marrow or peripheral blood samples were placed in RPMI 1640 supplemented with 15% fetal calf serum and sent by overnight carrier to the reference laboratory at the University of Alabama at

Birmingham. On arrival, cells were subjected to short-term culture, and karyotypic analysis was performed as previously described (Crist et al. 1990a).

Statistical Methods. Comparison of event-free survival was done by the log-rank method (Peto et al. 1978), and survival curves were generated by the Kaplan–Meier method (Kaplan and Meier 1958) with standard errors of Peto et al. (1978). Comparison of patient and leukemia cell characteristics was done using Fisher's exact test.

Results

Prognostic Factors for Risk Group Assignment: Pre-B and Ploidy Determinations

From 1986 to 1989, 510 patients with newly diagnosed B-precursor ALL were found to have clonal karyotypic abnormalities at the University of Alabama at Birmingham cytogenetic reference laboratory. Twenty-nine of 130 patients with clonal abnormalities and pre-B-ALL had the t(1;19)(q23;p13) translocation, compared to only five of 380 patients with early pre-B-ALL. Event-free survival of these 29 patients was much worse than that of patients with pre-B-ALL with other cytogenetic abnormalities, or those with normal karyotypes (Fig. 1) (Crist et al. 1990a). Outcome of patients with pre-B-ALL without the t(1;19) was not significantly different from that of children with early pre-B-ALL.

Because hyperdiploidy, measured either by cytogenetics or by a DI >1.6 by flow cytometry, was shown to be a favorable prognostic factor in a number of studies (Look et al. 1985; Williams et al. 1982), the POG has been measuring ploidy in all patients in its most recent studies. We have shown that patients with poor risk features defined by age and leukocyte count with DI >1.16 had a 91% 3-year event-free survival, compared to 61% among patients with similar clinical characteristics but DI ≤1.16 (Land et al. 1990). More recent data, now including 1535 children with newly diagnosed B-precursor ALL, have shown that DI >1.16 is the single most prognostic feature for event-free survival among age, white count, DI, race, sex, immunophenotype, and surface antigen expression (Trueworthy et al. 1992).

Based on the foregoing information, we have begun using laboratory criteria at diagnosis to help assign patients with B-precursor ALL to treatment protocols. A flow chart indicating our strategy is shown in Table 1. Patients are considered to be "good-risk" patients: (1) if they have clinical features of good risk, as defined by age, leukocyte count, and organomegaly, as previously described (Crist et al. 1990a); or (2) if their blasts have a DI >1.16, even in the setting of poor-risk clinical features. "Poor-

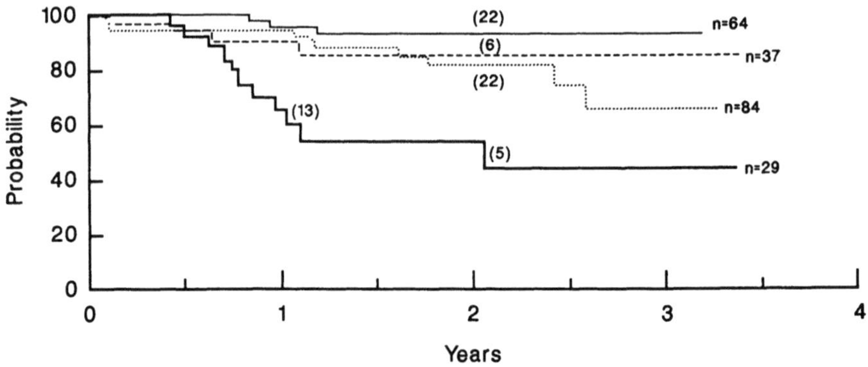

Fig. 1. Kaplan–Meier estimates of event-free survival in pre-B-ALL. ——, Group 1 with t(1;19); ...., group 2 with a normal karyotype; ------, group 3 with a translocation other than t(1;19); and ——, group 4 with a clonal abnormality but no t(1;19). Numbers in *parentheses* represent patients at risk of failure. Children with pre-B-ALL and t(1;19) (group 1) fare significantly worse than those in other groups ($p < 0.001$). (From Crist et al. 1990a; reprinted by permission)

Table 1. Schema for assignment of children to risk groups for therapy in most POG studies

Good risk
- Age/WBC favorable *or*
- Age/WBC unfavorable and DI >1.16

Poor risk
- Age/WBC unfavorable *and* DI <1.16 *or*
- t(1;19) *or*
- t(9;22) *or*
- CNS disease

Favorable clinical ("Age/WBC") criteria referred to are as follows:
- For children aged 3–5 years, leukocyte count $<100 \times 10^9$/l and no extramedullary or marked (below umbilicus) hepatomegaly or splenomegaly
- For children aged 1–2 or 6–10 years, leukocyte count $<10 \times 10^9$/l and no organomegaly or extramedullary disease.

All others are considered unfavorable (see Crist et al. 1990a)

risk" patients will be defined by those having both high-risk clinical features and DI ≤1.16. In addition, any patient with an unfavorable cytogenetic translocation – specifically the t(1;19), as discussed above, or the t(9;22) (i.e., Philadelphia chromosome) – or with central nervous system disease at diagnosis will also be considered poor risk.

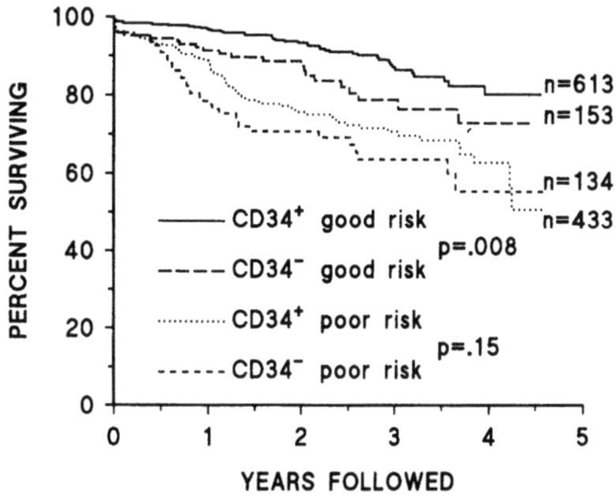

Fig. 2. Kaplan–Meier estimates of event free survival in B-precursor ALL based on CD34 expression and risk group. Note that the favorable prognostic effect of CD34 expression is seen in the clinically good risk subgroup of patients

Immunologic Markers as Prognostic Factors

Since 1986, the reference laboratory at Duke Medical Center has been immunophenotyping cases of B-precursor ALL with a panel of monoclonal antibodies. Using a traditional definition of 20% positive, we find that HLA-DR is the most frequently expressed antigen, and that the most sensitive and specific B marker is CD19, which is positive in greater than 98% of cases (Borowitz 1990). The rare CD19-negative cases can be recognized as being of B-cell lineage, based on expression of the B-specific marker CD22.

Recently, some of our results have called into question the appropriateness of using the arbitrary criterion of 20% to consider an antibody as positive. In particular, we have shown that for the case of CD34 antigen, which is normally expressed on about 1.5% of marrow cells (Civin et al. 1987), that a level of 10% expression is sufficient to be considered positive (Borowitz et al. 1990). This conclusion was reached because it was noted that patients with at least 10% positive cells exhibited clinical behavior that was more like those expressing higher levels of positivity than like those whose blasts were completely negative.

Patients whose blasts express CD34 antigen fare better than those whose blasts are CD34 negative (Borowitz et al. 1990). Although CD34 expression is positively correlated with hyperdiploidy, the favorable prognostic significance is maintained even after adjusting for ploidy. A partial explanation for this, as shown in Fig. 2, is that the poor prognosis effect of lack of CD34 antigen is restricted to patients who would be considered good risk based on clinical criteria. As noted above, the most dramatic effect of hyperdiploidy is found in patients who would be considered high risk by clinical criteria.

Table 2. Clinicopathologic characteristics of children with $CD19^+$, $CD10^-$, $CD24^{-/+}$ ALL

Patient characteristic	Percent of patients having characteristic		*p* value
	with this phenotype ($n = 53$)	with other phenotype ($n = 1609$)	
Age <1 year	57	1.6	<0.0001
WBC >50 × 10^9/l	74	16	<0.0001
CNS disease	10	3	0.03
$CD15^+$	53	8	<0.0001
$CD13^+$	9	9	0.92
$CD33^+$	2	8	0.18
$CD34^+$	76	80	0.29
t(4;11)	69	0.1	<0.0001
11q23 abnormal	89	1.1	<0.0001

Myeloid Antigen Expression

It has long been recognized that some cases of lymphoid leukemia express myeloid-associated antigens, although the significance of this is uncertain. We have included the antibodies CD13, CD15, and CD33 in our phenotyping panel. Expression of CD15 was found to correlate with age <1 year, and helps define a particular clinicopathologic syndrome (see below). Using the arbitrary criteria of 20% positive, and defining myeloid antigen positive (My^+) as expression of either CD13 or CD33, we find that 175/1141 (15.3%) of patients greater than 1 year of age are My^+. Among the My^+ patients, 23 (13.1%) have failed, compared to 151/966 (15.6%) in the My^- group ($p = 0.34$) (Borowitz et al. 1991). Similar lack of significance was found when we used different cutoffs to define the My^+ group.

Use of Immunophenotyping to Define Biological Subgroups of ALL

During the course of our phenotyping studies we noticed a small group of patients with a very distinctive phenotypic pattern. These patients had blasts that were uniformly negative for CD10 (CALLA) and uniformly positive for CD19, but examination of the CD24 histogram demonstrated lack of CD24 antigen on either all or some of the blasts. Fifty-three of 1662 children with B-precursor ALL were found to have this phenotype, which we refer to as $CD19^+$, $CD10^-$, and $CD24^{-/+}$. As shown in Table 2, children with the phenotype were more likely to be infants, and to have high leukocyte counts with central nervous system disease at presentation. As these clinical characteristics are commonly associated with cases of leukemia with the t(4;11) translocation, it is not surprising that this phenotype was correlated with the t(4;11), but the high degree of association is unexpected. Of 36 patients with this phenotype and satisfactory cytogenetic studies, 25 had the t(4;11). Moreover, 7/11 patients without t(4;11) had other abnormalities involving chromosome 11 band q23. By contrast, only one of 907 karyotyped patients with any other phenotype had the t(4;11) and only nine 907 had other 11q23 abnormalities. Thus, the predictive value of finding an 11q23 abnormality based on this phenotype is 89%; if we add to the phenotypic requirement the presence of CD15 antigen, the predictive value is 100% (data not shown).

Though many have considered leukemia with the t(4;11) to be a mixed lineage or "stem cell" leukemia, we believe that such terminology is potentially confusing. Table 2 shows that the phenotype we define is highly correlated with expression of CD15 antigen, but not with the other myeloid antigens CD33 or CD13 or the stem cell marker CD34.

Discussion

The POG has a long history of studying the biologic properties of leukemic cells in children with ALL (Pullen et al. 1981, 1984; Crist et al. 1986). Ultimately, the goal of such studies is to define distinct subgroups of children who might benefit from therapy designed based on the biologic characteristics of their disease. This principle has been followed in past POG protocols, in which children with B-ALL or T-ALL have been treated differently from the larger group of children with B-precursor ALL. The latter group, however, has, until now been assigned to therapeutic regimens based on traditional risk factors of age and leukocyte count.

Based on results presented here, and previous work by Look et al. (1985), we now consider children with hyperdiploid B-precursor ALL to be good risk, independent of considerations of age and leukocyte count. We have also shown that cytogenetics can be used to identify a subgroup of patients who might clinically be considered at low risk, but who are likely to fare poorly. One cytogenetic abnormality that has long been associated with poor prognosis is the Philadelphia (Ph) chromosome (Ribeiro et al. 1987; Crist et al. 1990b). Although recent studies have shown significant improvement in the overall outcome of children with ALL, patients with Ph^+ ALL continue to fare extremely poorly. Thus, children with the t(9;22) are being treated intensively independent of other risk features. In addition, based on the results presented above, children with the t(1;19) are also considered to have a high-risk form of leukemia. Though a large variety of nonrandom chromosomal translocations have been seen in ALL, no other marker has been shown to be an independent prognostic factor for poor outcome. While some might also consider children with the t(4;11) to be poor risk, it should be remembered that almost all of these children would be considered at high risk of treatment failure on clinical grounds alone, because of the strong association of the t(4;11) with hyperleukocytosis and infancy. Recently, Pui et al. (1991) have shown that children 1–9 years of age who have the t(4;11) fare relatively well.

The results presented here also shed light on the ability of immunophenotyping to define clinical and biologic entities. For many years, the t(1;19) was known to be associated with the pre-B phenotype, which was further associated with poor long-term survival. What we now know is that the pre-B group is heterogeneous, and contains a high-risk subgroup (the 25% of pre-B cases with the t(1;19)) that fare very poorly, combined with a larger number of cases lacking the t(1;19) that fare well. Thus, in a sense, the pre-B phenotype for many years served as a surrogate marker for the biologic entity that is better defined by cytogenetics, and preferably by molecular genetics.

Similarly, we now can define a phenotype, $CD19^{+}$, $CD10^{-}$, $CD24^{-/+}$, $CD15^{+/-}$, that serves as a surrogate marker for leukemias with abnormalities of chromosome 11q23. Unlike the association of the pre-B phenotype and t(1;19), which is only seen in about 25% of pre-B cases, this phenotype is highly associated with the karyotypic abnormality. In fact, the sensitivity and specificity of the phenotype for the 11q23 abnormality is probably the closest association of any karyotype with phenotype. Leukemias with 11q23 abnormalities, most commonly the t(4;11), have long been recognized as having interesting clinicopathologic features, and have often been considered "mixed lineage" leukemias (Arthur et al. 1982; Childs et al. 1988). We show no association of these leukemias with the myeloid antigens CD33 and CD13, which are the myeloid markers most commonly expressed in AML. Thus, we prefer not to include these cases with other diseases under the diagnostic term "mixed lineage leukemia," but rather to think of these "11q23" leukemias as a distinct entity which we can define phenotypically with great precision.

It is interesting to speculate about the significance of the small number of cases with these phenotypic or karyotypic abnormalities in which the karyotype and phenotype are discordant. It may be that these cases have different molecular abnormalities, even though they have identical karyotypes. In this regard, it is interesting to note that molecular studies have shown that patients with the t(1;19) who do not have pre-B-ALL have a different molecular defect than those who do have pre-B-ALL (Privitera et al. 1992). When tools for analyzing the molecular configuration of the 11q23 region become available it will be of interest to investigate these discordant cases.

Although immunophenotyping is particularly useful for identifying biologically distinct subgroups of leukemia, most immunophenotypic data are not yet mature enough to be used as independent means of assigning patients to protocols. Recently, Wiersma et al. (1991) suggested that myeloid antigen expression in ALL was the single best marker for predicting adverse outcome in children with ALL. Our results, and those of others (Pui et al.

1990), suggest that it may be premature to use myeloid antigen expression as a factor in stratifying patients in therapeutic studies, particularly because this marker is not a consistent indicator of poor prognosis.

We have shown a small but independently significant correlation between expression of CD34 antigen and patient outcome in B-precursor ALL. The fact that a relatively large number of patients are CD34 negative, and that the effect is small, suggests to us that the CD34-negative patient group is heterogeneous, comprising a subgroup which fares very poorly and a larger number of patients who fare well, much as was true of patients with pre-B-ALL. To date, we have not yet determined how to identify a very high risk subgroup within the group of CD34-negative patients. In preliminary studies (Borowitz et al. 1989), we had suggested that the combination of CD34 and CD10 negativity might define a small group with particularly poor prognosis. More recent data (not shown) fail to confirm these results, although they do indicate that CD10-negative patients also fare poorly.

One of the limitations of immunophenotyping has been that there have not been generally accepted criteria for interpretation of results. Traditionally, arbitrary criteria such as 20% positivity have been used to determine if an antigen is expressed in leukemia, and the prognostic significance of most markers has been evaluated by looking simply at whether each antigen is "positive" or "negative" on the blasts. Our results show that such an approach may miss important immunophenotypic information. First, 20% may not be an appropriate cutoff for all markers. For CD34, our results show that 10% is a better cutoff. By contrast, in the case of CD24, some patients with up to 60% or 70% positive blasts share clinical features with patients whose blasts completely lack CD24, and are different from patients whose blasts uniformly express CD24. If the arbitrary criterion of 20% reactivity were used to define cases as "positive," such patients would be misclassified. The most information will be obtained from immunophenotyping studies when combinations of markers are studied, and patient characteristics and biological parameters, rather than arbitrary analytical criteria, are used to help define immunophenotypic subgroups.

Acknowledgement. Supported in part by grants CA15525, CA21765 (CORE), CA31566, CA15989, CA05587, CA03161, CA29139 from the National Cancer Institute, National Institutes of Health, and by the American-Lebanese-Syrian Associated Charities.

References

Arthur DC, Bloomfield CD, Lindquist LL, Nesbit ME Jr (1982) Translocation 4;11 in acute lymphoblastic leukemia: clinical characteristics and prognostic significance. Blood 59:96

Borowitz MJ (1990) Immunologic markers in childhood acute lymphoblatic leukemia. Hematol Oncol Clin North Am 4:743–765

Borowitz MJ, Dowell BL, Boyett JM, Falletta JM, Pullen DJ, Crist WM, Humphrey GB, Metzger RS (1985) Monoclonal antibody definition of T cell leukemia. Blood 65:785
Borowitz M, Shuster J, Behm F, Look T, Carroll A, Land V, Pullen J, Crist W (1989) Prognostic significance of surface antigen phenotype in B-precursor ALL: a recursive partitioning analysis. Proc Am Assoc Cancer Res 30:230
Borowitz MJ, Shuster JJ, Civin CI, Carroll AJ, Look AT, Behm FG, Land VJ, Pullen DJ, Crist WM (1990) Prognostic significant of CD34 expression in childhood B-precursor acute lymphocytic leukemia: a Pediatric Oncology Group Study. J Clin Oncol 8:1389–1398
Borowitz MJ, Shuster JJ, Land VJ, Steuber CP, Pullen DJ, Viett TJ (1991) Clinical significant of myeloid antigen expression in pediatric acute lymphocytic leukemia. N Engl J Med 325:1379–1380
Childs CC, Hirsch-Ginsberg C, Culbert SJ, Ahearn M, Ruben J, Trujilo JM, Cork A, Walters RR, Freireich EJ, Stass SA (1988) Lineage heterogeneity in acute leukemia with the t(4;11) abnormality: implications for acute mixed lineage leukemia. Hematol Pathol 2:145
Civin CI, Banquerigo ML, Strauss LC et al. (1987) Antigenic analysis of hematopoiesis: VI. Flow cytometric characterization of My10 positive progenitor cells in normal human bone marrow. Exp Hematol 15:10–17
Crist W, Boyett J, Roper M, Pullen J, Metzgar R, van Eys J, Ragab A, Starling K, Vietti T, Cooper M (1984) Pre-B cell leukemia responds poorly to treatment: a Pediatric Oncology Group study. Blood 63:407
Crist W, Boyett J, Pullen J, van Eys J, Vietti T (1986) Clinical and biologic features predict poor prognosis in acute lymphoid leukemias in children and adolescents: a Pediatric Oncology Group Review. Med Pediatr Oncol 14:135
Crist W, Boyett J, Jackson J, Vietti T, Borowitz M, Chauvenet A, Winick N, Ragab A, Mahoney D, Head D, Iyer R, Wagner H, Pullen J (1989) Prognostic importance of the pre-B-cell immunophenotype and other presenting features in B-lineage children acute lymphoblastic leukemia: a Pediatric Oncology Group study. Blood 74:1252
Crist WM, Carroll AJ, Shuster JJ, Behm FG, Whitehead M, Vietti TJ, Look AT, Mahoney D, Ragab A, Pullen DJ, Land VJ (1990a) Poor prognosis of children with pre-B acute lymphoblastic leukemia is associated with the t(1;19)(q23;p13): a Pediatric Oncology Group study. Blood 76:117–122
Crist W, Carroll A, Shuster J, Jackson J, Head D, Borowitz M, Behm F, Link M, Steuber P, Ragab A, Hirt A, Brock B, Land V, Pullen J (1990b) Philadelphia chromosome positive childhood acute lymphoblastic leukemia: clinical and cytogenetic characteristics and treatment outcome – a Pediatric Oncology Group (POG) study. Blood 76:489–494
Gathings WE, Lawton AR, Cooper MD (1977) Immunofluorescent studies of the development of pre-B cells, B lymphocytes and immunoglboulin isotype diversity in humans. Eur J Immunol 7:804
Kaplan EL, Meier P (1958) Nonparametric estimation from incomplete observations. J Am Stat Assoc 53:457
Land VJ, Shuster JJ, Carroll AJ, Borowitz MJ, Harris MB, Pullen DJ, Look AT (1990) A DNA index (DI) greater than 1.16 in B-precursor childhood acute lymphoblastic leukemia (ALL) predicts a 95 percent 3-year event-free survival (EFS). Blood 76:292a
Look AT, Melvin SL, Williams DL, Brodeur GM, Dahl GV, Kalwinsky DK, Murphy SB, Mauer AM (1982) Aneupoloidy and percentage of S-phase cells determined by flow cytometry correlate with cell phenotype in childhood acute leukemia. Blood 60:959–967

Look AT, Roberson PK, Williams DK et al. (1985) Prognostic importance of blast cell and content in childhood acute lymphoblastic leukemia. Blood 65:1079–1085
Peto R, Pike MC, Armitage P, Breslow NE, Cox DR, Howard SV, Mantel N, McPherson K, Peto J, Smith PG (1978) Design and analysis of randomized clinical trials requiring prolonged observation of each patient: II. Analysis and examples. Br J Cancer 35:1
Privitera E, Kamps MP, Hayashi Y, Inaba T, Shapiro LH, Raimondi SC, Behm F, Hendershot L. Carroll AJ, Baltimore D, Look AT (1992) Different molecular consequences of the 1;19 chromosomal translocation in childhood B-cell precursor acute lymphoblastic leukemia. Blood 79:1781–1788
Pui C-H, Behm FG, Singh B et al. (1990) Myeloid-associated antigen expression lacks prognostic value in childhood acute lymphoblastic leukemia treated with intensive multiagent chemotherapy. Blood 75:198–202
Pui C-H, Frankel LS, Carroll AJ, Raimondi SC, Shuster JJ, Head DR, Crist WM, Land VJ, Pullen DJ, Steuber CP, Behm FG, Borowitz MJ (1991) Clinical characteristics and treatment outcome of childhood acute lymphoblastic leukemia with the t(4;11)(q21;q23): a collaborative study of 40 cases. Blood 77:440–447
Pullen DJ, Falletta JM, Crist WM, Vogler LB, Dowell B, Humphrey GB, Blackstock R, van Eys J, Cooper MD, Metzgar RS, Meydrech EF (1981) Southwest Oncology Group experience with immunologic phenotyping in acute lymphocytic leukemia of childhood. Cancer Res 41:4801
Pullen DJ, Sullivan MP, Falletta JM, Boyett JM, Humphrey GB, Starling KA, Land VJ, Dyment PG, Vats T, Duncan MH (1982) Modified LSA_2-L_2 treatment in 53 children with E-rosette-positive T-cell leukemia: results and prognostic factors (a Pediatric Oncology Group study). Blood 60:1159–1168
Pullen DJ, Crist WM, Falletta JM, Boyett JM, Roper M, Dowell B, van Eys J, Humphrey GB, Head D, Brock BL, Blackstock R, Metzgar RS, Cooper MD (1983) A Pediatric Oncology Group classification protocol of acute lymphocytic leukemia (ALinC 13): immunological phenotypes and correlation with treatment results. In: Murphy SB, Gilbert JR (eds) Leukemia research: advance in cell biology and treatment. Elsevier, New York, p 221
Pullen DJ, Boyett JM, Crist WM, Falletta JM, Roper M, Dowell B, van Eys J, Jackson JF, Humphrey GB, Metzgar RS, Cooper MD (1984) Pediatric Oncology Group utilization of immunologic markers in the designation of acute lymphocytic leukemia subgroups. Influence on treatment response. Ann NY Acad Sci 428:26
Ribeiro RC, Abromowitch M, Raimondi SC, Murphy SB, Behm F, Williams DL (1987) Clinical and biologic hallmarks of the philadelphia chromosome in childhood acute lymphoblastic leukemia. Blood 70:948–953
Sullivan MP, Pullin DJ, Crist WM, Brecher M, Ramirez I, Sabio H, Borowitz MJ, Head DR, Cerezo L, Shuster JJ, Murphy SB (1990) Clinical and biological heterogeneity of childhood B cell acute lymphocytic leukemia: implications for clinical trials. Leuk 4:6–11
Trueworthy R, Shuster J, Look T, Crist W, Borowitz M, Carroll A, Frankel L, Pullen J, Steuber P, Land V (1992) Ploidy of lymphoblasts is the strongest predictor of treatment outcome in B-progenitor cell acute lymphoblastic leukemia of childhood: a Pediatric Oncology Group study. J Clin Oncol 10:606–613
Wiersma SR, Ortega J, Sob el E, Weinberg KI (1991) Clinical importance of myeloid-antigen expression in acute lymphoblastic leukemia of childhood. N Engl J Med 324:800–808
Williams DL, Tsiatis A, Brodeur GMG et al. (1982) Prognostic importance of chromosome number in 136 untreated children with aucte lymphoblastic leukemia. Blood 60:864–871

Incidence and Prognostic Significance of Immunophenotypic Subgroups in Childhood Acute Lymphoblastic Leukemia: Experience of the BFM Study 86

W.-D. Ludwig[1], J. Harbott[2], C.R. Bartram[3], B. Komischke[1], C. Sperling[1], J.V. Teichmann[1], H. Seibt-Jung[1], M. Notter[1], E. Odenwald[4], A. Nehmer[4], E. Thiel[1], and H. Riehm[4]

[1] Department of Hematology and Oncology, Klinikum Steglitz, Free University of Berlin, W-1000 Berlin 45, Fed. Rep. of Germany
[2] Department of Pediatrics, University of Gießen, W-6300 Gießen, Fed. Rep. of Germany
[3] Section of Molecular Biology, Department of Pediatrics II, University of Ulm, W-7900 Ulm, Fed. Rep. of Germany
[4] Department of Pediatrics, Hannover Medical School, W-3000 Hannover, Fed. Rep. of Germany

Introduction

Due to the increasing availability of monoclonal antibodies (MAbs) recognizing lymphoid-, myeloid-, and progenitor-cell-associated antigens, immunophenotyping has greatly influenced studies on the biologic features of normal and leukemic hematopoietic progenitor cells (Greaves 1986). It has become possible to demonstrate the practical value of these data for the precise diagnosis and definition of clinically relevant immunophenotypic subsets of acute lymphoblastic leukemia (ALL) (Janossy et al. 1989). More recently, immunophenotyping has been supplemented by cytogenetic and molecular-genetic analyses in order to better characterize the biologic heterogeneity of ALL and to elucidate the mechanisms of lymphoid cell transformation and aberrant regulation of leukemic cell growth (Look 1988; Bain and Catovsky 1990; Pui et al. 1990c; van Dongen and Wolvers-Tettero 1991).

In childhood ALL, several studies have revealed an association between the maturational stage of B lymphoblasts and the treatment outcome, with a worse prognosis for patients whose leukemic blasts express immature CD10-negative or pre-B cell features (Pui et al. 1986; Béné et al. 1989; Crist et al. 1989). Though children with T-cell ALL generally have a poorer prognosis, this is mainly due to unfavorable clinical features (e.g., high leukocyte count, age), and attempts to identify subsets of T-cell malignancies in childhood ALL with prognostic relevance have hitherto been largely unsuccessful (Crist et al. 1988; Ludwig et al. 1989b; Garand et al. 1990). More recently, attention was focused on a subgroup of ALL patients whose blast cells

Recent Results in Cancer Research, Vol. 131

simultaneously express lymphoid- and myeloid-associated antigens (myeloid-antigen-positive ALL, My$^+$ ALL). However, results on the incidence and prognostic impact of My$^+$ ALL diverged markedly in both childhood and adult ALL (Drexler et al. 1991).

The paucity of controlled prospective studies on clinical and prognostic implications of immunophenotypic features has occasioned some uncertainty concerning the value of the immunophenotype as an independent predictor of treatment outcome (Chessells et al. 1987). More importantly, several recent studies have shown that the prognostic impact of many of the biologic and clinical features of childhood ALL is diminished by improved efficacy of chemotherapy, and prognostic factors must therefore be evaluated in the context of therapy delivered (Fletcher et al. 1989; Raimondi et al. 1990; Bleyer 1990).

In the ALL Berlin-Frankfurt-Münster (BFM) study 86, the vast majority of the protocol patients stratified for risk-adapted multidrug chemotherapy were prospectively examined by detailed immunophenotyping studies to evaluate the incidence, clinical behavior, and therapeutic sensitivity of B-cell precursor and T-lineage ALL subgroups. Additionally, leukemic cell karyotyping, DNA ploidy analysis, and Southern blotting were performed in a substantial proportion of these patients in order to identify numerical and/or structural chromosomal aberrations as well as to describe immunoglobulin (Ig) and T-cell-receptor (TCR) gene configuration of leukemic blast cells (Ludwig et al. 1990a; Harbott et al., this volume; Hiddemann et al., this volume). The present report summarizes some of the data from this study, focusing mainly on the prognostic impact of immunophenotyping in T-lineage ALL as well as on the blast-cell biologic features and treatment outcome of My$^+$ ALL.

Material and Methods

Patients. From October 1986 to March 1990, 895 previously untreated children with ALL were stratified according to their risk factors (e.g., tumor cell load and in vivo response to corticosteroids) and treated with intensive multidrug chemotherapy (Riehm et al. 1990). Complete immunophenotyping studies allowing both an affiliation with B- or T-lineage ALL and a characterization of the maturational stage of leukemic blasts were performed in 779 (87%) of these children in one central reference laboratory.

Immunophenotyping. Fresh bone marrow (BM) and/or peripheral blood (PB) samples containing >80% blasts were isolated by standard Ficoll-Hypaque density gradient centrifugation, and surface antigen expression was identified by an indirect immunofluorescence (IF) assay as previously described (Ludwig et al. 1988). Nonspecific binding was avoided by adding heat-inactivated 10% goat serum in both the first and second incubations.

Cells were evaluated for IF by an epi-illuminated fluorescence Zeiss microscope or by flow cytometry using a FACScan (Becton Dickinson Immunocytometry Systems, Mountain View, CA, USA).

For cytoplasmic and nuclear staining, cytospin preparations of leukemic blasts were fixed in acetone (cytoplasmic CD3, cyCD3, cyIgM) or methanol (terminal deoxynucleotidyl transferase, TdT) and subsequently assayed by direct (cyIgM) or indirect IF using MAb Leu-4 (cyCD3) or heterologous antisera (goat anti-mouse IgM, rabbit anti-TdT antiserum). The criterion for marker positivity was expression by ≥20% of the blast cells (surface antigens) or intracytoplasmic/intranuclear detection (cyCD3, cyIgM, TdT) in ≥10% of the leukemic cells.

In most My^+ ALL cases, two-color IF measurements were carried out on the FACScan flow cytometer using the direct/direct (fluorescein isothiocyanate/phycoerythrin) method as previously described (Ludwig et al. 1989a). The following panel of MAbs, all available from commercial sources, was applied for immunophenotyping: myeloid- (My7/CD13, My9/CD33, VIM-2/CD_W65), B-lineage- (HD37/CD19, B1/CD20, OKB2/CD24), and T-lineage-associated antigens (Na1 34/CD1a, OKT11/CD2, Leu-4/CD3, Leu-3a/CD4, Leu-1/CD5, Leu-9/CD7, OKT 8/CD8); non-lineage-specific reagents (OKIa1/HLA-DR, J5/CD10, My10/CD34).

Cytogenetic and DNA Analyses. Cytogenetic studies and Southern blot analyses were performed by standard methods as described in detail elsewhere (Harbott et al., this volume; Ludwig et al. 1989a).

Statistical Methods. All *p* values resulted from two-sided tests. Comparisons of event-free survival (EFS) were calculated using the log-rank test (Mantel 1966) and survival curves generated by the method established by Kaplan and Meier (1958).

Results

Incidence and Treatment Outcome of Immunophenotypic Subgroups

The reactivity patterns of leukemic cells with MAbs or heterologous antisera were taken as the basis for classifying patients into the following subgroups (van der Does-van den Berg et al. 1992):

1. *B-cell precursor ALL*: pre-pre-B ALL ($CD19^+$, $CD24^\pm$, cyIgM/surface Ig, $sIg/CD10^-$), common ALL ($CD19/CD24/CD10^+$, $cyIgM/sIg^-$); pre-B ALL ($cyIgM/CD19/CD24^+$, $CD10^\pm$, sIg^-).
2. *B-ALL*: $sIg/CD19/CD24^+$, $CD10^\pm$, $cyIgM^-$.
3. *T-lineage ALL*: early T-ALL ($CD7/cyCD3^+$, CD1a/membrane $CD3^-$); intermediate T-ALL ($CD1a/CD7^+$, cy or membrane $CD3^+$); mature T-ALL (membrane $CD3/CD7^+$, $CD1a^-$).

Table 1. Distribution and response to induction therapy of immunophenotypic subgroups

Immunophenotype	Patients		CR rate (%)
	(*n*)	(%)	
Pre-pre-B-ALL	38	4.9	94.7
Common ALL	507	64.9	99.0
Pre-B-ALL	114	14.6	100
B-ALL	24	3.1	95.8
T-ALL	96	12.3	98.6

CR, complete remission

Table 1 summarizes the incidence of immunophenotypic subgroups and their response to induction therapy in the ALL-BFM study 86. The vast majority of children with ALL achieved complete remission (CR), and no significant differences were observed between the immunophenotypic subgroups. After a median follow-up of 33 months, children with common and pre-B-ALL had a significantly longer duration of EFS than patients with immature CD10-negative pre-pre-B-ALL or T-lineage ALL (Fig. 1). A remarkable prognostic improvement was observed for B-ALL patients (Fig. 1).

Clinical Characteristics and Prognosis of T-Lineage ALL Classified According to Its Maturational Stage

The distribution and presenting clinical features of T-lineage subgroups classified according to a presumptive sequence of T-cell differentiation are shown in Table 2. Three patients with T-lineage ALL did not fit into the T-cell differentiation stages as defined above. No significant differences were found between these subgroups with respect to the main clinical risk factors (i.e., age and leukocyte counts). The incidence of hepatomegaly was significantly higher in children with an immature T-lineage phenotype, and the vivo response to corticosteroids was significantly worse with an early or mature T-cell phenotype than with a CD1a-positive intermediate T-ALL. Life-table analyses of T-lineage subgroups disclosed a significantly longer EFS for intermediate than for early or mature T-ALL (Fig. 2).

Incidence, Blast-Cell Biologic Features, and Prognosis of My$^+$ ALL

Myeloid-antigen expression was determined in 734 protocol patients entering the ALL-BFM 86 trial, and in 50 of them (6.8%) ≥20% of blast cells

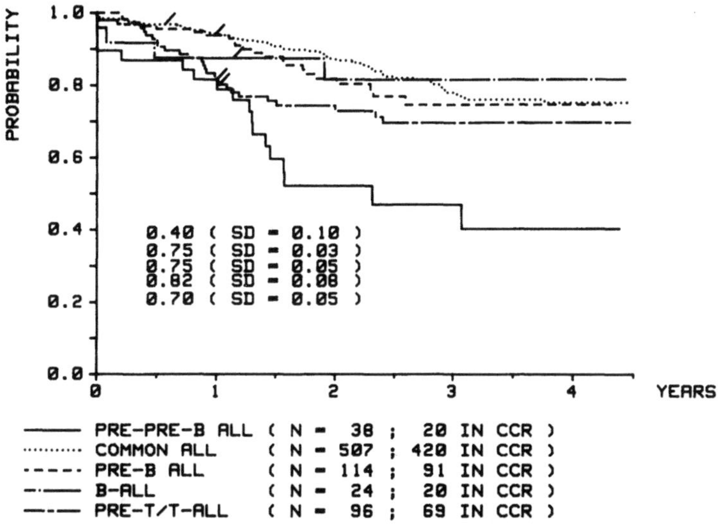

Fig. 1. Probability of event-free survival for 779 children with acute lymphoblastic leukemia (ALL) according to immunophenotypic subgroups. Median follow-up 33 months. *Slashes* indicate last patient entering the group, as in Figs. 2 and 4. *p* values: pre-pre-B ALL vs common, pre-B-, B-, and pre-T/T-ALL, <0.01; common ALL vs pre-T/T-ALL, <0.001. *CCR*, continuous complete remission

disclosed simultaneous expression of at least one myeloid-lineage-associated antigen. In most of these patients (45/50, 90%), leukemic blasts could be analyzed for all three myeloid antigens ($CD13/CD33/CD_w65$). Coexpression of two myeloid markers was detected in 7/45 and positivity of all three antigens in none of the My^+ ALL cases. The vast majority of My^+ ALL patients had a B-cell-precursor ALL (45/50, 90%) with an immature CD10-negative pre-pre-B phenotype being significantly more often associated with myeloid-antigen coexpression (mostly CD_w65) than common or pre-B-ALL (Fig. 3).

Analyses of Ig and TCR gene configuration could be performed in 42 of 50 My^+ ALL patients and demonstrated rearrangement of Ig heavy-chain genes in 40 of 41 children with B-cell precursor ALL or of both TCRγ and TCRδ genes in all three patients with My^+ T-lineage ALL. Patients with My^+ ALL and My^- ALL did not differ significantly in their incidence of cross-lineage (e.g., rearranged TCRβ, TCRγ, and TCRδ genes in B-cell precursor ALL) or oligoclonal rearrangements (data not shown).

Cytogenetic studies were successfully carried out in 30 of 50 (60%) My^+ ALL patients and revealed a strong correlation between an immature, usually CD_W65-positive, pre-pre-B phenotype and rearrangements involving chromosome 11 band q23, whereas no clear-cut associations were detected between the other My^+ ALL subgroups and specific chromosomal aberrations (Table 3).

Table 2. Presenting clinical and hematologic features and response to induction therapy of T-lineage subgroups (therapy study ALL-BFM 86)

Characteristics analyzed	Subgroups						*p* value
	Early (*n* = 37)		Intermediate (*n* = 45)		Mature (*n* = 11)		
	(*n*)	(%)	(*n*)	(%)	(*n*)	(%)	
Age (years)							
<1	1	2.7	0		0		
1–9	21	56.8	26	57.8	6	54.5	N.S.
⩾10	15	40.5	19	42.2	5	45.5	
Male sex	27	72.9	33	73.3	11		N.S.
WBC ($\times 10^9$/l)							
⩾50	25	67.6	24	53.3	5	45.5	N.S.
Hemoglobin							
⩽8.0 g/dl	7	18.9	6	13.3	1	9.1	N.S.
Platelet count ($\times 10^9$/l)							
⩽100	16	43.2	28	62.2	8	72.7	N.S.
Hepatomegaly[a]	24	64.8	21	46.7	2	18.2	<0.05
Splenomegaly[a]	18	48.6	23	51.1	4	36.4	N.S.
Mediastinal mass	23	62.1	35	77.8	9	81.4	N.S.
CNS disease	2	5.4	7	15.6	1	9.1	N.S.
Prednisone-poor response	13	35.1	1	2.2	5	45.5	<0.001
CR	35	94.5	45		11		N.S.

NS, not significant (chi square).
[a] >4 cm below the costal margin.

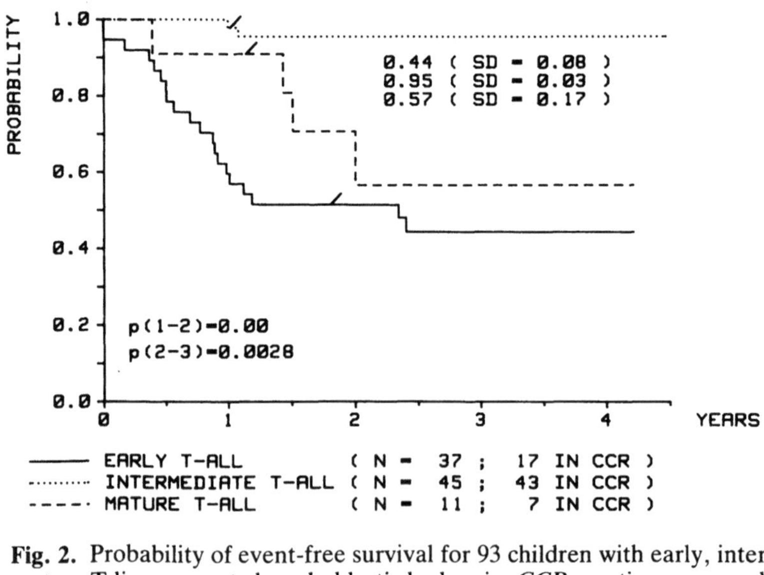

Fig. 2. Probability of event-free survival for 93 children with early, intermediate, and mature T-lineage acute lymphoblastic leukemia. *CCR*, continuous complete remission

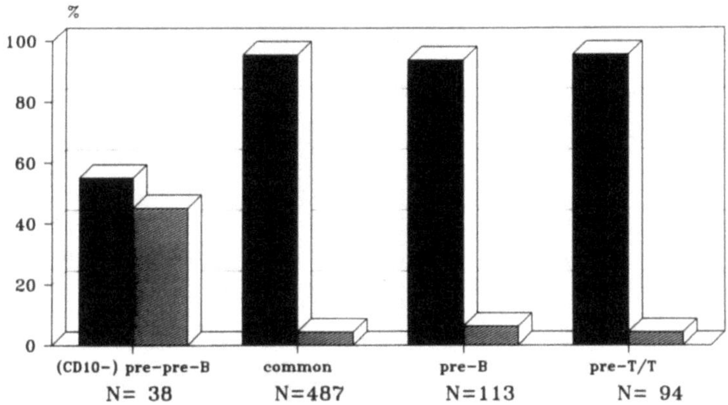

Fig. 3. Distribution of immunophenotypes in 684 patients with myeloid-antigen-negative (*black bars*, My^-) and 50 with myeloid-antigen-positive (*hatched bars*, My^+) ALL. Shown here are the percentages of My^- and My^+ cases in B-cell precursor subtypes and T-lineage acute lymphoblastic leukemia

The comparison of presenting clinical features and response to induction chemotherapy between My^+ and My^- ALL patients showed that a significantly higher percentage of those with My^+ ALL were infants under 1 year of age and presented with a leukocyte count exceeding 50×10^9/l (Table 4). These two groups exhibited no significant differences in sex distribution or other clinical and hematologic features such as extramedullary organ involvement, in vivo response to corticosteroids, and CR rate. Life-table analyses did not reveal any significant EFS differences between My^+ and My^- ALL patients (Fig. 4).

Discussion

During the last decade, several studies have described the immunophenotypic features of childhood ALL and stressed the relationship of immunologically defined entities to chromosomal aberrations, DNA content, clinical characteristics, and prognosis (Crist et al. 1988, 1989, 1990; Ludwig et al. 1989b; Pui et al. 1990c; Garand et al. 1990). With the exception of B-ALL, however, none of the immunophenotypic subgroups has been generally accepted as an independent risk factor for stratification of childhood ALL patients, and more recent studies have suggested that intensive chemotherapeutic protocols may lessen the negative prognostic implications of both biologic and clinical features in childhood ALL (Fletcher et al. 1989; Riehm et al. 1990; Raimondi et al. 1990). Furthermore, the unfavorable prognosis associated with certain immunophenotypic subgroups (e.g., CD10-negative B-cell precursor ALL, pre-B-ALL) was found to be primarily attributable to

Table 3. Immunophenotype and cytogenetic features in 30 myeloid-antigen-positive ALL cases

Patient no.	Immuno-phenotype	Karyotype
1	Pre-pre-B	46,XY
2	Pre-pre-B	46,XX,t(4;11)(q21;q23)
3	Pre-pre-B	46,XX
4	Pre-pre-B	46,XY,-3,-12,der(3)t(3;?)(q29;?),del(12)(p13)
5	Pre-pre-B	46,XY
6	Pre-pre-B	46,XX,t(4;11)(q21;q23)
7	Pre-pre-B	46,XX,t(4;11)(q21;q23)
8	Pre-pre-B	46,XY,t(1;11)(q21;q23)
9	Pre-pre-B	46,XY,t(4;11)(q21;q23)
10	Pre-pre-B	46,XX,t(1;11)(p32;q23)
11	Pre-pre-B	46,XY
12	Pre-pre-B	46,XX
13	Pre-pre-B	46,XX,der(14q)
14	Common	46,XY,t(2;15)(p21;q24),inv(3)(p25;q21)
15	Common	hyperdiploid (>50 chromosomes)
16	Common	tetraploid
17	Common	46,XY
18	Common	46,XY,del(12)(p12.2)
19	Common	46,XX
20	Common	46,XX
21	Common	46,XY,+mar
22	Common	46,XX
23	Common	hyperdiploid (>50 chromosomes)
24	Common	47,XX,+mar
25	Common	46,XX
26	Pre-B	46,XX
27	Pre-B	46,XX,der(19)t(1;19)(q23;p13)
28	T	46,XX,del(6q)
29	T	45,XY,-9,-10,-14,del(9)(p22),der(10),t(10;14)(q24;q11)
30	T	46,XX,del(2)(p23)

the presence of specific chromosomal translocations and adverse clinical features within these subsets (Chessells et al. 1987; Katz et al. 1988; Ludwig et al. 1989b; Crist et al. 1990; Pui et al. 1991a). Therefore, only a combined analysis including the characterization of immunophenotypic, karyotypic, and molecular-biologic features and their associations with clinical risk factors may allow a more precise definition of biologically relevant entities and the identification of high-risk subgroups in ALL that may profit by more intensive treatment strategies.

In children with B-cell precursor ALL, several immunophenotypic features, including CD10 or CD34 negativity, the detection of cytoplasmic μ chain, and surface expression of CD20, have been linked with a poorer prognosis (Pui et al. 1986; Ludwig et al. 1989b; Crist et al. 1989; Borowitz et al. 1990).

Table 4. Comparison of presenting clinical and hematologic features and response to induction therapy between My$^+$ and My$^-$ ALL (therapy study ALL-BFM 86)

Characteristics analyzed	Myeloid antigen expression				p value[a]
	No (n = 684)		Yes (n = 50)		
	(n)	(%)	(n)	(%)	
Age (years)					
<1	17	2.5	8	16.0	
1–9	532	77.8	32	64.0	<0.01
≥10	135	19.7	10	20.0	
Male sex	383	56.0	22	44.0	N.S.
WBC (×10^9/l)					
≥50	138	20.2	16	32.0	<0.05
Hemoglobin					
≤8.0 (g/dl)	382	55.8	27	54.0	N.S.
Platelet count (×10^9/l)					
≤100	490	71.6	41	82.0	N.S.
Hepatomegaly[a]	255	37.3	15	30.0	N.S.
Splenomegaly[a]	209	30.6	16	32.0	N.S.
CNS disease	19	2.8	2	4.0	N.S.
Prednisone-poor response	62	9.1	5	10.0	N.S.
CR	676	98.8	48	96.0	N.S.

NS, not significant (chi square).
[a] >4 cm below the costal margin.

In the ALL-BFM 86 study, children with an immature CD10-negative pre-pre-B phenotype had a significantly worse treatment outcome than those with common or pre-B ALL. This difference, however, could be largely attributed to the strong association of this immunophenotype with both unfavorable biologic features (e.g., high incidence of rearrangements involving chromosome 11 band q23, see below) and adverse clinical characteristics (i.e., age under 1 year, high initial leukocyte count). In contrast to other reports (Crist et al. 1989; Borowitz et al. 1990), life-table analyses of patients with B-cell precursor ALL did not reveal any significant difference in the duration of EFS between common or pre-B-ALL and CD34-negative or CD34-positive subsets (data not shown), suggesting that these immunophenotypic features may not be useful as predictive factors for childhood ALL within the context of intensive multidrug treatment protocols.

In T-lineage ALL, different immunophenotypic features, including an immature pre-T-ALL phenotype, membrane expression of CD3, and negativity of CD5, THY antigen (similar to CD1), or CD10, were found to involve an increased risk of treatment failure (Thiel et al. 1989; Garand et al. 1990; Ludwig et al. 1990b; Pui et al. 1990b; Shuster et al. 1990). The prognostic impact of these factors, however, differed according to the treat-

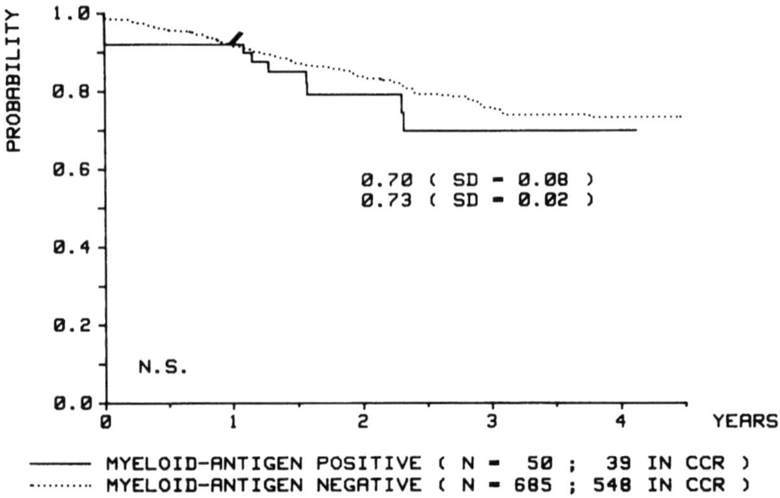

Fig. 4. Probability of event-free survival for 684 children with myeloid-antigen-negative and 50 with myeloid-antigen-positive B-cell precursor or T-lineage acute lymphoblastic leukemia (non-B-ALL). *N.S.*, *p* value not significant; *CCR*, continuous complete remission

ment strategies used, and risk assignment in T-lineage ALL based on immunophenotypic criteria has not yet been accepted.

In the ALL-BFM 86 study, life-table analyses of T-lineage subgroups classified according to their maturational stage provided strong evidence for clinically relevant differences in treatment outcome between these subgroups. Children with a CD1a-positive intermediate T-cell phenotype disclosed a significantly better in vivo response to corticosteroids and a longer duration of EFS than those with an immature early (including pre-T) or more mature (membrane CD3-positive) phenotype. These differences could not be explained by unequal distribution of the well-established clinical risk factors age and leukocyte count. Further investigations aimed at better defining the correlation between immunophenotypes and other biological features (e.g., chromosomal abnormalities, growth factor activation, expression of proteins serving as transcriptional regulatory factors) are therefore clearly warranted to elucidate the biologic heterogeneity in T-lineage ALL (Raimondi et al. 1988; Brown et al. 1990; O'Connor et al. 1991; Sawyers et al. 1991).

Our data on the incidence and prognostic impact of My^+ ALL are in clear contrast to a recent study reporting My^+ ALL in 22% of childhood ALL and suggesting that myeloid-antigen expression is an important independent predictor of a poor response to chemotherapy (Wiersma et al. 1991). The incidence of My^+ ALL observed in the ALL-BFM 86 study was substantially lower (7%) and comparable to that reported by most other studies on childhood ALL (Pui et al. 1990a; Borowitz et al. 1991; Pui et al. 1991b;

Cantù-Rajnoldi et al. 1991). Interestingly, almost 50% of patients with an immature B-precursor cell phenotype had myeloid-antigen expression (usually CD_w65), whereas much less than 10% disclosed myeloid-antigen positivity in the other B-cell precursor or T-lineage ALL subgroups. Possible explanations for these discrepancies in the incidence and prognosis of My^+ ALL (e.g., differences in definitions of My^+ ALL, immunophenotyping methods, study populations, or treatment strategies) have been discussed in detail elsewhere (Drexler et al. 1991; Borowitz et al. 1991).

In keeping with our results, other recent studies have also failed to demonstrate any prognostic value for myeloid-antigen expression in childhood ALL and have suggested that highly effective therapy will abolish the prognostic impact of My^+ ALL (Pui et al. 1990a; Borowitz et al. 1991; Pui et al. 1991b; Cantù-Rajnoldi et al. 1991). It should be noted that, within the group of pediatric My^+ ALL patients, we and others have recently described a distinct clinicopathologic entity with poor treatment outcome characterized by unique biologic (i.e., CD15- and/or CD_w65-positive pre-pre-B phenotype, rearrangements of chromosome 11 band q23) and clinical (i.e., age under 1 year, hyperleukocytosis) features (Katz et al. 1988; Ludwig et al. 1989a; Pui et al. 1991a). Further studies based on consistent diagnostic criteria and applying more detailed immunophenotypic and genotypic characterization as well as ultrastructural cytochemistry are clearly needed to elucidate the biologic heterogeneity and to establish the clinical importance of other My^+ ALL subtypes.

Acknowledgments. We are indebted to Stefanie Böttcher, Mathilde Martin, and Annette Sindram for skillful technical assistance. We thank the participants in the German multicenter trial ALL-BFM 86 for their fruitful cooperation. This work was supported in part by the Deutsche Krebshilfe and by the Deutsche Leukämie-Forschungshilfe.

References

Bain B, Catovsky D (1990) Current concerns in haematology 2: classification of acute leukaemia. J Clin Pathol 43:882–887

Béné MC, Boumsell L, Vannier JP, Garand R, Solary E, Faure G, Bernard A, French Groupe d'Etude Immunologique des Leucémies (GEIL) (1989) Immunologic analysis of a thousand cases of acute leukemia. Nouv Rev Fr Hematol 31:133–136

Bleyer WA (1990) Acute lymphoblastic leukemia in children. Advances and prospectus. Cancer 65:689–695

Borowitz MJ, Shuster JJ, Civin CI, Carroll AJ, Look AT, Behm FG, Land VJ, Pullen DJ, Crist WM (1990) Prognostic significance of CD34 expression in childhood B-precursor acute lymphocytic leukemia: a Pediatric Oncology Group study. J Clin Oncol 8:1389–1398

Borowitz MJ, Shuster JJ, Land VJ, Steuber CP, Pullen DJ, Vietti T (1991) Myeloid-antigen expression in childhood acute lymphoblastic leukemia. N Engl J Med 325:1379–1380

Brown L, Cheng JT, Chen Q, Siciliano MJ, Crist W, Buchanan G, Baer R (1990) Site-specific recombination of the *tal*-1 gene is a common occurrence in human T cell leukemia. EMBO J 9:3343–3351
Cantù-Rajnoldi A, Putti C, Saitta M, Granchi D, Foà R, Schirò R, Castagni M, Valeggio C, Jankovic M, Miniero R, Paolucci P, Basso G (1991) Co-expression of myeloid antigens in childhood acute lymphoblastic leukaemia: relationship with the stage of differentiation and clinical significance. Br J Haematol 79:40–43
Chessells JM, Hardisty RM, Richards S (1987) Long survival in childhood lymphoblastic leukemia. Br J Cancer 55:315–319
Crist WM, Shuster JJ, Falletta J, Pullen DJ, Berard CW, Vietti TJ, Alvarado CS, Roper MA, Prasthofer E, Grossi CE (1988) Clinical features and outcome in childhood T-cell leukemia-lymphoma according to stage of thymocyte differentiation: a Pediatric Oncology Group Study. Blood 72:1891–1897
Crist W, Boyett J, Jackson J, Vietti T, Borowitz M, Chauvenet A, Winick N, Ragab A, Mahoney D, Head D, Iyer R, Wagner H, Pullen J (1989) Prognostic importance of the pre-B-cell immunophenotype and other presenting features in B-lineage childhood acute lymphoblastic leukemia: a Pediatric Oncology Group study. Blood 74:1252–1259
Crist WM, Carroll AJ, Shuster JJ, Behm FG, Whitehead M, Vietti TJ, Look AT, Mahoney D, Ragab A, Pullen DJ, Land VJ (1990) Poor prognosis of children with pre-B acute lymphoblastic leukemia is associated with the t(1;19)(q23;p13): a Pediatric Oncology Group study. Blood 76:117–122
Drexler HG, Thiel E, Ludwig WD (1991) Review of the incidence and clinical relevance of myeloid antigen-positive acute lymphoblastic leukemia. Leukemia 5:637–645
Fletcher JA, Kimball VM, Lynch E, Donnelly M, Pavelka K, Gelber RD, Tantravahi R, Salla SE (1989) Prognostic implications of cytogenetic studies in an intensively treated group of children with acute lymphoblastic leukemia. Blood 74:2130–2135
Garand R, Vannier JP, Béné MC, Faure G, Favre M, Bernard A, Groupe d'Etude Immunologique des Leucémies (1990) Comparison of outcome, clinical, laboratory, and immunological features in 164 children and adults with T-ALL. Leukemia 4:739–744
Greaves MF (1986) Differentiation-linked leukemogenesis in lymphocytes. Science 234:697–704
Janossy G, Coustan-Smith E, Campana D (1989) The reliability of cytoplasmic CD3 and CD22 antigen expression in the immunodiagnosis of acute leukemia: a study of 500 cases. Leukemia 3:170–181
Kaplan EL, Meier P (1958) Nonparametric estimation from incomplete observations. J Am Stat Assoc 53:457–481
Katz F, Malcolm S, Gibbons B, Tilly R, Lam G, Robertson ME, Czepulkowski B, Chessells J (1988) Cellular and molecular studies on infant null acute lymphoblastic leukemia. Blood 71:1438–1447
Look AT (1988) The cytogenetics of childhood leukemia: clinical and biologic implications. Pediatr Clin North Am 35:723–741
Ludwig WD, Bartram CR, Ritter J, Raghavachar A, Hiddemann W, Heil G, Harbott J, Seibt-Jung H, Teichmann JV, Riehm H (1988) Ambiguous phenotypes and genotypes in 16 children with acute leukemia as characterized by multiparameter analysis. Blood 71:1518–1528
Ludwig WD, Bartram CR, Harbott J, Köller U, Haas OA, Hansen-Hagge T, Heil G, Seibt-Jung H, Teichmann JV, Ritter J, Knapp W, Gadner H, Thiel E, Riehm J (1989a) Phenotypic and genotypic heterogeneity in infant acute leukemia: I. Acute lymphoblastic leukemia. Leukemia 3:431–439
Ludwig WD, Seibt-Jung H, Teichmann JV, Komischke B, Gatzke A, Gassner G, Odenwald E, Hofmann J, Riehm H (1989b) Clinicopathological features and

prognostic implications of immunophenotypic subgroups in childhood ALL: experience of the BFM-ALL study 83. In: Neth R, Gallo RC, Greaves MF, Gaedicke G, Gohla S, Mannweiler K, Ritter J (eds) Modern trends in human leukemia VIII. Springer, Berlin Heidelberg New York, pp 51–57 (Haematology and blood transfusion, vol 32)

Ludwig WD, Bartram CR, Raghavachar A, Harbott J, Thiel E, Riehm H (1990a) Clinical relevance of immunoglobulin (Ig) and T-cell receptor (TCR) gene rearrangements in childhood B-cell precursor (BCP)-ALL. Blood 76 [Suppl 1]: 298a

Ludwig WD, Thiel E, Bartram CR, Kranz BR, Raghavachar A, Löffler H, Ganser A, Büchner T, Hiddemann W, Heil G, Freund M, Maschmeyer G, Reiter A, Messerer D, Riehm H, Hoelzer D (1990b) Clinical importance of T-ALL subclassification according to thymic or prethymic maturation stage. In: Büchner T, Schellong G, Hiddemann W, Ritter J (eds) Acute Leukemias: II. Prognostic factors and treatment strategies. Springer, Berlin Heidelberg New York, pp 419–247 (Haematology and blood transfusion, vol 33)

Mantel N (1966) Evaluation of survival data and two new rank order statistics arising in its consideration. Cancer Chemother Rep 50:163–170

O'Connor R, Cesano A, Lange B, Finan J, Nowell PC, Clark SC, Raimondi SC, Rovera G, Santoli D (1991) Growth factor requirements of childhood acute T-lymphoblastic leukemia: correlation between presence of chromosomal abnormalities and ability to grow permanently in vitro. Blood 77:1534–1545

Pui CH, Williams DL, Raimondi SC, Melvin SL, Behm FG, Look AT, Dahl GV, Rivera GK, Kalwinsky DK, Mirro J, Dodge RK, Murphy SB (1986) Unfavorable presenting clinical and laboratory features are associated with CALLA-negative non-T, non-B lymphoblastic leukemia in children. Leuk Res 10:1287–1292

Pui CH, Behm FG, Singh B, Rivera GK, Schell MJ, Roberts WM, Crist WM, Mirro J (1990a) Myeloid-associated antigen expression lacks prognostic value in childhood acute lymphoblastic leukemia treated with intensive multiagent chemotherapy. Blood 75:198–202

Pui CH, Behm FG, Singh B, Schell MJ, Williams DL, Rivera GK, Kalwinsky DK, Sandlund JT, Crist WM, Raimondi SC (1990b) Heterogeneity of presenting features and their relation to treatment outcome in 120 children with T-cell acute lymphoblastic leukemia. Blood 75:174–179

Pui CH, Crist WM, Look AT (1990c) Biology and clinical significance of cytogenetic abnormalities in childhood acute lymphoblastic leukemia. Blood 76:1449–1463

Pui CH, Frankel LS, Carroll AJ, Raimondi SC, Shuster JJ, Head DR, Crist WM, Land VJ, Pullen J, Steuber CP, Behm FG, Borowitz MJ (1991a) Clinical characteristics and treatment outcome of childhood acute lymphoblastic leukemia with the t(4;11)(q21;q23): a collaborative study of 40 cases. Blood 77:440–447

Pui CH, Raimondi SC, Head DR, Schell MJ, Rivera GK, Mirro J, Crist WM, Behm FG (1991b) Characterization of childhood acute leukemia with multiple myeloid and lymphoid markers at diagnosis and at relapse. Blood 78:1327–1337

Raimondi SC, Behm FG, Roberson PK, Pui CH, Rivera GK, Murphy SB, Williams DL (1988) Cytogenetics of childhood T-cell leukemia. Blood 72:1560–1566

Raimondi SC, Behm FG, Roberson PK, Williams DL, Pui CH, Crist WM, Look AT, Rivera GK (1990) Cytogenetics of pre-B-cell acute lymphoblastic leukemia with emphasis on prognostic implications of the t(1;19). J Clin Oncol 8:1380–1388

Riehm H, Gadner H, Henze G, Kornhuber B, Lampert F, Niethammer D, Reiter A, Schellong G (1990) Results and significance of six randomized trials in four consecutive ALL-BFM studies. In: Büchner T, Schellong G, Hiddemann W, Ritter J (eds) Acute Leukemias: II. Prognostic factors and treatment strategies. Springer, Berlin Heidelberg New York, pp 439–450 (Haematology and blood transfusion, vol 33)

Sawyers CL, Denny CT, Witte ON (1991) Leukemia and the disruption of normal hematopoiesis. Cell 64:337–350

Shuster JJ, Falletta JM, Pullen DJ, Crist WM, Humphrey GB, Dowell BL, Wharam MD, Borowitz M (1990) Prognostic factors in childhood T-cell acute lymphoblastic leukemia: a Pediatric Oncology Group study. Blood 75:166–173

Thiel E, Kranz BR, Raghavachar A, Bartram CR, Löffler H, Messerer D, Ganser A, Ludwig WD, Büchner T, Hoelzer (1989) Prethymic phenotype and genotype of pre-T ($CD7^+/ER^-$)-cell leukemia and its clinical significance within adult acute lymphoblastic leukemia. Blood 73:1247–1258

Van der Does-van den Berg A, Bartram CR, Basso G, Benoit Y, Biondi A, Debatin K, Haas O, Harbott J, Kamps WA, Köller U, Lampert F, Ludwig WD, Niemeyer C, van Wering ER (1992) Minimal requirements for the diagnosis, classification and evaluation of the treatment of childhood acute lymphoblastic leukemia (ALL) in the "BFM family" cooperative group. Med Pediatr Oncol 20:497–505

Van Dongen JJM, Wolvers-Tettero ILM (1991) Analysis of immunoglobulin and T cell receptor genes: II. Possibilities and limitations in the diagnosis and management of lymphoproliferative diseases and related disorders. Clin Chim Acta 198:93–171

Wiersma SR, Ortega J, Sobel E, Weinberg KI (1991) Clinical importance of myeloid-antigen expression in acute lymphoblastic leukemia of childhood. N Engl J Med 324:800–808

Incidence, Clinical and Laboratory Features, and Prognostic Significance of Immunophenotypic Subgroups in Acute Lymphoblastic Leukemia: The GEIL Experience

R. Garand[1], M.C. Béné[2], and the GEIL*

[1] Laboratoire d'Hématologie du CHU, Rue Gaston Veil, 44000 Nantes, France
[2] Laboratoire d'Immunologie du CHU, Faculté de Médecine, BP184, 54500 Vandoeuvre les Nancy, France

Introduction

Extensive immunophenotyping of hematologic proliferations has been made possible by the availability of monoclonal antibodies to surface or intracellular molecules. The four workshops dedicated to leukocyte typing have moreover helped classifying the molecules identified and reagents used in developing an internationally adopted nomenclature for clusters of differentiation (CD) (Bernard et al. 1984). The extensive immunophenotypic variety of acute lymphoblastic leukemias (ALL) has thus become apparent (Foon and Todd 1986), and questions have been raised as to the clinical and prognostic significance of these new biological parameters. In France, a group of hematologists, immunologists, and clinicians has been interested in the definition of leukemias since November 1983. Their major concern is to obtain maximal immunophenotypic information on as many proliferations as

*GEIL is composed of Drs.: J. Gardais (Angers), M.C. Leglise, G. Lecalvez (Brest), M. Bernier, M. Massy (Brussels), A.M. Griveau, P. Boutard, C. Lebrun (Caen), J. Bonhomme, B. Chassagne, F. Demeocq, C. Rapatel (Clermont-Ferrand), H. Jouault (Créteil Mondor), F. Lelong (Créteil Intercommunal), E. Solary, O. Cassasnovas, M. Maynadié (Dijon), J.C. Bensa, M. Favre, M.C. Jacob (Grenoble), C. Sartiaux (Lille), M. Drouet (Limoges), L. Campos, A. Larese (Lyon), P. Poncelet, C. Brunet (Marseille), T. Lavabre-Bertrand, J. Taib (Montpellier), G. Kandel, G. Jung (Mulhouse), R. Garand (Nantes), P. Philip, F. Monpoux, I. Sudaka, F. Baudouin, C. Caldani, A. Bernard (Nice), M. Reguer, H. Schill (Paris Val de Grâce), G. Schaison, L. Boumsell (Paris Saint Louis), D. Vanhaecke, L. Douay (Paris Trousseau), A. Brizard (Poitiers), J.P. Roualet, T. Tabary (Reims), N. Genetet (Rennes), O. Lees, B. Lenormand, J.P. Vannier (Rouen), J.C. Le Petit, S. Acquart, O. Sabido (Saint-Etienne), A. Falkenrodt (Strasbourg), J.L. Bremond, A.M. Masy (Tours), F. Roubinet, E. Kuhlein (Toulouse), F. Lebaron, P. Duthilleul, B. Reumaux (Valenciennes), M.C. Bene, G. Faure, P. Bordigoni, F. Witz (Vandoeuvre les Nancy), C. Bayle, J. Antonini (Villejuif).

Recent Results in Cancer Research, Vol. 131

possible. What cannot be achieved by a single institution becomes possible if several teams gather their data. Thirty-two teams have now joined this informal federation, exchanged information, developed homogeneous methods for extensive immunophenotyping, and collected data from more than 2000 patients, validated by internal workshops. The multicentric strategy appears to have worked since significant numbers of rare phenotypes and follow-up data on large numbers of more classical proliferations have been collected (Vannier et al. 1989; Béné et al. 1989; Garand et al. 1987, 1990). Because each group retained its autonomy, similar patients have benefited from many different treatment protocols, thus reducing the possible therapeutic bias and increasing the significance of immunophenotypic features.

In this paper, we report on a selected group of 882 ALL patients at diagnosis, describing the distribution, characteristics, and outcome of the immunophenotypic groups observed.

Patients and Methods

Inclusion Criteria

The series includes only ALL cases identified as such on morphological criteria using the FAB proposals (Bennet et al. 1981). All patients were examined at diagnosis, and no cases of secondary or relapsing leukemia were included. Special attention was given to the composition of the blood or bone marrow sample used for the immunophenotyping. Only cases with more than 50% of blast cells and less than 20% of lymphocytes were retained. The immunophenotyping had to be as extensive as possible, including at least the markers allowing the identification of the immunophenotypic subtype without ambiguity.

Immunophenotypes

Immunophenotyping techniques were performed in each center for its respective patients. Direct or indirect immunofluorescence on purified cell suspensions was applied to fresh or sometimes thawed cells. The latter were mainly used for the investigation of additional molecules, in order to complete the immunophenotypic definition of the proliferation. All laboratories used UV light microscopy until 1987, and progressively became equipped for flow-cytometry analysis, now used everywhere. Three internal workshops confirmed the similarity of immunophenotyping techniques in the various centres. The latest yielded 94% consistency.

Positivity thresholds were defined as follows: expression on more than 30% of the cells for B- and T-lineage markers, more than 20% for myeloid-lineage-associated molecules, and more than 10% for intracytoplasmic μ chains.

The immunophenotypes observed were classified according to a working scheme derived from previously reported models of lymphoid differentiation (Reinherz et al. 1980; Roper et al. 1983; Nadler et al. 1984; Campana et al. 1985; Foon and Todd 1986; Loken et al. 1987; Haynes et al. 1988; Uckun 1990). ALL cells with B-cell markers were denominated pre-B-ALL, unless they expressed surface immunoglobulins (sIg), in which case they were called B-ALL.

Pre-B-ALL was further divided into four subtypes:

- Pre-B1 ("early") was defined by the expression of CD19, in the absence of CD10 and of the B-cell maturation-associated molecules CD20 and intracytoplasmic μ chains (cμ).
- Pre-B2 ("common") corresponded to a $CD10^{+}/CD20^{-}/c\mu^{-}$ immunophenotype, together with at least one of the B-cell associated antigens CD19, CD22, or CD24.
- Pre-B3 was defined by the membrane expression of CD20, in the absence of cytoplasmic μ chains;
- Pre-B4 or true pre-B cells contained intracytoplasmic μ chains ($c\mu^{+}$).

ALL expressing T-lineage markers was similarly divided into four subtypes:

- T1 or pro-T-ALL ("pro-thymocytic") expressed at least one of the pan-T molecules CD2, CD5, and CD7 but none of the thymocyte-associated antigens CD1, CD3, CD4, and CD8 on the cells' surface.
- T2- and T3-ALL were defined as cells expressing an immunophenotype similar to those of cortical ($CD1^{+}$ and/or $CD4^{+}/CD8^{+}$) or medullary ($CD4^{+}$ or $CD8^{+}$) thymocytes, respectively.
- T4-ALL defined less frequently encountered cells expressing CD3 in the absence of CD4 and CD8, and likely to have a functional T-cell receptor γδ (TCRγδ).

ALLs expressing only myeloid (CD13, CD11b, CD14, CD15, and/or CD33) antigens, yet displaying morphological characteristics of ALL, were termed M0. Finally, cases most extensively investigated and without any B, T, or myeloid marker were called "undifferentiated" (A-LL).

Data Collection

Clinical and laboratory data and all immunophenotypic information were collected for each patient and forwarded to the group's secretariat. All information was fed to a computerized data base specifically developed using Myosotis (Coultronics France, Margency, France) software. Follow-up information was updated regularly, on December 1990 for this study.

Statistics

Statistical analysis was performed with either D-Base IV (Ashton-Tate, Torrance, CA, USA) or Myosotis (Coultronics France) software, using the χ^2 test, the Yates correction for the χ^2 test, and Student's t test. Outcome evaluation was performed for a selected subgroup of patients, excluding those who had benefited from allogenic bone marrow transplantation while in first complete remission. Life tables for event-free survival were constructed by the method of Kaplan and Meier (1958), with differences compared by the log-rank test (Peto et al. 1977).

Results

Immunophenotypes Are Distributed According to Age

Table 1 shows the distribution of the various subtypes observed, in relation to age. Infants are children less than 1 year old, and the adult group stretches between 16 and 87 years of age. The incidence of pre-B-ALL subtypes decreased while those of T-ALL, B-ALL, M0-AL, and U-AL significantly increased in correlation with age ($p < 0.00001$): 96% of the infants had pre-B-ALL, versus 75% of the children and only 50% of the

Table 1. Immunophenotypic distribution of 882 ALL patients at diagnosis

Type/subtype	Infants			Children			Adults		
	n	AG%	ST%	*n*	AG%	ST%	*n*	AG%	ST%
Pre-B (total)	22	96		415	75		154	50	
Pre-B1	10	44	45	32	6	8	37	12	24
Pre-B2	10	44	45	262	47	63	67	22	43.5
Pre-B3	1	4	5	98	18	23.5	44	14	28.5
Pre-B4	1	4	5	23	4	5.5	6	2	4
B	0			15	2.5		19	6	
T (total)	1	4		114	21		106	35	
T1	1			35	6.5	31	49	16	46
T2	0			53	9.5	46	40	13	38
T3	0			18	3	16	10	3.5	9.5
T4	0			8	1.5	7	7	2.5	6.5
MO	0			2	0.5		12	4	
Undifferentiated	0			6	1		15	5	
Total	23			552			306		

AG%, percentage in age group; ST%, percentage in in subtype.

adults; by contrast, T-ALL was found in 35% of the adults versus only 21% of the children. Twelve out of 14 cases of M0-ALL were adult patients, U-ALL was very rare, most likely because of the extensive panel used in the immunophenotypic studies. The 21 cases reported here were thoroughly investigated. An additional percentage expressed CD24 and could perhaps be related to B-lineage ALL. Only 17 could not be assigned to any lineage.

Infants displayed a high incidence of pre-B1-ALL (45%), and the most mature forms of pre-B-ALL were seldom observed in infants. The distributions of the pre-B- and T-ALL subgroups appeared more homogeneous between children and adults, although pre-B2 was more frequent in the former. Interestingly, pre-B1-ALL (lacking CD10 expression) accounted for nearly 1 in 4 adult pre-B-ALL. Lineage infidelity was observed in 25% of infant ALL, 13% of childhood ALL, and 16 % of adult ALL. Myeloid markers (My^+ ALL) were associated with 14% of the pre-B-ALL and 9% of the T-ALL phenotypes. My^+ T-ALL was significantly more frequent in adults (13%) than in children (4%) ($p = 0.05$).

B-Lineage ALL

Immunophenotypes and Clinical and Laboratory Features at Diagnosis

Table 2 shows the incidence of the clinical and laboratory factors known to be associated with a poor prognosis (Hammond et al. 1986) according to the age and immunophenotypic subgroup in B-lineage ALL.

Pre-B1-ALL in infants appeared to be a clinically distinct entity characterized by a female prevalence (80%), a high incidence of tumoral syndrome (80%) and, in 70% of the cases, leukocyte counts higher than $100 \times 10^9/l$ ($p = 0.04$ when compared to other infant ALL). High leukocyte counts were also more frequent in childhood pre-B1-ALL than in childhood pre-B-ALL ($p < 0.01$), while adult pre-B subtypes were characterized by a lower frequency of tumoral masses and anemia than childhood pre-B-ALL.

B-ALL was associated with a higher frequency (26%) of central nervous system involvement than pre-B-ALL (3%). Its clinical features did not differ significantly between children and adults, save for the less frequent liver involvement in the latter ($p = 0.04$).

Immunophenotypes and Karyotypic Abnormalities

Cytogenetic analyses were available in 231 patients with B-lineage ALL. The proportion of abnormal karyotypes was similar in all subtypes, ranging between 73% and 92%. Hyperdiploidy was significantly less frequent in pre-B1-ALL and B-ALL, which, however, displayed a higher incidence of structural abnormalities than other pre-B subtypes. These observations

Table 2. Age-related clinical and biological features in B-lineage ALL subtypes

	Pre-B1	Pre-B2	Pre-B3	Pre-B4	B
Males (%)					
Infants	20		50[a]		
Children	56	50	50	48	80
Adults	51	55	61		58
Adenomegaly (%)					
Infants	60		50[a]		
Children	56	55	57	50	47
Adults	27	4	36		53
Splenomegaly (%)					
Infants	80		42[a]		
Children	69	56	63	52	60
Adults	46	46	39		37
Hepatomegaly (%)					
Infants	80		50[a]		
Children	50	56	57	43	60
Adults	16	21	32		26
Anemia: Hb < 100 g/l (%)					
Infants	70		83[a]		
Children	84	76	62	78	67
Adults	49	54	50		37
High WBC: $> 10^{11}$/l (%)					
Infants	70		17[a]		7
Children	22	4	4	9	5
Adults	22	15	9		

[a] For pre-B2, pre-B3, and pre-B4 together.

are of interest since hyperdiploidy has been shown to be a favorable pronostic feature when the number of chromosomes is higher than 50. By contrast structural abnormalities appear to identify high-risk ALL patients (Bloomfield et al. 1986; Pui et al. 1990).

Some karyotypic abnormalities appeared strongly associated with specific subtypes:

- The t(4;11) translocation was more frequent in pre-B1-ALL (8 out of 9 cases) than in any other subtype, which is consistent with previous reports (Vannier et al. 1989; Pui et al. 1990).
- The now classical association between t(8;14) and B-ALL (Berger et al. 1979) was observed in 6 out of 8 patients displaying this translocation.

Conversely, the t(9;22)/Philadelphia chromosome, the most frequent translocation described in adult ALL (Pui et al. 1990), did not appear to be

Table 3. Distribution of leukocyte differentiation markers in B-lineage ALL Data are reported as percentage and (number of cases investigated)

	Pre-B1		Pre-B2		Pre-B3		Pre-B4		B	
	(%)	(*n*)	(%)	(*n*)	(%)	(*n*)	(%)	(*n*)	(%)	(*n*)
CD19	100	80	96	299	96	129	93	27	83	30
CD20	0	76	0	339	100	143	41	29	88	34
CD21	21	47	18	175	9	65	20	15	25	16
CD22	43	21	36	53	76	27			50	4
CD24	61	54	85	220	97	87	86	22	86	22
HLA-DR	70	44	91	154	95	58	83	18	100	17
CD9	77	65	82	268	90	103	83	24	88	23
CD10	0	80	100	339	96	139	77	31	31	32
CD34	52	25	61	77	65	43	50	6	17	12

restricted to a particular pre-B subtype. However, none of the 13 patients with a t(9;22) were phenotypically classified as pre-B1-ALL or B-ALL.

Expression of Leukocyte Differentiation Antigens

Table 3 shows the positivity of individual markers among pre B and B-ALL. CD19 appeared to be one of the best B-lineage markers, being present in 93%–100% of the cases. Of the pre-B1-ALL cases, 61% and 43% expressed the B-cell-associated CD24 and CD22 molecules, respectively, confirming their B-lineage origin. Surprisingly, CD10 expression was noted in one third of B-cell ALL cases. The hematopoietic progenitor CD34 antigen was present in more than half of pre-B1-ALL cases, and also unexpectedly remained in a significant proportion of more mature pre-B-ALL, as well as in 17% of B-cell ALL. CD34 has been reported to disappear from the surface of normal maturing B cells before the acquisition of CD20 and surface immunoglobulin (sIg) molecules (Loken et al. 1987). The $CD34^+/CD20^+$ or $CD34^+/sIg^+$ ALL reported here could thus be regarded as resulting from an abnormal asynchronous differentiation process characterizing leukemogenesis. A similar interpretation could be given for the persistence of an aberrant expression of myeloid markers in the most mature forms of pre-B- and B-ALL, even though their incidence is higher in pre-B1-ALL.

Clinical Evolution (Fig. 1)

Comparison of the event-free survival (EFS) of infant ALL according to the immunophenotype showed the pre-B1-ALL subtype to be associated with a

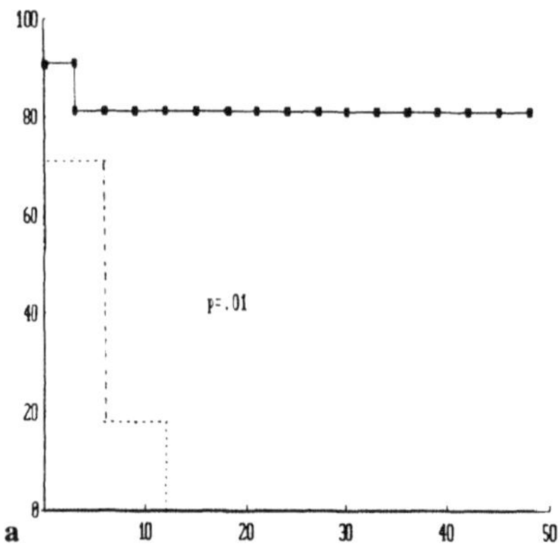

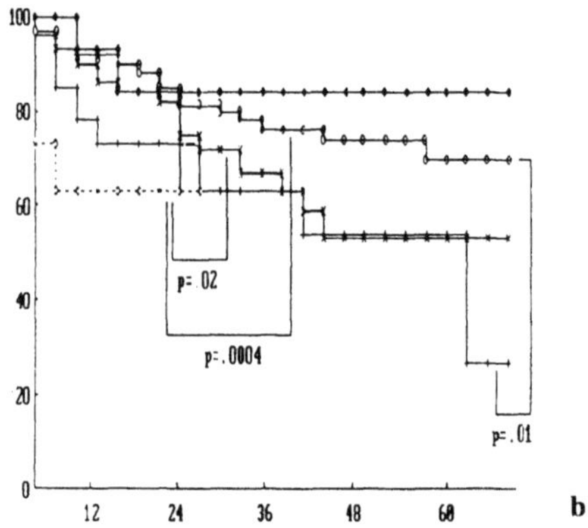

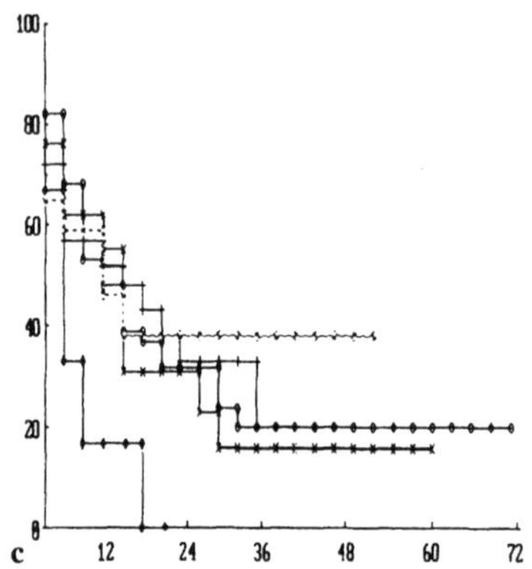

Fig. 1. Event-free survival curves of infants (**a**), children (**b**), and adults (**c**) with pre-B- or B-ALL. The percentages of individuals still in first complete remission are indicated on the *abcissa*. Months of follow-up are on the *ordinate*. Frequencies and statistical significance were established using the log-rank test. *Symbols* are as follows: B-ALL, ○, *dotted* line; pre-B1-ALL, +; pre-B2-ALL, ○; pre-B3-ALL, ×; pre-B4-ALL, ◆. Pre-B1-ALL were compared to the pool of other pre-B-ALL in the group of infants

dramatically bad prognosis. Evolution of the four pre-B-ALL subgroups and B-ALL could be compared in the larger group of children. Pre-B1- and B-ALL were associated with a significantly shorter EFS than other pre-B subtypes. None of the individual membrane markers accounted for these differences by itself, and prognostic criteria thus derive only from the complete immunophenotype. Lineage infidelity in both children and adults with pre-B-ALL was not associated with a significantly different prognosis. The outcome of adult patients was significantly worse than that of children, and did not appear to be associated with a specific subtype.

T-Lineage ALL

More than 15 different phenotypes were observed in the subgroup of 222 cases of ALL in this study, and it was decided to collect them in the two larger groups of T1 (pro-T) ALL and T2-T4 (late-T) ALL. The age of the patients was only taken into account in this study for outcome evaluation.

Table 4. Clinical and biological features in T-lineage ALL subtypes

	Pro-T-ALL (n = 86)	Late-T-ALL (n = 136)
Age, median (range) (years)	19 (1–81)	14 (1–64)
Males (%)	74	80
Adenomegaly (%)	65	79
Splenomegaly (%)	49	75
Hepatomegaly (%)	44	56
Mediastinal mass (%)	44	55
CNS involvement (%)	6	8
Pleural effusion (%)	10	9
Anemia (Hb < 100 g/l) (%)	42	28
High WBC (>10^{11}/l) (%)	22	46

Immunophenotypes and Clinical Features at Diagnosis

As shown in Table 4, pro-T-ALL patients differed from those with late-T-ALL by having a lower incidence of lymph node ($p < 0.02$) and splenic ($p < 0.001$) involvement. Anemia was observed twice as often in this group, whereas leukocyte counts were significantly lower ($p < 0.001$). However, classic T-ALL-associated features, i.e., male prevalence, mediastinal mass (Sen and Borella 1975), and polar acid phosphatase positivity in blast cells (Catovsky et al. 1974), were found with similar frequencies in both T-ALL subgroups.

Phenotypic Characteristics of Pro-T-ALL

The CD7 antigen was found positive on the leukemic cells from 82 out of 84 pro-T-ALL patients. Less than half of these $CD7^+$ cases coexpressed CD2. Conversely, CD34 (43%), HLA-DR (32%), CD9 (34%), and aberrant myeloid-associated markers (16%) were significantly associated with the pro-T phenotype.

Intracytoplasmic expression of CD3 (cCD3) was observed in 81% of late-T-ALL cases, but in only half of the pro-T-ALL cases tested. However, cCD3 was found in 60% of $CD7^+/CD2^-$ pro-T-ALL cases, 30% of which also expressed surface CD5, thus suggesting that these apparently very immature ALL indeed belong to the T-lineage (Van de Velde et al. 1991).

Southern blot analysis of the TCR genes could be performed in 18 cases of pro-T-ALL, and seven of late-T-ALL. All the latter showed both the TCRβ and TCRγ genes to be rearranged. In the pro-T-ALL subgroup, rearrangments of TCRβ were observed in seven out of 18 cases and of

TCRγ in seven out of 16 cases studied. At least one of these genes had been rearranged in ten cases, again suggesting their involvement in T-cell differentiation.

CD34 was found to be expressed in 16 out of 38 cases with a pro-T-ALL phenotype; however, these patients only differed from $CD34^-$ patients in their lower incidence of adenomegaly. Mediastinal masses and acid phosphatase positivity were observed in both groups with a similar frequency as in patients with late-T-ALL. In the pro-T-ALL subgroup, CD34 expression appeared to be associated with a distinct phenotype including CD9 and HLA-DR expression. The expression of myeloid markers also appeared highly linked to the expression of CD34 since 47% of $CD34^+$ pro-T-ALL patients were My^+ versus only 5% of $CD34^-$ cases.

Southern blot analysis showed the TCRβ gene to be in germline configuration in seven out of eight $CD34^+$ pro-T-ALL cases. TCRγ also was in germline configuration in five out of seven of these cases. Conversely, TCRβ and TCRγ rearrangements were observed in six of ten and five of nine $CD34^-$ pro-T-ALL cases, respectively. TCR gene rearrangement thus appears to correlate with the loss of CD34 expression. Positivity for cCD3, however, was observed with a similar incidence in $CD34^+$ (58%) and $CD34^-$ (47%) pro-T-ALL patients, suggesting that cCD3 expression precedes TCR gene rearrangements.

Clinical Evolution of Pro-T-ALL (Fig. 2)

As shown in Fig. 2, EFS is significantly shorter in adult patients with a pro-T-ALL ($p < 0.05$), but this difference is not true for children. Comparison of the outcome according to the expression of the antigens more often expressed in pro-T-ALL showed a major detrimental influence of HLA-DR expression on the response to therapy. The median EFS of HLA-DR^+ pro-T-ALL patients was only 6 months, versus 18 for HLA-DR^- cases ($p < 0.02$).

No significant prognostic value appeared to be associated with CD2, CD34, or myeloid antigen expression.

Conclusions

The data reported in this study indicate that immunophenotypic criteria help define subgroups of ALL patients with significantly different clinical, biological, and evolutionary features. Such partitions are mostly relevant when the age of the patient is taken into account. Phenotypic discrimination appears to be significant in children. Should they take these differences into account, appropriate therapeutic protocols could in the future efficiently improve the outcome of children with B- and pre-B1-ALL and of infants

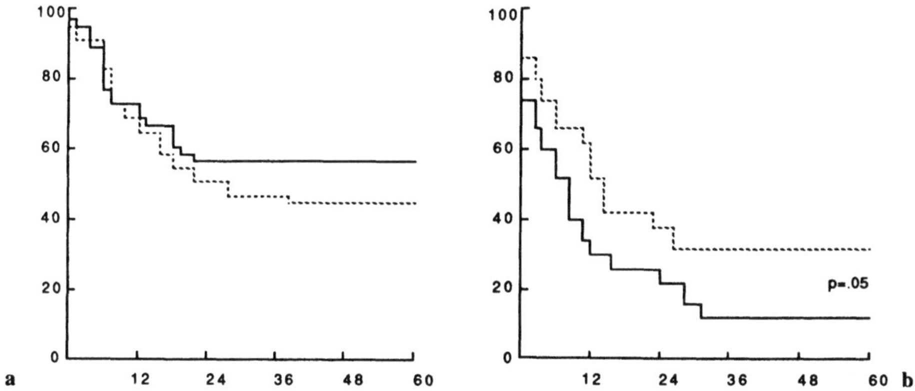

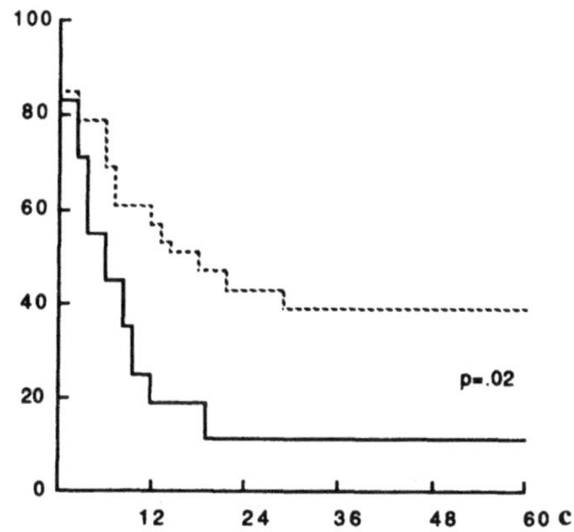

Fig. 2. Event-free survival curves of untransplanted children (**a**) and adults (**b**) with pro-T-ALL (*unbroken line*) or late-T-ALL (*dotted line*) and of pro-T-ALL patients (**c**) with blast cells expressiong (*unbroken line*) class II antigens or not (*dotted line*). The percentages of individuals still in first complete remission are indicated on the *abcissa*. Months of follow-up are on the *ordinate*. Frequencies and statistical significance were established using the log-rank test

with pre-B1-ALL. The latter would likely benefit most from an early allogeneic bone marrow transplantation.

From a more fundamental point of view, analysis of T-ALL phenotypes and characteristics suggest that a large subset of pro-T-ALL cases indeed belong to the group of T-lineage ALL. MHC class II expression appears to be the most significant marker associated with a bad prognosis in T-ALL, perhaps, however, because some of these cells behave more like undifferentiated or multipotent cells than true T cells, and do not respond to the classical T-ALL therapy. Finally, this work supports the validity of multicentric studies, allowing the collection of significant series of ALL cases with unusual phenotypes in a relatively short time.

References

Béné MC, Boumsell L, Bernard A, Vannier JP, Garand R, Solary E, Faure G, GEIL (1989) Immunologic analysis of a thousand cases of acute leukemia. Nouv Rev Fr Hematol 31:133–136

Bennet JM, Catovsky D, Daniel MT, Flandrin G, Galton DAG, Granlick HR, Sultan C, the FAB Cooperative Group (1981) The morphological classification of acute lymphoblastic leukaemia: concordance among observers and clinical correlations. Br J Haematol 47:553–561

Berger R, Bernheim A, Brouet JC, Daniel MT, Flandrin G (1979) t(8; 14) translocation in a Burkitt's type of lymphoblastic leukemia (L3). Br J Haematol 43:87–90

Bernard A, Boumsell L, Hill C (1984) Joint report of the first international workshop on human leukocyte differentiation antigens by the investigators of the participating laboratories. In: Bernard A, Boumsell L, Dausset J, Milstein C, Schlossman SF (eds) Leucocyte typing. Springer, Berlin Heidelberg New York, pp 9–143

Bloomfield CD, Goldman AI, Alimena G, Berger R, Borgstrom GH, Brandt L, Catovsky D, De la Chapelle A, Dewald GW, Garson OM, Garwicz S, Golomb HM, Hossfeld DK, Lawler SD, Mitelman F, Nilsson P, Pierre RV, Philip P, Prigogina E, Rowley JD, Sakurai M, Sandberg AA, Secker Walker LM, Tricot G, Van den Berghe H, Van Orshoven A, Vuopio P, Whang Peng J (1986) Chromosomal abnormalities identify high-risk and low-risk patients with acute lymphoblastic leukemia. Blood 67:415–420

Campana D, Janossy G, Boffil M, Trejdosiewicz LK, Ma D, Hoffbrand AV, Mason DY, Lebacq AM, Forster HK (1985) Human B-cell development: I. Phenotypic differences of B lymphocytes in bone marrow and peripheral lymphoid tissues. J Immunol 134:1524–1530

Catovsky D, Galetto J, Okos A, Miliani E, Galton DAG (1974) Cytochemical profile of B and T leukaemic lymphocytes with special reference to acute lymphoblastic leukaemia. J Clin Pathol 27:767–771

Foon KA, Todd RF (1986) Immunological classification of leukemia and lymphoma. Blood 68:1–31

Garand R, Vannier JP, Béné MC, Faure G, Bernard A, GEIL (1987) Correlations between acute lymphoid leukemia (ALL) immunophenotype and clinical and laboratory data at presentation: a study of 350 patients. Cancer 59:2020–2026

Garand R, Vannier JP, Béné MC, Faure G, Favre M, Bernard A, GEIL (1990) Comparison of outcome, clinical, laboratory and immunological features in 164 children and adults with T-ALL. Leukemia 4:739–744

Hammond D, Sather H, Nesbit M, Miller D, Coccia P, Bleyer A, Likens J, Siegel S (1986) Analysis of prognostic factors in acute lymphoblastic leukemia. Med Pediatr Oncol 14:124–134

Haynes BF, Martin ME, Kay HH, Kurtzbzerg J (1988) Early events in human T-cell ontogeny. Phenotypic characterization and immunohistologic localization of T-cell precursors in early human fetal tissues. J Exp Med 168:1061–1080

Kaplan EL, Meier P (1958) Non-parametric estimation from incomplete observations. J Am Stat Assoc 53:457–481

Loken MR, Shah VO, Dattilio KL, Civin CI (1987) Flow cytometric analysis of human bone marrow: II. Normal B lymphocyte development 70:1316–1324

Nadler LM, Korsmeyer SJ, Anderson KC, Boyd AW, Slaughenhoupt B, Park E, Jensen J, Coral F, Mayer RJ, Sallan SE, Ritz J, Schlossmann SJ (1984) B cell origin of non-T cell acute lymphoblastic leukemia: a model for discrete stages of neoplastic and normal pre-B cell differentiation. J Clin Invest 74:332–340

Peto R, Pike MC, Armitage T (1977) Design and analysis of random and clinical trials requiring prolonged observations of each patient: 2. Analysis and examples. Br J Cancer 35:1–3

Pui CH, Crist WM, Look T (1990) Biology and clinical significance of cytogenetic abnormalities in childhood acute lymphoblastic leukemia. Blood 76:1449–1463

Reinherz EL, Kung PC, Goldstein G, Levey RH, Schlossmann SF (1980) Discrete stages of human intrathymic differenciation: analysis of normal thymocytes and leukemic lymphoblasts of T cell lineage. Proc Nat Acad Sci USA 77:1588–1592

Roper M, Crist WM, Metzgar R, Ragad AH, Smith S, Starling K, Pullen J, Leventhal B, Bartolucci AA, Cooper MD (1983) Monoclonal antibody characterization of surface antigens in childhood T cell lymphoid malignancies. Blood 61:830–837

Sen L, Borella L (1975) Clinical importance of lymphoblasts with T markers in childhood acute leukemia. N Engl J Med 292:828–832

Uckun FM (1990) Regulation of human B-cell ontogeny. Blood 76:1908–1923

Van de Velde H, Von Hoegen I, Luo W, Parnes JR, Thielemans K (1991) The B-cell surface protein CD72/Lyb2 is the ligand for CD5. Nature 351:662–665

Vannier JP, Béné MC, Faure G, Bastard C, Garand R, Bernard A (1989) Investigation of the CD10 (cALLA) negative acute lymphoblastic leukemia: further description of a group with a poor prognosis. Br J Haematol 72:156–160

Incidence and Prognostic Significance of Immunophenotypic Subgroups in Childhood Acute Lymphoblastic Leukemia: The Experience of the AIEOP Cooperative Study

G. Basso[1], R. Rondelli[2], M.C. Putti[1], A. Cantù Rajnoldi[3], D. Granchi[2], M.G. Cocito[1], M. Saitta[4], T. Santostasi[5], C. Guglielmi[7], A. Lippi[8], N. Santoro[6], M.G. Russo[9], A. Pession[2], M. Aricò[10], and A. Biondi[3]

[1] Department of Pediatrics, University of Padova, Via Giustiniani, 3, Padova, Italy
[2] Department of Pediatrics, University of Bologna, Bologna, Italy
[3] Department of Pediatrics, University of Monta-Milan, Milan, Italy
[4] Department of Pediatrics, University of Turin, Turin, Italy
[5] Department of Pediatrics, University of Bari I, Bari, Italy
[6] Department of Pediatrics, University of Bari II, Bari, Italy
[7] Department of Pediatrics, University of Rome, Rome, Italy
[8] Department of Pediatrics, University of Florence, Florence, Italy
[9] Department of Pediatrics, University of Catania, Catania, Italy
[10] Department of Pediatrics, University of Pavia, Pavia, Italy

The role of immunological phenotype in childhood acute lymphoblastic leukemias (ALL) is important in classifying the different origins of ALL, but the identification of different subgroups of clinical relevance is still under discussion. In fact, frequent discrepancies are observed in the prognostic value of immunological subgroups in individual series. A poor outcome was seen in immunophenotype T in the first clinical studies (Greaves et al. 1981), but these results have not always been confirmed and now the T origin of ALL is not considered a prognostic factor (Hammond et al. 1986).

Other immunological markers have sometimes correlated with the negative response to the treatment, in particular the presence of cytoplasmic immunoglobulins (Crist et al. 1989), the positivity for CD20 (Ludwig et al. 1989a) and the coexpression of myeloid antigens (MyAg) in lymphoid blast cells (Sobol et al. 1987). These results have not always been confirmed by other studies. The nonreproducibility of immunological results observed between different series of patients could be due to various factors, but we suggest that the different therapeutic protocols used for the treatment are a very important variable. To overcome these variables we examined, individually and in combination, the immunological features of 892 patients treated by two different regimens during the same period of time by the *Associazione Italiana Ematologia Oncologia Pediatrica* (AIEOP). The analyses of the immunological subgroups were correlated to the therapy response and to the event-free survival (EFS) and the results suggest the possible role of immunophenotype in drawing the future therapeutic protocols.

Recent Results in Cancer Research, Vol. 131

Materials and Methods

Some 892 children affected by ALL were analyzed for this study; 528 were treated according to 1987 and 364 to 1988 protocols of AIEOP.

Morphological and cytochemical diagnoses of ALL were performed on bone marrow smears using widely adopted criteria (Bennett et al. 1976). Immunological diagnoses were made by indirect immunofluorescence according to previously described methods (Basso et al. 1985). A panel of monoclonal antibodies and heterologous antisera were utilized in immunological diagnoses; CD1/2/3/5/7 and cytoplasmic CD3 (CyCD3) identifying T-lineage ALL; CD10/19/20/24, cytoplasmic (CyIg) and surface immunoglobulins (sIg) identifying B-lineage ALL; TdT and HLA-DR, non-lineage-restricted. To identify MyAg, CD11b/13/14/15/33/w65 were employed. All analyses were performed in the center where the patient was initially examined. Results were then reviewed by a committee and the diagnosis confirmed on the basis of the tests carried out. The immunophenotype were considered adequate when at least CD19, 10, 7, CyCD3, HLA-DR, and sIg tests were performed. The definition of immunological subgroups was based on the criteria of Nadler et al. (1984).

The AIEOP 1987 protocols were formulated on the basis of CCSG experience (Steinherz et al. 1986). Briefly, there was an induction phase with vincristine, prednisone, daunomycin, and l-asparaginase; the first three drugs were used in the reinforced reinduction phase and maintenance therapy consisted of methotrexate and 6-mercaptopurin with a monthly pulse of prednisone and vincristine (Vecchi et al. 1991).

The AIOEP 1988 protocols were oriented according to those of BFM (Schrappe et al. 1987b), with the induction phase comprising vincristine, prednisone, daunomycin, l-asparaginase, cyclophosphamide, and ara-C, a consolidation phase followed by high-dose methotrexate, and a reinduction phase similar to the initial one. Maintenance therapy was with methotrexate and 6-mercaptopurin (Rossi et al. 1991). The enlistment of patients in the protocols was different; infants with ALL were excluded in the 1987 protocols but included in the 1988 ones. Both protocols were performed in the same period of time, from 1987 to 1990; the 1988 protocols were performed in the eight largest AIEOP centers to evaluate their feasibility, while the 1987 protocols were applied in the remaining centers.

In analyzing the clinical outcome of immunophenotype T and of positivity of CyIg, CD20, and MyAg, we considered as parameters good response to prednisone (less than 1000 blasts/mm^3 in the peripheral blood smears after 7 days of prednisone therapy; Schrappe et al. 1987b) the achievement of complete remission after the first induction cycle, and EFS.

Data were collected with patient-oriented and protocol-specific forms. All the information was stored, controlled, and analyzed by VENUS, an integrated software facilities system running on an IBM mainframe at the Italian Interuniversity Computing Center (CINECA). The EFS analysis was estimated by Kaplan-Meier method. Differences in survival curves were assessed by long-rank test.

Results

The treatment results have previously been reported (Vecchi et al. 1991; Rossi et al. 1991), and global EFS was similar in the populations of both protocols (67.6% vs. 66.3%, respectively).

The distribution of the different immunological subgroups in the two protocols are referred to in Table 1. Numerous differences have been found regarding the distribution of various immunological subgroups in the two protocols. An important difference has been found in the percentage of C-ALL (75.0% in 1987 vs. 65.9% in 1988), and pre-B ALL (7.9% vs. 13.1%) but CyIg were tested only in 211/528 (39.9%) cases in 1987 protocols and in 226/364 (62.0%) in the 1988 ones (Table 2). More T-ALL were found in the 1988 (13.1% vs. 11.4%) and also the CD10 negative B-oriented ALL (pre-pre-B and AUL), (7.8% vs. 5.6%). Regarding the other immunological

Table 1. Distribution of different immunophenotypic subgroups in the 1987 and 1988 protocols

Immunophenotypic subgroup	1987		1988		
	(*n*)	(%)	(*n*)	(%)	
CALL	396	75.0	239	65.9	
pre-B	42	7.9	48	13.1	
pre-pre-B	17	3.2	25	6.8	
AUL	13	2.4	4	1.0	
T	60	11.4	48	13.1	
Total	528		364		892

Table 2. Positivity of immunological markers in the 1987 and 1988 protocols

Marker		1987		1988	
		(*n*)	(%)	(*n*)	(%)
CyIg	Tested	211		226	
	Positive	42	19.9	48	21.2
CD20	Tested	101		201	
	Positive	31	30.6	65	32.3
MyA	Tested	153		321	
	Positive	10	6.5	22	6.8

Table 3. Correlation of good prednisone response (GPR) and achievement of complete remission (CR) after induction with immunophenotype

Good prednisone response							
Protocols	GPR	T-ALL		non-T-ALL		Total	
		(*n*)	(%)	(*n*)	(%)		
1987 + 1988	Yes	74		644		718	$p < 0.005$
	No	34	31.4	140	17.8	174	
1987	Yes	39		368		407	$p < 0.025$
	No	22	36.0	100	21.3	122	
1988	Yes	35		276		311	
	No	12	25.5	40	12.6	52	$p < 0.05$
Complete remission achievement after induction							
Protocols	CR	T-ALL		non-T-ALL		Total	
		(*n*)	(%)	(*n*)	(%)		
1987 + 1988	Yes	98		766		864	
	No	10	9.2	18	2.3	28	$p < 0.001$
1987	Yes	56		460		516	
	No	4	6.6	9	1.9	13	p ns
1988	Yes	42		306		348	
	No	6	12.5	9	2.9	15	$p < 0.01$

Table 4. Correlation of good prednisone response (GPR) and complete remission (CR) after induction with myeloid antigen positivity (MyAg)

Good prednisone response							
Protocols	GPR	MyAg+		MyAg−		Total	
		(*n*)	(%)	(*n*)	(%)		
1987 + 1988	Yes	27		372		399	
	No	5	15.6	70	15.8	75	ns
1987	Yes	9		113		122	
	No	1	10.0	30	20.9	31	ns
1988	Yes	18		259		277	
	No	4	18.1	40	13.3	44	ns
Complete remission after induction							
	CR	MyAg+		MyAg−		Total	
		(*n*)	(%)	(*n*)	(%)		
1987 + 1988	Yes	27		424		451	
	No	5	15.6	18	4.0	23	$p < 0.025$
1987	Yes	9		142		151	
	No	1	10.0	1	0.69	2	ns
1988	Yes	18		282		300	
	No	4	18.1	17	5.6	21	ns

markers considered for this study, CD20 and MyAg, the percentage of positivity was similar in both protocols even if these tests were performed in nonidentical numbers of cases (Table 2; CD20: 30.6% in 1987 protocols, 32.3% in 1988 protocols) (MyAg: 6.5% in 1987 protocols, 6.8% in 1988).

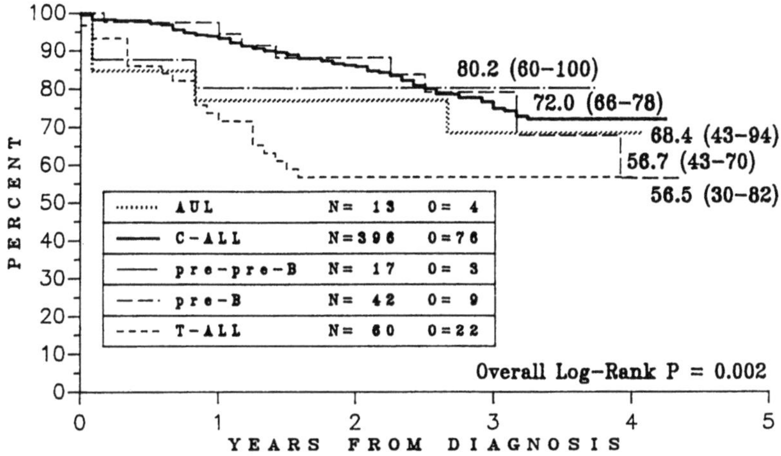

Number of patients at risk:

13	10	10	8	1	AUL
396	316	224	119	7	C-ALL
17	10	8	6	0	pre-pre-B
42	31	20	15	4	pre-B
60	34	22	12	0	T-ALL

Fig. 1. Event-free survival by immunophenotype: AIEOP protocols 1987

An important difference appeared when examining the good response to prednisone and immunological subgroups, considering the protocols both together and separately. In fact the percentage of poor response was higher in T-ALL (31.4%) than in other subgroups (17.8%). This difference showed a statistical relevance (Table 3). Analogous results were obtained examining the achievement of CR after the first induction cycle (at day 28 for 1987 protocols and at day 35 for 1988 ones). Some 9.2% of T-ALL did not achieve CR while the percentage was lower in the non-T-ALL (2.3%). These differences demonstrated a statistical value in examining the protocols together ($p < 0.001$) and in 1988 alone ($p < 0.01$) (Table 3). The positivity for CyIg and for CD20 have not revealed any difference regarding the good prednisone response and achievement of CR. The MyAg coexpression (7/131 in 1987 and 18/294 in 1988 protocols) was not correlated to good prednisone response but demonstrated a statistically significant correlation with CR achievement in both protocols examined in combination (Table 4).

The evaluation of EFS demonstrated a statistical difference among the immunological subgroups in both protocols (Figs. 1, 2). No difference was noted between those with CyIg-positive ALL and those negative for CyIg (pre-B, 55.7%; non-pre-B 57.9%). Analogous behavior was observed for the coexpression of MyAg, being EFS 65.5% in MyAg-negative and 60.1% in MyAg-positive ALL. The difference did not demonstrate any statistical significance.

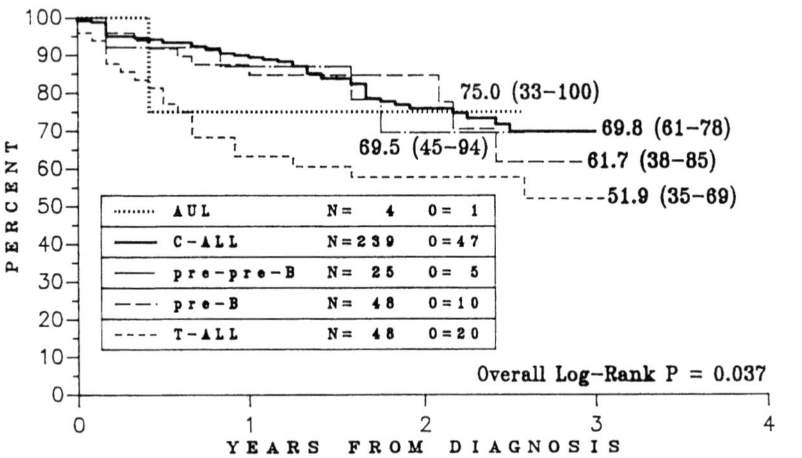

Number of patients at risk:

4	3	2	0	AUL
239	162	65	0	C-ALL
25	17	7	0	pre-pre-B
48	29	12	0	pre-B
48	25	17	1	T-ALL

Fig. 2. Event-free survival by immunophenotype: AIEOP protocols 1988

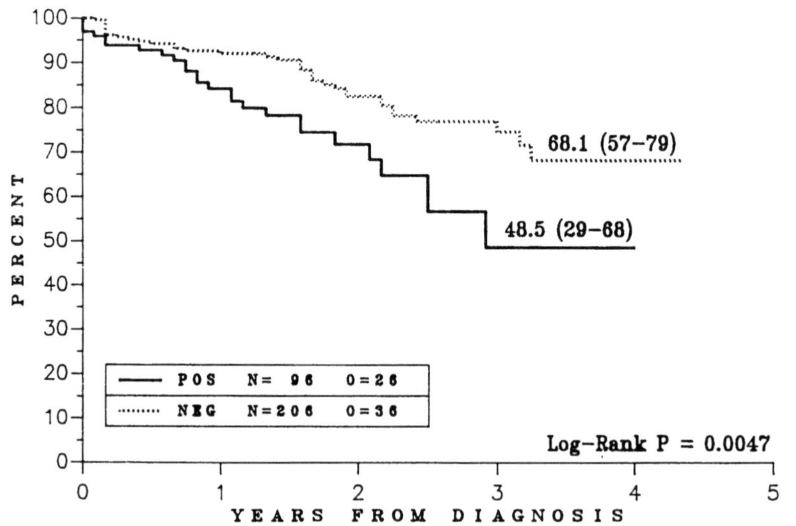

Number of patients at risk:

96	60	21	4	0	POS
206	150	82	30	4	NEG

Fig. 3. Event-free survival by CD20: AIEOP protocols 1987–1988

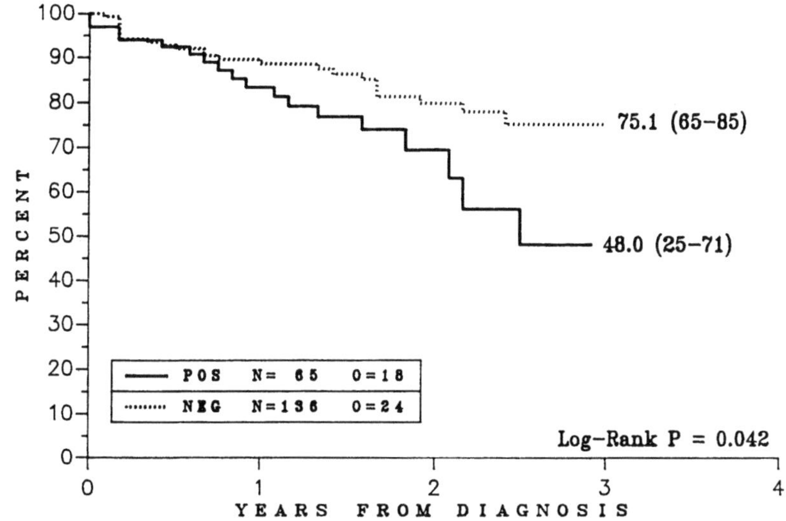

Number of patients at risk:

65	41	11	0	POS
136	92	44	0	NEG

Fig. 4. Event-free survival by CD20: AIEOP protocols 1988

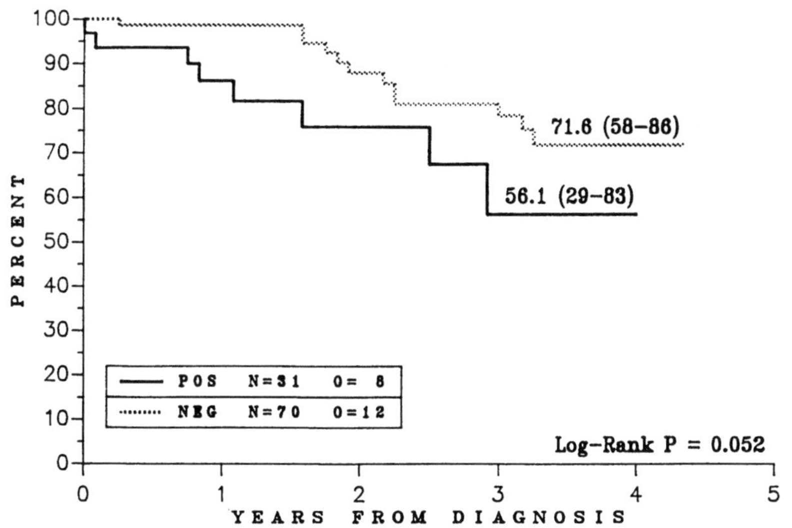

Number of patients at risk:

31	19	10	4	0	POS
70	58	38	30	4	NEG

Fig. 5. Event-free survival by CD20: AIEOP protocols 1987

The analysis of EFS in non-T-ALL examining the CD20 reactivity showed a statistically significant difference in the 1987 and 1988 protocols taken together (68.1% vs. 48.5%) (Fig. 3) and in 1988 protocols (75.1% vs. 48.0%; Fig. 4). The difference (71% vs. 56%) was not statistically significant in the 1987 protocols when examined alone, but only 101 cases were tested (Fig. 5).

Discussion

Prognostic factors in childhood ALL have been analyzed in various clinical trials in the past. However, the results are controversial as far as the value of immunophenotype is concerned (Hammond et al. 1986). Different parameters demonstrated prognostic relevance in individual series. The presence of T antigens was first affirmed in this field as an important factor (Sen and Borella 1975). Also our analysis showed clinical relevance of T immunophenotype. This was evaluated not only as EFS but also as therapy response. The T-ALL highlighted a worse prednisone response than other immunological subgroups. The non-complete response to prednisone is now considered such an important negative signal as to force the change in therapeutic protocol. The poor efficacy of chemotherapy in these cases of ALL was also confirmed by the lower percentage of CR after the first induction cycle, even if 106/108 T-ALL were treated by a more aggressive chemotherapy regimen (high risk protocols; Vecchi et al. 1991; Rossi et al. 1991). These results could indicate that induction therapy was inadequate for T-ALL treatment in both protocols. The difference in incidence of T immunophenotype in the two series is not due to an inadequate immunological characterization but probably to a selection of patients with high risk leukemia in the 1988 protocols, which were performed in the main Italian centers. Other important differences in the distribution of immunological subgroups regard the lower percentage of pre-B-ALL in the 1987 protocols that might be due to the low percentage of tests performed in the peripheral centers. In fact the percentage of positivity in the tested cases was similar. The pre-B phenotype was an independent negative prognostic factor in various trials of the Pediatric Oncology Group (Crist et al. 1989), but recently the poor outcome was restricted to the pre-B with t(1;19), which are also associated to some classical high risk factors, including black race, high white blood cell count and a DNA index below 1.16 (Crist et al. 1990). In our study there were not any differences between CyIg-positive and CyIg-negative ALL in therapy response and in EFS, even if only one third of patients were evaluated for this test.

The coexpression of MyAg in ALL was reported to be a negative prognostic factor (Sobol et al. 1987); furthermore, the incidence of these leukemias is higher in infants and frequently associated with some specific cytogenetic translocations (Ludwig et al. 1989b). In this group of patients we recently demonstrated the clinical relevance of these immunological markers (Basso et al. 1992).

In contrast, in this study we did not find any difference in prednisone response in either protocol, but a statistical correlation was noted in the achievement of CR after the first induction cycle in the 1987 and 1988 protocols examined together. This difference could probably be due to the low number of patients tested in these series (474/864); in fact, in the 1988 results, in which about 90% of cases were tested, there was no statistical correlation. But as already noted, infants were excluded from the 1987 protocol and included in the 1988 ones and that could explain the higher percentage of CD10-negative ALL in 1988 protocols. Therefore, it should have been more probable to find some differences in the 1988 protocols for the higher percentage of cases with MyAg positivity in these patients (Basso et al. 1992). Moreover, there was not any statistical difference in EFS between the ALL with and those without coexpression of MyAg in the protocols, even if considered single and associated. That could suggest that the clinical relevance of myeloid markers should be limited to younger patients in which this could indicate a possible non-lymphoid origin of these leukemias (Zaki et al. 1989).

We did not analyze the single myeloid marker to evaluate whether some of these might have prognostic significance, because there was no homogeneity in the analysis performed, and it was not possible to exclude the importance of single markers such as the CD14 and the CD33 in this evaluation, as suggested by Sobol et al. (1987).

The CD20-positive ALL showed a poor outcome in BFM analyses (Ludwig et al. 1989a), but the significance of this difference is not always demonstrated. We found a great difference between CD20-negative and CD20-positive ALL, independent of the protocol used; the absence of statistical value in considering the 1987 protocol alone might be due only to the low number of cases evaluated (n = 101). Even if a multivariate analysis was not attempted, the high significance ($p < 0.005$) of the observed difference might suggest this to be an important prognostic parameter in the subgroup of non-T-ALL. The absence of a difference regarding the prednisone response and achievement of CR in this group suggest that the CD20-positive ALL could need more intensive reinductions in future protocols.

This analysis is limited by the fact that the immunological characterizations were performed at many different centers by different methods (flow cytometry or microscope). This is not important in T-ALL, whose diagnosis is relatively simple and noncontroversial, and the difference in the clinical outcome is evident in both protocols. However, the significance of the expression of various antigens (CyIg and MyAg) might suffer from technical problems and from the limited number of tests performed in the peripheral centers even if the clinical relevance of CD20 positivity has been demonstrated. These data suggest that the immunological markers have relevance in the identification of various subgroups of ALL that for best results may require an intensification of therapy at different times during the protocols, induction for T-ALL and reinduction for CD20-positive ALL. Moreover, for the optimum evaluation of the clinical relevance of immunological markers in a cooperative study, a central laboratory is necessary.

Acknowledgments. This work was partly supported by CNR "Progetto Finalizzato Applicazioni Cliniche della Ricerca Oncologica"; MURST 40% e 60%.

References

Basso G, Capuzzo F, Simioni E et al (1985) Immunocytochemical evidence of common ALL antigen in null ALL. Scand J Haematol 35:536–542

Basso G, Putti MC, Cantù-Rajnoldi A et al (1992) The immunophenotype in infant acute lymphoblastic leukaemia: correlation with clinical outcome. An italian multicentre study (AIEOP). Br J Haematol 81:184–191

Bennett JM, Catovsky D, Daniel MT et al (1976) Proposals for the classification of the acute leukemias. Br J Haematol 33:451–458

Crist W, Boyett J, Jackson J et al (1989) Prognostic importance of the pre-B-cell immunophenotype and other presenting features in B-lineage childhood acute lymphoblastic leukemia. A Pediatric Oncology Group Study. Blood 74:1252–1259

Crist WM, Carroll AJ, Shuster JJ et al (1990) Poor prognosis of children with pre-B acute lymphoblastic leukemia in children: their relationship to presentation features and prognosis. Br J Haematol 48:179–197

Greaves MF, Janossy G, Peto J, Kay H (1981) Immunologically defined subclasses of acute lymphoblastic leukemia in children: their relationship to presentation features and prognosis. Br J Haematol 48:179–197

Hammond D, Sather H, Nesbit M et al (1986) Analysis of prognostic factors in acute lymphoblastic leukemia. Med Ped Oncol 19:28–32

Henze G, Fegler R, Reiter A et al (1990) Impact of early intensive reinduction therapy on event-free survival in children with low-risk acute lymphoblastic leukemia. Haematol Blood Transfusion 2:483–488

Ludwig WD, Seibt-Jung H, Teichmann JV et al (1989a) Clinicopathologic features and prognostic implications of immunophenotypic subgroups in childhood ALL: experience of the BFM-ALL study 83. In: Neth R, Gallo RC, Greaves MF, Gaedicke G, Gohla S, Mannweiler K, Ritter J (eds) Modern Trends in Human Leukemia VIII. Springer, Berlin Heidelberg New York, pp 51–57 (Haematology and blood transfusion, vol 32)

Ludwig WD, Bartram CR, Harbott J et al (1989b) Phenotypic and genotypic heterogeneity in infant acute leukemia I. Acute lymphoblastic leukemia. Leukemia 6:431–439

Miller DR, Coccia PF, Bleyer WA et al (1989) Early response to induction therapy as a predictor of disease-free survival from Children Cancer Study Group. J Clin Oncol 7:1807–1815

Nadler LM, Korsmeyer SJ, Anderson KC et al (1984) B cell origin of non-T cell acute lymphoblastic leukemia. A model for discrete stages of neoplastic and normal pre-B cell differentiation. J Clin Invest 74:332–340

Rossi MR, Valsecchi MG, Testi AM et al (1991) Preliminary report on AIEOP protocol 88 for childhood acute lymphoblastic leukemia (ALL). Haematologica 76 [Suppl 4]:174 (abstr)

Schrappe M, Beck J, Brandeis WE et al (1987a) Die Behandlung der akuten lymphoblastischen Leukaemie im Kindes- und Jugendalter: Ergebnisse der multizentrischen Therapiestudie ALL-BFM81. Klin Paediatr 199:133–150
Schrappe M, Henze G, Ludwig R et al (1987b) The in vivo corticosteroid response and its prediction for early therapy failure in childhood ALL: a report from the BFM study group. Fourth International Symposium on Therapy of Acute Leukemias. Rome, February 1987, p 167
Sen L, Borella L (1975) Clinical importance of lymphoblast with T markers in childhood acute leukemia. N Engl J Med 292:828
Sobol RE, Mick R, Royston I et al (1987) Clinical importance of myeloid antigen expression in adult acute lymphoblastic leukemia. N Engl J Med 316:1111–1117
Steinherz PG, Gaynon P, Miller DR et al (1986) Improved disease free survival of children with acute lymphoblastic leukemia at high risk for early relapse with the New York regimen – a new intensive therapy protocol: a report from the CCSG. J Clin Oncol 4:744–752
Vecchi V, Rondelli R, Rosati D et al (1991) 87-AIEOP protocol for non-B newly diagnosed childhood acute lymphoblastic leukemia. Haematologica 76 [Suppl 4]: 178 (abstr)
Zaki SR, Austin GE, Swan D et al (1989) Human myeloperoxidase gene expression in acute leukemia. Blood 6:2096–2102

Mutations in the Regulatory Domains of bcr/abl-*Positive Leukemias Detected by Solid-Phase Automated DNA Sequencing*

J. Maurer[1], R. Reinhardt[2], G. Kuhlenbäumer[1], and E. Thiel[1]

[1] Department of Internal Medicine, Hematology and Oncology, Klinikum Steglitz, Free University of Berlin, Hindenburgdamm 30, W-1000 Berlin 45, Fed. Rep. of Germany
[2] Max Planck Institute of Molecular Genetics, Abt. Wittmann, Ihnestr. 73, W-1000 Berlin 33 (Dahlem), Fed. Rep. of Germany

Introduction

The Philadelphia (Ph) chromosome translocation is present in up to 96% of chronic myeloid leukemia (CML) cases and in 35% of adult acute lymphoblastic leukemia (ALL) cases, in which it is associated with a poor prognosis (Maurer et al. 1991). At the molecular level of this reciprocal translocation t(9;22)(q34;q11), the c-*abl* oncogene on chromosome 9 is translocated to a gene on chromosome 22, called *bcr* (Heisterkamp et al. 1985). This fusion of the *bcr* and *abl* genes results in the expression of a leukemia specific chimeric protein (Shtivelmann et al. 1986). The molecular anatomy of the *abl* part of this protein shows a protein tyrosine kinase domain and further upstream (5′) the SH3 and SH2 domains which are also present in other oncogenes with protein tyrosine kinase activity (Fig. 1). Both regions seem to play an important role in regulating enzyme activity. The SH2 region may function as a tyrosine kinase regulatory domain in *abl*, whereas SH3 seems to be important for the exact cellular location of the Abl protein by interacting with the cytoskeleton (Pawson 1988). For example, a deletion mutant of mouse c-*abl* protooncogene lacking the SH3 region becomes oncogenically activated and causes lymphoid transformation in newborn mice (Jackson and Baltimore 1989). Point mutations in the SH3 region are able to enhance oncogenic activation in murine c-*abl* N-terminal deletion mutants (Shore et al. 1990) and, furthermore, mutations in the SH3 domain of a myristylated form of murine c-*abl* result in oncogenic activation (Franz et al. 1989). Recently, Pendergast et al. (1991) have shown that part of the first *bcr* exon binds specifically to the SH2 domain of *abl*, thereby deregulating tyrosine kinase activity. To look for an involvement of SH3 and SH2 domains in human *bcr-abl* positive leukemias, especially in the transition of CML from chronic phase to blast crisis, we decided to sequence these domains, using a new solid-phase DNA-sequencing method, from different patient samples to detect subtle point mutations.

Recent Results in Cancer Research, Vol. 131

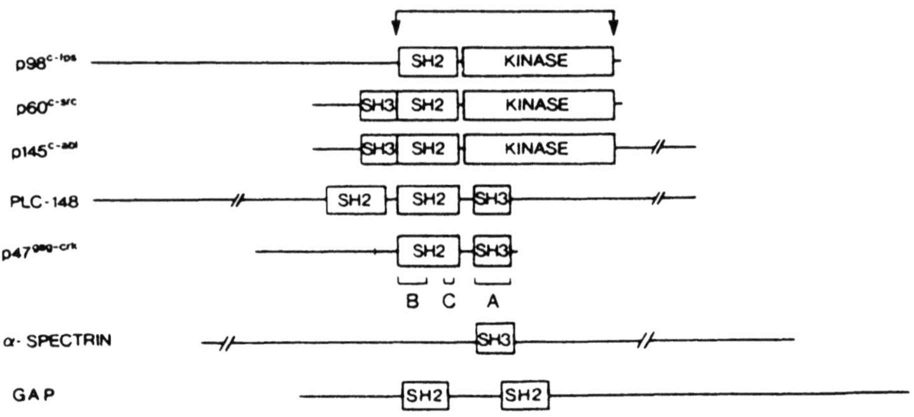

Fig. 1. SH3 and SH2 motifs in other oncogenes (Pawson 1988)

Methods

RNA was isolated according to the AGPC method (Chomczynski and Sacchi 1987). Starting from RNA the nucleic acid was reverse transcribed into complementary (cDNA) using Moloney murine leukemia virus (MMLV) reverse transcriptase (BRL) and random nonamer primers. Subsequently, the cDNA was polymerase chain reaction (PCR) amplified with *Taq* polymerase using a nested primer approach with a set of internal primers (SH3(4)NB, 5′CML or 5′ALL) for a second amplification round to enhance specificity and yield of amplified DNA.

Oligonucleotides (Table 1) were synthesized according to published sequence data on a Cyclone Plus DNA Synthesizer (Milligen). Purification of the oligonucleotides was carried out by electrophoresis over a 20% polyacrylamide/7 *M* urea gel. After staining the oligonucleotide bands with the dye methylene blue, the oligonucleotide-containing bands were excised and the DNA was electroeluted. Biotin-labeling of the primer (SH3(4)B) was done either by using a reactive group (Aminolink 2, ABI) at the 5′ end and subsequent attachment of biotin (biotin-X-NHS-ester, Clontech) or by using a biotin-phosphoamidite (DMT-Biotin-C6-PA, Cambridge Research Biochemicals). Synthesis of the primers for sequencing requires a fluorescent dye at the 5′ end. This was achieved either by attaching fluorescein isothiocyanate (FITC) according to the biotinylation-method via aminolinker or by using FITC phosphoamidite (Pharmacia).

After amplification the PCR products are then coupled to streptavidin-coated magnetic beads (Dynal) and strand-separated with 8 µl 0.1 *M* sodium hydroxide (Fig. 2). After washing and neutralization of the unbound strand with 4 µl 0.2 *M* hydrochloric acid, both solid-phase bound and separated DNAs were sequenced according to the dideoxy chain termination method:

Table 1. Oligonucleotide primers used for amplification and sequencing

Oligonucleotide	Sequence
5′ALL	5′-ACCATCGTGGGCGTCCGCAAGA-3′
5′ALL il	5′-ATCTGGCCCAACGATGGCGAGGGCGCCT-3′
5′CML	5′-GAAGTGTTTCAGAAGCTTCTCC-3′
5′CML il	5′-TGGAGCTGCAGATGCTGACCAACTCGTGTG-3′
SH3(2)	5′-TGTGCTTCATGGTGATGTCCGTGC-3′
SH3(4)NB[a]	5′-TGCGTTCCATCTCCCACTTGTCGTAGT-3′
SH3 FF[b]	5′-AGCCGCTCGTTGGAACTCCAA-3′
SH2 RF[b]	5′-CGCTTTGGGGCTGGATAATGG-3′

[a] Biotin-labeled at the 5′ end.
[b] FITC-labeled at the 5′ end.

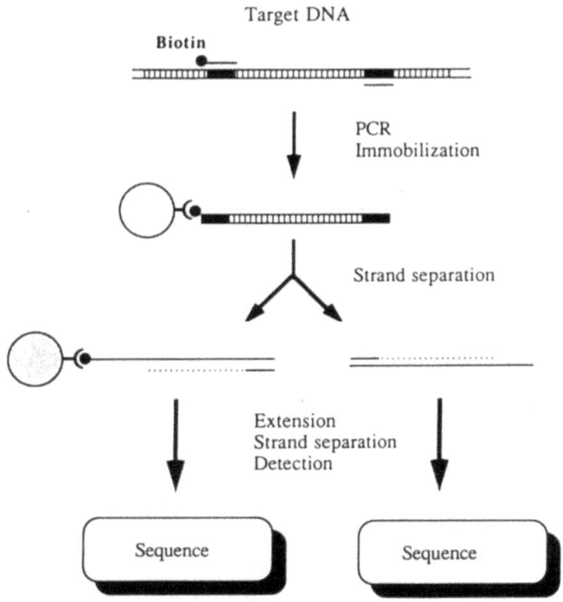

Fig. 2. Scheme of solid-phase sequencing (Hultmann et al. 1991)

DNA was dissolved in 12 µl H_2O, 3 µl of a manganese-containing buffer system (buffer 1, Tris HCl (pH 7.5) 670 m*M*; buffer 2, DTT 380 m*M*; buffer 3, $MnCl_2$ 132 m*M*, isocitrate 1 *M*; equal volumes of all three buffers were mixed immediatedly before sequencing) and 2 µl of the sequencing primer; SH3 FF for the solid-phase bound strand, SH3 RF for the unbound strand were added. The concentration of the sequencing primers was adjusted to 1 pmol/µl. Annealing of primer and template was 3 min at 65°C and 10 min at T_m −5°C of the sequencing primer. After annealing, 4 U T7 polymerase

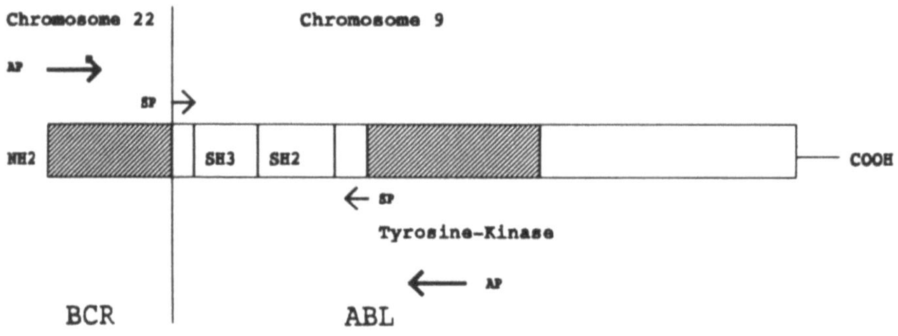

Fig. 3. Amplification and sequencing strategy of the SH3 and SH2 domains of the translocated allele

(Sequenase Version 2.0, USB) was added and 4.5 µl of this reaction mixture was mixed with 2.5 µl of the respective termination mix (1 m*M* dNTPs, 4.5 µ*M* ddNTPs) on microtiter plates and incubated at 42°C for 5–10 min. The reaction was stopped with formamide, denatured at 83°C for 3 min, and loaded on a 6% polyacrylamide/7 *M* urea denaturing sequencing gel. Electrophoresis and on-line detection of sequencing signals was done in an automated sequencing device (A.L.F., automated laser fluorescent, Pharmacia). After editing the sequences the data were downloaded to DNASIS to screen for point mutations. The amplification and sequencing strategy is shown in Fig. 3.

Results

In contrast to the oncogenic activation of v-*abl* by deletion of N-terminal sequences, including SH3, and replacement by *gag* sequences, providing a myristylation signal, the *bcr-abl* forms lack all these features (Mes-Masson et al. 1986). We have investigated whether the SH3 domain is also involved in the *bcr-abl* leukemia, not by gross genetic alterations or deletions, but by point mutations. We have now sequenced both regions in 26 patients with *bcr-abl*-positive CML and ALL (8 CMLs in chronic phase, 12 CMLs in blast crisis, and 6 ALLs), using a new nonradioactive solid-phase DNA-sequencing approach.

So far, only in one case (CML in blast crisis) was a point mutation seen in the SH3 region (Fig. 4). This mutation resulted in an amino acid exchange from Ala to Asp. These data do not support the hypothesis that mutations in the SH2 or SH3 regions play a major role in the pathogenesis or progression towards a more malignant state (CML: chronic phase to blast crisis) of *bcr-abl* positive leukemias. However, SH3 mutations may contribute to disease progression in some cases of CML.

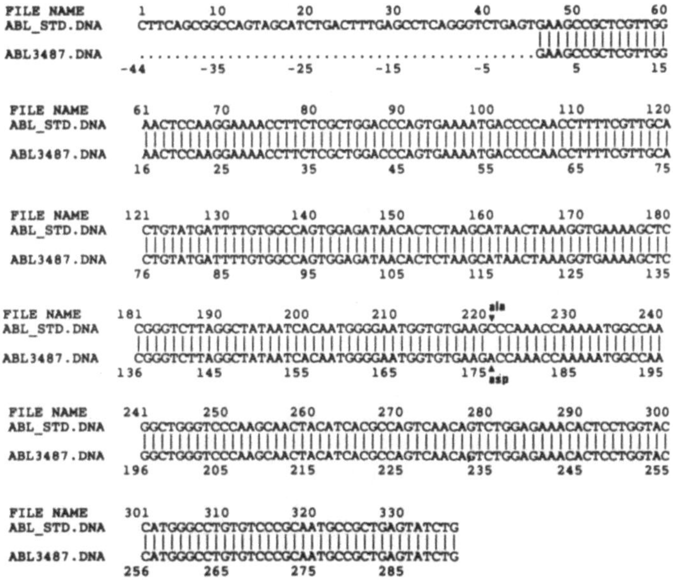

Fig. 4. Sequence comparison of published sequence data of SH3 and SH2 (abl_std. DNA) with CML in blast crisis (abl3487.DNA), showing a point mutation in SH3 with a resulting amino acid exchange

The new solid-phase-based automated sequencing method gives 650–800 base pairs (bp) of sequence information of a symmetrically amplified PCR product. Furthermore, the use of magnetic beads circumvents any precipitation steps, which also makes the method more suitable for automation. A critical point in DNA sequencing is the purity of the template. Coupling of the template to the magnetic beads allows washing away of any impurities. The technique also makes it easy to change buffers and enzymes between the PCR and the sequencing steps. The whole procedure outlined above, starting from RNA, yields sequencing data the same day. We believe that automated solid-phase DNA sequencing will soon be a valuable diagnostic method not only in large human genome sequencing projects, but also in clinical oncology.

References

Chomczynski P, Sacchi N (1987) Single-step method of RNA isolation by acid guanidinium thiocyanate-phenol-chloroform extraction. Anal Biochem 162:156–159

Franz WM, Berger P, Wang JYJ (1989) Deletion of an N-terminal regulatory domain of the c-abl tyrosine kinase activates its oncogenic potential. EMBO J 8:137–147

Heisterkamp N, Stam K, Groffen J, de Klein A, Grosveld G (1985) Structural organization of the bcr gene and its role in the Ph-Translocation. Nature 315:758

Hultman T, Bergh S, Moks T, Uhlen M (1991) Bidirectional solid phase sequencing of in vitro amplified plasmid DNA. Biotechniques 10:84–93

Jackson P, Baltimore D (1989) N-terminal mutations activate the leukemogenic potential of the myristoylated form of c-abl. EMBO J 8:449–456

Maurer J, Janssen JWG, Thiel E, van Denderen J, Ludwig WD, Aydemir Ü, Heinze B, Fonatsch C, Harbott J, Reiter A, Riehm H, Hoelzer D, Bartram CR (1991) Detection of chimeric BCR-ABL genes in acute lymphoblastic leukaemia by the polymerase chain reaction. Lancet 337:1055–1058

Mes-Masson AM, McLaughlin J, Daley GQ, Paskind M, Witte ON (1986) Overlapping cDNA clones define the complete coding region for the $P210^{c\text{-}abl}$ gene product associated with chronic myelogenous leukemia cells containing the Philadelphia-chromosome. Proc Natl Acad Sci USA 83:9768–9772

Pawson T (1988) Non-catalytic domains of cytoplasmic protein-tyrosine kinases: regulatory elements in signal transduction. Oncogene 3:491–495

Pendergast AM, Muller AJ, Havlik MH, Maru Y, Witte ON (1991) BCR sequences essential for transformation by the BCR-ABL oncogene bind to the ABL SH2 regulatory domain in a non-phosphotyrosine-dependent manner. Cell 66:161–171

Shore SK, Bogart SL, Reddy RE (1990) Activation of murine c-abl protooncogene: effect of a point mutation on oncogenic activation. Proc Natl Acad Sci USA 87:6502–6506

Shtivelmann E, Lifshitz B, Gale RP, Rose BA, Canaani E (1986) Alternative splicing of m-RNA's transcribed from the bcr-abl fused gene. Cell 47:277–284

VI. Leukemic Cell Characterization in Acute Myeloid Leukemia: Biological and Clinical Implications

*Clonal Analysis of n-*ras *Gene Activation in Acute Myeloid Leukemia*

M. Lübbert[1], W. Oster[2], F. McCormick[3], R. Mertelsmann[1], and F. Herrmann[4]

[1] Department of Internal Medicine 1, University of Freiburg Medical Center, Hugstetter Str. 55, W-7800 Freiburg, Fed. Rep. of Germany
[2] Behringwerke AG, W-3550 Marburg, Fed. Rep. of Germany
[3] Cetus Corporation, Emeryville, CA 94608, USA
[4] Department of Medical Oncology and Applied Molecular Biology, UKRV, Free University of Berlin, 1115 Berlin, Germany

Introduction

Members of the *ras* gene family code for 21-kDa proteins (p21) located at the inner cellular membrane. Several lines of evidence suggest that p21 proteins are involved in intracellular signal transduction pathways, thus regulating cellular growth and differentiation. Ras proteins bind and hydrolyze GTP (Gibbs et al. 1984; Sweet et al. 1984) and show sequence homology to G proteins (Hurley et al. 1984) which are thought to participate in the action of some cytokines. The p21 of n-*ras* has been shown to couple receptor binding of hematopoietic growth factors to inositol lipid hydrolysis in fibroblasts (Wakelam et al. 1986). Conversely, activation of G proteins by sodium fluoride in the presence of Al^{3+} results in expression of cytokines (Yamato et al. 1989), and expression of an activated *ras* gene transfected into normal cells or cell lines can induce cytokine expression by these cells (Yiagnisis and Spandidos 1987; Demetri et al. 1988; Andrejauskas and Moroni 1989) and change their responsiveness towards growth factors (Kelekar and Cole 1987; Leof et al. 1987). Point mutations leading to an activated p21 occur in numerous human malignancies (for a review, see Bos 1988). Activating mutations of n-*ras* have been reported to occur in 25%–40% of cases of acute myelogenous leukemia (AML). (Bos et al. 1985; Janssen et al. 1987; Farr et al. 1988). However, the presence of these mutations can be restricted to subpopulations (subclones) of leukemic cells (Toksoz et al. 1987). It has been suggested that the biological role of subclonal presence of *ras* activation in leukemias should be viewed differently than monoclonal activation (Toksoz et al. 1987; Yunis et al. 1989). We

Recent Results in Cancer Research, Vol. 131

characterized a population of patients with AML for the presence of (monoclonal or subclonal activating) n-*ras* point mutations. The presence of strongly clonal n-*ras* activation was correlated with the ability of these cells to express IL-6, an interleukin that is transcribed at very high levels in about 30% of primary AML blasts (Oster et al. 1989). A strong correlation was found between n-*ras* activation and expression of IL-6 messenger (m)RNA ($p < 0.001$). Growth and differentiation properties of different subpopulations of leukemic cells that either did or did not harbor n-*ras* mutations were dissected using soft agar culture.

Material and Methods

Cells and Cell Lines

Leukemic cells were isolated from peripheral blood or bone marrow of patients with different types of AML after obtaining informed consent. Diagnosis was based on morphology, cytochemistry, and immunofluorescence analysis. The low-density mononuclear cell fraction was isolated by density centrifugation using Ficoll-Hypaque (Sigma, Munich, FRG). T-cell depletion was achieved by rosetting with 2-aminoethylisothiouronium bromide-treated sheep red blood cells (5% v/v solution). Monocytes were removed by repeated adherence to plastic surfaces. The resulting blast-enriched cell fractions contained >90% leukemic blasts as estimated by inspection of Wright–Giemsa-stained slide preparations.

Cell lines used included PA-1 teratocarcinoma cells, MOLT-4 T-lymphoid cells (kindly provided by E. Reinherz, Dana Faber Cancer Institute, Boston, USA) and HL-60 promyelocytic cells (kindly provided by H.P. Koeffler, UCLA, Los Angeles, USA). Cells were cultured in 1640 RPMI medium supplemented with 10% low endotoxin fetal calf serum (Hazelton Laboratories, Vienna, VA, USA), glutamine, and antibiotics at 37°C, 7% CO_2 in a humidified atmosphere.

Colony Forming Assay

For analysis of colony growth by leukemic colony-forming cells (L-CFC), a standard double-layer soft agar assay was performed in quadruplicate as described previously (Oster et al. 1989). Leukemic cells were seeded at 10^5 cells/ml in the presence or absence of recombinant human (rh) granlocyte–macrophage colony-stimulating factor GM-CSF (25 ng/ml) and rhIL-3 (25 ng/ml) (both kindly provided by D. Krumwieh, Behringwerke AG, Marburg, FRG) and rh grannlocyte colony-stimulating factor (G-CSF; 20 ng/ml, kindly provided by L. Souza, Amgen, Thousand Oaks, CA, USA). At days 10–14, individual colonies were isolated by aspiration with glass capillaries and were processed for polymerase chain reaction

(PCR). Colonies were classified as blast-type (dense, homogeneous colonies composed entirely of blast cells), mature-type (disperse, heterogeneous colonies composed of cells with the ability to migrate into the agar), and intermediate-type colonies (heterogeneous, large colonies containing both immature and mature cells).

DNA and RNA Isolations

Cells were lysed in guanidinium/isothiocyanate followed by separation of nucleic acids on a cesium chloride (CsCl) gradient. DNA was precipitated in the presence of 2 *M* ammonium acetate, redissolved, digested with proteinase K (100 μg/ml) overnight at 50°C and further purified by repeated isopropanol precipitations in the presence of 2 *M* ammonium acetate as described (Hardy et al. 1985). Following CsCl gradient centrifugation, RNA was dissolved in TES (10 m*M* Tris 7.4, 1 m*M* EDTA, 0.1% sodium dodecylsulfate, SDS) and precipitated twice in the presence of 300 m*M* sodium acetate.

Northern and Southern Blot Analyses

For northern blot analysis, total RNA was electrophoresed on denaturing formaldehyde gels and blotted onto nylon membrane (Nytran, Schleicher, and Schuell, Dassel, FRG). Prehybridization was carried out at 42°C overnight in the presence of 5× SSC (1× SSC = 0.15 *M* NaCl, 0.015 *M* sodium citrate), 0.5% SDS, 1× Denhardt's solution, 100 μg/ml denatured salmon sperm DNA. Hybridization took place in the presence of 2× SSC, 10% dextran sulfate, 0.5% SDS, 1× Denhardt's solution, 100 μg/ml denatured salmon sperm DNA, and ^{32}P-labeled (Feinberg and Vogelstein 1983) 440-base pair (bp) *Taq*I/*Ban*II restriction fragment of the pBSF2.38.1 IL-6 complementary (c)DNA (Hirano et al. 1986) as probe.

For Southern blot analysis, genomic DNA was restricted, electrophoresed on a 1% agarose gel, and blotted onto nylon membrane (GeneScreen Plus, Dupont de Nemours, Wilmington, DE, USA). Prehybridization and hybridization took place at 42°C in the presence of 5× SSC, 10% dextran sulfate, 1% SDS, 1× Denhardt's solution, 100 μg/ml denatured salmon sperm DNA. The 414-bp *Pst*I/*Pst*I fragment of exon 2 of human *myc* gene (Dalla-Favera et al. 1982) was radiolabeled by random priming (Feinberg and Vogelstein 1983) and used as probes.

In Vitro Amplification of DNA by PCR

DNA isolated from leukemic blasts was in vitro amplified for either n-*ras* exon 1 or exon 2 sequences (sequences of oligonucleotides available upon request). In brief, 25–32 cycles of PCR were performed as described by Saiki et al. (1985) with modifications published by us (Lübbert et al. 1990). For analysis of cell colonies grown in soft agar culture, individual colonies were isolated, resuspended in 20 µl H_2O and boiled for 10 min. Cell debris was pelleted and 10 µl of supernatant was used in the PCR (35–38 cycles). Amplified products were electrophoresed (5 µl) on 4% agarose gels (NuSieve, FMC, Rockland, ME, USA) and transferred to nylon membrane (Zetaprobe, Bio-Rad, Laboratories, Richmond, CA, USA) by alkaline blotting. Filters were sequentially hybridized with a panel of oligonucleotide probes (sequences available upon request) designed to recognize all possible activating point mutations at n-*ras* codons 12, 13, and 61. Hybridizations took place in the presence of 5× SSPE (1× SSPE = 10 m*M* sodium phosphate, 0.18 *M* NaCl, 1 m*M* EDTA, pH 7.0), 5× Denhardt's solution, 100 mg/ml denatured sonicated salmon sperm DNA, 10 m*M* EDTA and 1% SDS. Hybridization and rinsing conditions were chosen which allowed only fully matched hybrids to remain thermally stable. A prehybridization step was omitted. Autoradiography was performed for 2–12 h.

Results

*Analysis of n-*ras *Activation in Myeloid Leukemic Cells*

Leukemic cells from 50 patients with different types of newly diagnosed AML were screened for point mutations of the n-*ras* gene involving the first and second nucleotides of codons 12 and 13 and each nucleotide of codon 61 of this gene. By sequential hybridization of mutation-specific oligonucleotide probes to these sequences after amplification by PCR, 16 different cases (34%) were shown to carry mutations. These involved each of the seven nucleotide positions tested (Fig. 1). Both the incidence and distribution pattern of mutations are in line with studies by others (Bos et al. 1985; Janssen et al. 1987; Farr et al. 1988). The mutations were verified by reamplification of the DNAs and repeat hybridizations. All mutations were heterozygous, as indicated by hybridization of the normal allele to the wild-type probes (panels wt N-1 and N-2 in Fig. 1). Comparison of the intensity of hybridization signals in samples carrying mutations to that of several positive controls (cell lines) carrying known n-*ras* mutations as well as to signal intensity obtained with wild-type specific probe revealed comparably very strong signal intensity in six cases of AML (patients 12, 17, 23, 29, 30, 39), indicating highly clonal presence of the mutations in the leukemic blasts. In 11 patients, hybridization signals indicating presence of the mutated alleles were significantly weaker than in the controls (subclonal presence of the mutation), and in four patients (17, 27, 29, 43) signal was obtained with more than one mutation-specific probe (oligoclonality of the mutations).

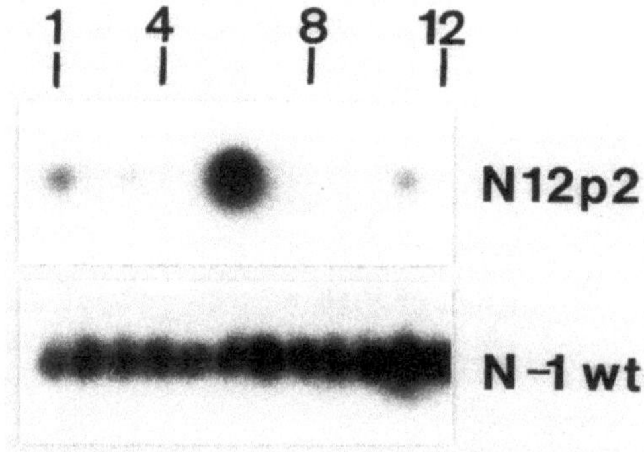

Fig. 1. Clonal and suabclonal activating point mutations of n-*ras* in AML blasts. DNA from primary leukemic cells of 11 patients with AML was amplified for n-*ras* exon 1, electrophoresed, blotted, and sequentially hybridized to either an oligonucleotide probe matching the unmutated, "wild type" sequence encompassing codon 12 (*lower panel*: *N-1 wt*) or a mixture of oligonucleotide probes matching all three possible base pair substitutions at the second nucleotide of codon 12 of N-ras (*upper panel*: *N12p2*) as described in "Material and Methods." *Lanes 1–11*, DNA from patients with AML; *lane 12*, DNA from normal peripheral blood lymphocytes. *Lane 6* contains DNA from patient 39; *lanes 1, 3, 11* contain DNA from patients with subclonal presence of heterozygous n-*ras* codon 12, second nucleotide substitions

*Correlation Between Clonal Activation of n-*ras *and Expression of IL-6 mRNA by Myeloid Leukemic Cells*

Activation of n-*ras* in blasts from those patients who exhibited strongly clonal presence of the mutation was correlated with the ability of these cells to express mRNA for IL-6, a cytokine that is expressed at abnormally high levels by about 25% of primary AML blasts (Oster et al. 1989). As shown in Fig. 2, all of the cell samples exhibiting highly clonal presence of n-*ras* mutation (patients 12, 17, 23, 29, 30, 39) also expressed moderate to high levels of IL-6 mRNA (lanes 1–5, 9). Statistical analysis by Fisher's exact test revealed a highly significant correlation between activation of n-*ras* in AML cells and the ability of these cells to express the interleukin ($p < 0.001$). Expression patterns of other cytokines that are expressed by some AMLs (GM-CSF, G-CSF) did not correlate with activation of n-*ras* (results not shown).

*Clonal Analysis of Subpopulations of Myeloid Leukemic Cells Carrying n-*ras *Mutations*

Leukemic cells from peripheral blood of two patients showing only faint signal in the analysis for mutations at the second nucleotide of n-*ras* codon

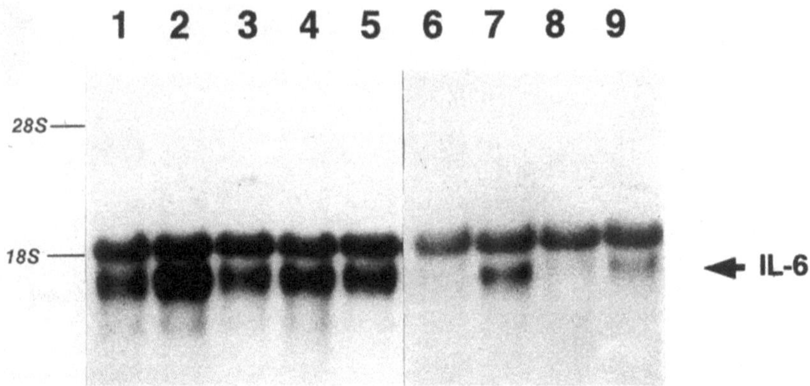

Fig. 2. Expression of IL-6 mRNA in myeloid leukemic blasts with n-*ras* mutations. RNA was extracted from leukemic blasts from patients 29 (*lane 1*), 39 (*lane 2*), 30 (*lane 3*), 12 (*lane 4*), 23 (*lane 5*), 4 (*lane 6*), 9 (*lane 8*), and 17 (*lane 9*), as well as from normal human diploid embryonal lung fibroblasts (FH 109) treated with TPA (10^{-8} *M* for 24 h) (*lane 7*, positive control). RNA was then extracted, electrophoresed, blotted to nylon-based membrane, and hybridized to an IL-6 cDNA as described in "Materials and Methods." Autoradiography followed. Inspection of the 28*S* and 18*S* ribosomal RNAs ensured intactness and equal loading of the RNA in each lane

12 (patients 33, 48; Fig. 1, panel N12p2, lanes 13, 27, respectively) and no signal with the other mutation-specific probes were subjected to clonal analysis. The signal intensity obtained in the mutation-specific hybridization when examining DNA from bulk leukemic cells from these patients was compared to signal observed in a dilution series of DNA from PA-I cells (also with known mutation at codon 12 of n-*ras*). The results suggested presence of the mutations in a subclone(s) comprising about 10% of bulk leukemic cells in both cases (data not shown). Bulk leukemic cells were therefore cultured in soft agar in the presence or absence of a combination of IL-3 plus GM-CSF plus G-CSF. Cells from both patients formed colonies in the presence of CSFs; cells from one patient (33) formed several colonies in the absence of these factors. Individual colonies were examined for presence of a mutation at N12p2, as described in "Material and Methods." About half the colonies formed by cells from patient 33 (acute myelomonocytic leukemia) showed hybridization signal that was comparable to that of a control cell line, and thus about tenfold stronger than signal obtained with DNA from the patient's total blast cells (Fig. 3a). The other colonies showed only very faint or no signal in the hybridization assay. The majority of colonies strongly positive for the mutation at N12p2 were dispersed and composed of mature elements, as judged by inspection. Cells not carrying this mutation gave rise to predominantly blast-type colonies (Table 1). Cells from a second patient (48) formed colonies only in the

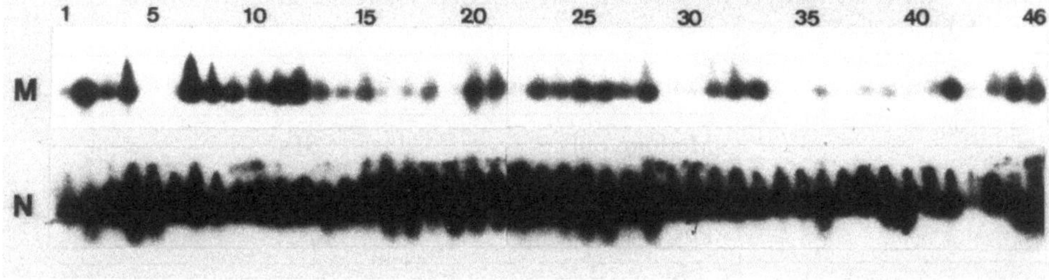

a

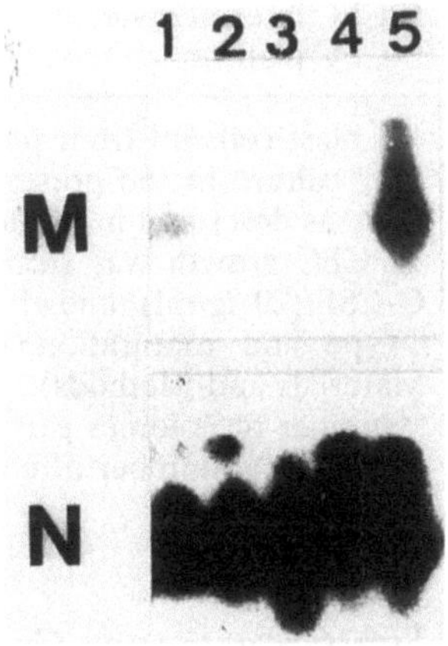

b

Fig. 3a,b. Analysis of n-*ras* gene activation in subclones of leukemic colony-forming cells. Peripheral blood cells from patients 33 (**a**) and 47 (**b**) were subjected to a standard colony- forming assay in soft agar in the presence and absence of CSFs (IL-3, 25 ng/ml, plus GM-CSF, 25 ng/ml, plus G-CSF, 20 ng/ml). Individual colonies were isolated and analyzed for presence of a mutation at n-*ras* codon 12, second nucleotide, by PCR and differential oligonucleotide hybridization as described in "Material and Methods." *Panels M*, filters were hybridized with a probe detecting all possible nucleotide substitutions at N12p2; *panels N*, filters were hybridized with a probe detecting unmutated (wild-type) sequences at exon 1 of n-*ras*. **a** *Lane 1*, normal PBLs; *lane 2*, PA-I cells; *lane 3*, total blast cells from patient 33; *lanes 4, 6–15, 17–39, 42–46*, colonies formed by leukemic blasts of patient 33 in the presence of CSFs; *lanes 5, 16, 40, 41*, colonies formed in the absence of CSFs. **b** *Lane 1*, total blast cells from patient 47; *lanes 2–5*, colonies formed by leukemic blasts of patient 47 in the presence of CSFs

presence of CSFs; of these, one colony showing presence of the mutation at N12p2 was composed of mature cells, whereas the colonies scoring negative for this mutation were composed of blast-like cells (Fig. 3b).

Leukemic cells from patient 33 that had formed several colonies in the absence of CSFs (autonomous growth) were also examined. Surprisingly, none of the resulting colonies showed strong prevalence of the RAS mutation at position N12p2 (Table 1 and Fig. 3a, lanes 5, 16, 40, 41).

Table 1. n-*ras* activation in subclones of myeloid leukemic colony-forming cells (L-CFC)

Colony type[b]	Culture stimulation			
	Medium only n-*ras* mutation (N12p2)[c]		CSFs[a] n-*ras* mutation (N12p2)[c]	
	Pos.	Neg.	Pos.	Neg.
L-CFC blast	–	1/1	5/17	12/17
L-CFC intermediate	–	–	5/10	5/10
L-CFC mature	–	3/3	11/15	4/15

10^5 blast cells/ml from peripheral blood of patient 33 were seeded in standard soft agar culture in the presence or absence of CSFs. Analysis for n-ras activation was done as described in the legend to Fig. 3.
[a] L-CFC growth was stimulated with a combination of rh GM-CSF (25 ng/ml), rh G-CSF (20 ng/ml), and rh IL-3 (25 ng/ml).
[b] Type and maturation degree of colonies were estimated by inspection (see Materials and Methods).
[c] Number of colonies carrying mutation at n-*ras* codon 12, second nucleotide (N12-2), per total number of colonies.

Structure of the myc *Gene in AML Blasts Carrying n-*ras *Mutations*

In several leukemic cell lines, alterations of the *myc* protooncogene have been reported to coincide with an activated n-*ras* gene (Collins and Groudine 1982; Murray et al. 1983; Ernst et al. 1988; Mallet et al. 1989). The copy number and structure of the *myc* gene were examined in all patients showing highly clonal presence of a mutated n-*ras* allele. As shown in Fig. 4, the 12.5-kilobase (kb) *Eco*RI band encompassing the entire coding region of *myc* was unaltered and present as single copy in all patients investigated. In contrast, HL-60 cells (heterozygous mutation at N61p2) showed the reported strong amplification of *myc*.

Discussion

The role of activated *ras* oncogenes in the scenario of multistep carcinogenesis is only poorly understood. The p21 *ras* proteins share several features with G proteins and may thus be similarly involved in ligand-mediated signal transduction, with the ligands being for instance cytokines. The patterns of growth, cytokine-dependent proliferation, and expression of cytokines following transfection of activated *ras* genes have been studied in different cell models. Expression of a transfected human *ras* oncogene can induce abrogation of IL-3 dependence and expression of IL-3 and GM-CSF in

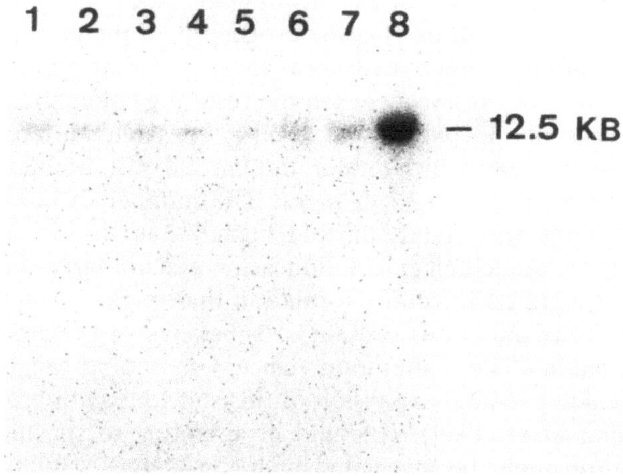

Fig. 4. Gene structure and copy number of *myc* gene of patients with activating point mutations of n-*ras*. DNA from patients 39 (*lane 1*), 12 (*lane 2*), 17 (*lane 3*), 23 (*lane 4*), 30 (*lane 5*), 29 (*lane 6*), from normal PBL (*lane 7*), and from HL-60 cells (known amplification of myc, *lane 8*) was digested with *Eco*RI, electrophoresed (10 μg/lane), blotted, and hybridized to the 414 bp *Pst*I/*Pst*I cDNA fragment covering exon 2 of the human *myc*

murine mast cells (Andrejauskas and Moroni 1989), an IL-3-like activity in rat fibroblasts (Yiagnisis and Spandidos 1987), expression of G-CSF, GM-CSF, and IL-1β in human fibroblasts (Demetri et al. 1988). Thus, it is conceivable that in primary leukemic cells, presence of an activated *ras* gene may influence the patterns of growth and differentiation of these cells.

By screening leukemic cells from 50 patients with AML, we identified several cases in which activation of *ras* involved the large majority of cells, as well as a number of cases where *ras* mutations were present in only a subpopulation of the leukemic cells. Leukemic cells that showed strongly clonal activation of n-*ras* uniformly expressed high levels of IL-6 mRNA, a cytokine that is expressed in about 25% of primary myeloid leukemic blasts (Oster et al. 1989). This statistically significant correlation suggests that in some cases of myeloid leukemia, activation of *ras* may mediate turning-on of expression of IL-6 (this question is pursued further by our laboratory using transfection techniques). Secretion of IL-6 might in turn mediate a growth advantage to leukemic cells via a paracrine loop: IL-6 stimulates bone marrow stromal cells to secrete cytokines such as CSFs, which in turn are known to stimulate the proliferation of some AML blasts (Griffin et al. 1986).

We also addressed the question of whether the subpopulations of leukemic cells carrying n-*ras* activation showed distinct biological features. A northern blot analysis of these cells as a means of studying their patterns of cytokine expression would not be meaningful, since the patterns of *ras* activation already demonstrate clear heterogeneity of the blast populations. Therefore, we combined clonal analysis of these different populations in soft agar with detection of *ras* oncogenes in the resulting colonies using PCR. This allowed analysis of the patterns of proliferation and differentiation of clonogenic leukemic cells which either did or did not harbor a particular *ras* gene mutation at codon 12 of n-*ras*. The number of colonies positive for these mutations was about fourfold higher than the number of cells within the total leukemic cell population estimated to carry the mutation, suggesting a net increase in colony formation that might be mediated by activation of *ras*. n-*ras* mutations present in subclones of preleukemic blasts have been termed a "late" alteration, since longitudinal analyses of these patients revealed eventual expansion of this subclone with progression of the disease (Yunis et al. 1989). It would be tempting to speculate that this biological feature might be associated with the increased plating efficiency observed by us.

Colonies composed of mature cells and forming in the presence of CSFs were predominantly positive for activation of *ras*, whereas blast-type colonies generated thus were predominantly of a clone not carrying this mutation. The mature morphology of most colonies formed by cells carrying an activated n-*ras* suggests that expression of this oncogene does not necessarily result in a block in maturation that cannot be overcome by the addition of CSFs. This is in line with the observation that HL-60 cells, which have a mutation at the second nucleotide of codon 61, can be induced by G-CSF or GM-CSF to differentiate into more mature myeloid cells (Tomonaga et al. 1986; Begley et al. 1987). In fact, the high number of mature colonies formed in the presence of exogenously added CSFs by cells harboring an n-*ras* oncogene compared to those composed of cells not carrying this oncogene might reflect an increased responsiveness of the cells carrying the *ras* oncogene towards the differentiation-inducing effect of the CSFs. It should be noted that in some studies examining the incidence of n-*ras* activation in AML, preferential involvement of more mature leukemias was noted (see Yunis et al. 1989; Bartram et al. 1989). In different systems, *ras* oncogenes seem to have either inducing or inhibitory effects upon cellular differentiation. Introduction of an activated *ras* gene into PC12 pheochromocytoma cells (Noda et al. 1985) or into Epstein-Barr virus-transformed B cells (Seremetis et al. 1989) results in differentiation of the respective cells. Conversely, in myoblast cells, presence of a *ras* oncogene is associated with a blockade of differentiation (Olson et al. 1987).

Cells from one patient exhibiting an n-*ras* activation in only a fraction of leukemic blasts formed colonies in soft agar in the absence of CSFs (autonomous growth). Surprisingly, of these colonies, none was composed of cells carrying the particular point mutation of n-*ras*, suggesting that in cells giving rise to these colonies, a transforming event other than the n-*ras* point mutation is associated with autonomous stimulation of colony growth.

It is highly unlikely that activation of a *ras* gene alone is sufficient in causing leukemic transformation of cells. In vitro studies have shown that cotransfection using both a cytoplasmic oncogene like *ras* and a nuclear oncogene such as *myc* can lead to transformation of primary rodent cells (Land et al. 1983). Similarly, some leukemic cell lines show concomitant activation of n-*ras* and amplification or rearrangement of *myc* (Collins and Groudine 1982; Murray et al. 1983; Ernst et al. 1988; Mallet et al. 1989). However, the AML patients we analyzed did not exhibit alterations of their *myc* gene, implying that concomitant alteration of both genes may occur only infrequently in myeloid cells in vivo.

Acknowledgements. We are grateful to A. Müller for expert technical assistance and to T. Forsthuber, M.D., for statistical analysis of the data. Also, thanks to A. Lindemann, M.D., and D. Jonas, M.D., for helpful discussions. This work was supported by Deutsche Forschungsgemeinschaft (He 1380-2/1) and BMFT 0319012 B.

References

Andrejauskas E, Moroni C (1989) Reversible abrogation of IL-3 dependence by an inducible H-*ras* oncogene. EMBO J 8:2575–2581

Bartram CR, Ludwig WD, Hiddemann W, Lyons J, Buschle M, Ritter J, Harbott J, Fröhlich A, Janssen JWG (1989) Acute myeloid leukemia: analysis of Ras gene mutations and clonality defined by polymorphic x-linked loci. Leukemia 3:247–256

Begley CG, Metcalf D, Nicola NA (1987) Purified colony stimulating factors (G-CSF and GM-CSF) induce differentiation in human HL-60 leukemic cells with suppression of clonogenicity, Int J Cancer 39:99–105

Bos JL (1988) The RAS gene family and human carcinogenesis. Mutation Res 195:255–271

Bos JL, Toksoz D, Marshall CJ, Verlaan-de Vries M, Veeneman GH, van der Eb AJ, van Boom JH, Janssen JWG, Steenvorden ACM (1985) Amino-acid substitutions at codon 13 of the N-RAS oncogene in human acute myeloid leukemia. Nature 315:726–730

Collins S, Groudine M (1982) Amplification of endogenous *myc*-related DNA sequences in a human myeloid leukemia cell line. Nature 298:679–681

Dalla-Favera R, Gelman EP, Martinotti S, Franchini G, Papas TS, Gallo RC, Wong-Staal F (1982) Cloning and characterization of different human sequences related to the onco gene (*v-myc*) of avian myelocytomatosis virus (MC29). Proc Natl Acad Sci USA 79:6497–6501

Demetri GD, Ernst TJ, Pratt ES, Zenzie BW, Rheinwald JG, Griffin JD (1990) Expression of *ras* oncogenes in cultured human cells alters the transcriptional and posttranscriptional regulation of cytokine genes. J Clin Invest 86:1261–1269

Ernst TJ, Gazdar A, Ritz J, Shipp MA (1988) Identification of a second transforming gene, RAS^n, in a human multiple myeloma line with a rearranged c-*myc* allele. Blood 72:1163–1167

Farr CJ, Saiki RK, Erlich HA, McCormick F, Marshall CJ (1988) Analysis of RAS gene mutations in acute myeloid leukemia by polymerase chain reaction and oligonucleotide probes. Proc Natl Acad Sci USA 85:1629–1633

Feinberg AP, Vogelstein B (1983) A technique for radiolabelling DNA restriction endonuclease fragments to high specific activity. Ann Biochem 132:6–13
Gibbs JB, Sigal IS, Poe M, Scolnick EM (1984) Intrinsic GTPase activity distinguishes normal and oncogenic *ras* p21 molecules. Proc Natl Acad Sci USA 81:5704–5708
Griffin JD, Young DC, Herrmann F, Wiper D, Wagner K, Sabbath KD (1986) Effects of recombinant human GM-CSF on proliferation of clonogenic cells in acute myeloblastic leukemia. Blood 76:1448–1453
Hardy KJ, Peterlin BM, Atchinson RE, Stobo JD (1985) Regulation of expression of the human interferon alpha gene. Proc Natl Acad Sci USA 82:8173–8177
Hirano T, Taga T, Yasukawa K, Harada H, Taga T, Watanabe Y, Matsuda T, Kashiwamura S, Nakajima K, Koyama K, Iwamatu A, Tsunasawa S, Sakiyama F, Matsui H, Takahara Y, Taniguchi T, Kishimoto T (1986) Complementary DNA for a novel human interleukin (BSF-2) that induces B lymphocytes to produce immunoglobulin. Nature 324:73–75
Hurley JB, Simon MI, Teplow DB, Robishaw JD, Gilman AG (1984) Homologies between signal transducing G proteins and ras gene products. Science 226:860–862
Janssen JWG, Steenvoorden ACM, Lyons J, Anger B, Böhlke JU, Bos JL, Seliger H, Bartram CR (1987) RAS gene mutations in acute and chronic myelocytic leukemias, chronic myeloproliferative disorders, and myelodysplastic syndromes. Proc Natl Acad Sci USA 84:9228–9232
Kelekar A, Cole MD (1987) Immortalization by c-*myc*, H-*ras*, and Ela oncogenes induces differential cellular gene expression and growth factor responses. Mol Cell Biol 7:3899–3907
Land H, Parada LF, Weinberg RA (1983) Tumorigenic conversion of primary embryo fibroblast requires at least two cooperating oncogenes. Nature 304: 596–602
Leof EB, Proper JA, Moses HL (1987) Modulation of transforming growth factor type beta action by activated *ras* and c-*myc*. Mol Cell Biol 7:2649–2652
Lübbert M, Mirro Jr J, Kahan J, Miller CW, Isaac G, Kitchingman G, Mertelsmann R, Herrmann F, McCormick F, Koeffler HP (1990) N-*ras* gene point mutations in childhood acute lymphocytic leukemia correlate with a poor prognosis. Blood 75:1163–1169
Mallet M, Mane SM, Meltzer S, Needleman SW (1989) C-*myc* amplification coexisting with N-*ras* point mutation in the biphenotypic cell line RED-3. Leukemia 7:511–515
Murray MJ, Cunningham JM, Parada LF, Duatry F, Lebowitz P, Weinberg RA (1983) The HL-60 transforming sequence: a RAS oncogene coexisting with altered *myc* genes in hematopoietic tumors. Cell 33:749–757
Noda M, Ko M, Ogura A, Liu DG, Amano T, Takano T, Ikawa I (1985) Sarcoma viruses carrying ras oncogenes induce differentiation-associated properties in a neuronal cell line. Nature 318:73–75
Olson EN, Spizz G, Tainsky MA (1987) The oncogenic forms of N-*ras* or H-*ras* prevent skeletal myoblast differentiation. Mol Cell Biol 7:2104–2111
Oster W, Cicco NA, Klein H, Hirano T, Kishimoto T, Lindemann A, Mertelsmann RH, Herrmann F (1989) Participation of the cytokines Interleukin 6, tumor necrosis factor-alpha, and Interleukin 1-beta secreted by acute myelogenous leukemia blasts in autocrine and paracrine leukemia growth control. J Clin Invest 84:451–457
Saiki R, Scharf S, Faloona F, Mullis K, Horn G, Erlich HA, Arnheim N (1985) Enzymatic amplification of β-globin genomic sequences and restriction site analysis for diagnosis of sickle cell anemia. Science 230:1350–1353
Seremetis S, Inghirami G, Ferrero D, Dalla-Favera R (1989) Transformation and plasmacytoid differentiation of EBV-infected human B lymphoblasts by RAS oncogenes. Science 243:660–663

Sweet RW, Yokoyama S, Kamata T, Feramisco JR, Rosenberg M, Gross M (1984) The product of RAS is a GTPase and the T24 oncogenic mutant is deficient in this activity. Nature 311:273–275

Toksoz D, Farr CJ, Marshall CJ (1987) *ras* gene activation in a minor proportion of the blast population in acute myeloid leukemia. Oncogene 1:409–413

Tomonaga M, Golde DW, Gasson JC (1986) Biosynthetic (recombinant) human granulocyte-macrophage colony stimulating factor: effect on normal bone marrow and leukemic cell lines. Blood 67:31–36

Wakelam MJO, Davies SA, Houslay MD, McKay I, Marshall CJ, Hall A (1986) Normal $p21^{N\text{-}ras}$ couples bombesin and other growth factor receptors to inositol phosphate production. Nature 323:173–176

Yamato K, El-Hajjaoui Z, Kuo JF, Koeffler HP (1989) Granulocyte-macrophage colony-stimulating factor: signals for its mRNA accumulation. Blood 74:1314–1320

Yiagnisis M, Spandidos DA (1987) Interleukin-3 like activity secreted from human RAS or MYC transfected rodent cells. Anticancer Res 7:1293–1298

Yunis JJ, Boot AJM, Mayer MG, Bos JL (1989) Mechanisms of ras mutation in myelodysplastic syndrome. Oncogene 4:609–614

Human Stem Cell Factor Is a Growth Factor for Myeloid Leukemia Cells

T. Pietsch[1], U. Kyas[1], H.G. Drexler[2], and K. Welte[1]

[1] Department of Pediatric Hematology and Oncology, Hanover Medical School, Konstanty-Gutschow-Str.8, W-3000 Hanover 61, Fed. Rep. of Germany
[2] German Collection of Microorganisms and Cell Cultures (DSM), W-3300 Brunswick, Fed. Rep. of Germany

Introduction

Recently, the ligand of the myeloid surface receptor encoded by the proto-oncogene c-*kit* (Yarden et al. 1987; Zsebo et al. 1990b) was identified to be a novel hematopoietic growth factor that stimulates primitive progenitor cells (Zsebo et al. 1990a,c). This stem cell factor (SCF) is a multipotent hematopoietic colony-stimulating factor acting on early progenitors of the different hematopoietic lineages. The complementary (c)DNA for human SCF has been cloned and expressed in mammalian cells, and the recombinant factor purified to homogeneity (Zsebo et al. 1990c; Martin et al. 1990). Whereas SCF itself has only a low capacity for inducing colony formation in progenitor assays in vitro [colony-forming unit–granulocyte, macrophage (CFU-GM), burst-forming unit–erythrocyte (BFU-E), CFU–granulocyte, erythrocyte, macrophage, megakaryocyte (CFU-GEMM), and CFU–lymphocyte (CFU-L)] on normal bone marrow cells, it has strong synergistic activities with other factors. It synergizes with granulocyte colony-stimulating factor (G-CSF), granulocyte-macrophage CSF (GM-CSF), and interleukin-3 (IL-3) in myelopoiesis (McNiece et al. 1991a), with erythropoietin (EPO) in erythropoiesis (McNiece et al. 1991a), with IL-6 in megakaryopoiesis, with IL-7 in lymphopoiesis (McNiece et al. 1991b), and with IL-3 in mast cell growth (Medlock et al. 1990). In this study we investigated the mitogenic potential of SCF alone or in synergy with other factors on myeloid leukemia lines as well as the expression of its specific receptors on the cell surface.

Material and Methods

Cell Lines. Most human myeloid leukemia cell lines were obtained from the American Tissue Culture Collection (ATCC) and the German Collection of Microorganisms (DSM; Deutsche Sammlung für Mikroorganismen, Brunswick, FRG). The GM-CSF-dependent cell line GM/SO was kindly provided by Dr. S. Oez, Universitätsklinikum, Nuremberg, FRG (Oez et al. 1990). The cell line GM-153 was provided by Dr. M. Freund, Medizinische Hochschule, Hanover, FRG. The cell lines were cultured in RPMI 1640 (Gibco, Berlin, FRG) with 10% fetal calf serum (FCS) and 1 m*M* L-glutamine. All cultured cell lines were tested and found free of mycoplasma contamination by DNA staining and culture methods.

Human Recombinant Factors. Recombinant human (rh) SCF and rhG-CSF were kindly provided by Dr. K. Zsebo and Dr. L. Souza, AMGEN, Thousand Oaks, California, USA; rhGM-CSF, rhIL-3, and rhEPO were from Behringwerke, Marburg, FRG, and M-CSF from Alpha Therapeutics, Japan.

Antibodies. The monoclonal anti-*kit* antibody YB5.B8 (Ashman et al. 1989) was kindly provided by Dr. L. Ashman, University of Adelaide, South Australia. This antibody was in the form of ascites and used in a 1:1000 dilution for FACS analysis.

Binding Studies with ^{125}I-rhSCF. rhSCF was radiolabeled by the lactoperoxidase/glucose oxidase method using Enzymobeads (Bio-Rad) following the instructions of the manufacturer. Briefly, 10 µg rhSCF was labeled by incubation with 1 mCi Na ^{125}I (Amersham, Brunswick, FRG) in the presence of enzymobeads to a specific activity of 20 µCi/µg. Free iodide was removed by passage through a desalting column (P6-DG; Biorad, Richmond, VA, USA) and equilibrated with phosphate-buffered saline (PBS) containing 0.02% Tween 20 (Biorad) and 0.01% NaN_3. Binding assays were performed on 4×10^6 leukemic blasts in a volume of 500 µl RPMI 1640 with 0.1% gelatin with various concentrations of ^{125}I-rhSCF ranging between 100 and to 30000 pmol/l. The incubation was performed at 37°C for 1 h. Identical incubations were also performed in the presence of 2.5 µmol/l unlabeled rhSCF. Aliquots of 125 µl of the cell suspension were then layered onto silicon oil and centrifuged. The radioactivity in the pellet (bound) and the supernatant (free) was determined seperately in a gamma-counter. The specific binding was calculated from the difference between the radioactivity bound in the absence and presence of unlabeled rhSCF. The dissociation constant and the number of binding sites per cell were determined using Scatchard analysis (Scatchard 1949). Prior to the assays the cells were treated for 20 s with sodium citrate buffer (10 mmol/l, pH 4.0) and subsequently washed with RPMI 1640 prior to the binding assay in order to remove bound natural SCF.

Chemical Crosslinking. 2.5×10^7 leukemic cells were incubated with 0.1 µCi (0.05 µg) ^{125}I-rhSCF for 1 h on ice in the presence or absence of a 100-fold excess of unlabeled rhSCF. Unbound rhSCF was then removed by three washes with ice-cold PBS. Subsequently, the cells were treated with the bifunctional crosslinking reagent DSS (0.5 m*M*; Pierce, Geisenheim, FRG) and lysed with ice-cold PBS containing 1% Triton X-100 and 1 m*M* phenyl methyl sulfonylfluoride (PMSF). The soluble proteins were separated by sodium dodecylsulfate polyacrylamide gel electrophoresis (SDS-PAGE) with subsequent autoradiography of the dried gels for 72 h at −80°C.

Flow Cytometry. Indirect immunofluorescence for staining with the anti-*kit* antibody YB5.B8 (Ashman et al. 1989) was performed as described (Hadam 1985) using commercial immunoglobulin (Gammonativ; Kabi, Munich, FRG) to competetively block Fc receptors and fluoresceinated goat immunoglobulin $F(ab')_2$ fragments directed against mouse immunoglobulin G (IgG) and IgM (Dianova, Hamburg, Germany) as developing reagent. All incubations were carried out in PBS with 0.1% bovine serum albumin and 0.02% NaN_3. Flow cytometry was performed on a FACS 440 cell sorter (Becton-Dickinson, Heidelberg, FRG).

Preparation of RNA and Polymerase Chain Reaction After Reverse Transcription (RT-PCR) for c-kit Messenger RNA. Total RNA from cell lines was isolated as described (Sambrook et al. 1989). RNA from 10^8 cells was extracted by guanidinium thiocyanate (5.0 m) followed by centrifugation through a cesium chloride (5.0 m) cushion. Single-stranded complementary (c)DNA synthesis and the PCR were carried out as described (Kawasaki 1990). Briefly, 2 µg total RNA was used as a template for cDNA synthesis in 40 µl reaction mixture containing 1 µg random hexamer and 20 units of avian myeloblastosis virus reverse transcriptase (Boehringer, Mannheim, FRG). An aliquot (2.5 µl) of the reaction mixture was then diluted with 25 µl PCR buffer (Kawasaki 1990) containing 7.5 pmol of the upstream and downstream primers and 1 m*M* $MgCl_2$. The primers for the PCR reaction for c-*kit* were chosen using the Oligo software (Med Probe, St. Hanshaugen, Norway). The sets of primers for c-*kit* were 21-mers starting at nucletide positions 653 (upstream) and 1168 (downstream). Individual control PCR reactions were done without cDNA and with cDNA and aldolase-specific primers (23-mers at nucleotide positions 141 and 583, respectively). The reaction was started by the addition of 1 unit *Taq* polymerase (Boehringer) and was performed in a DNA thermal cycler (Forschungswerkstatt der MHH, Hanover, FRG). The conditions for the PCR were 65 s at 94°C, 100 s at 57°C, and 70 s at 72°C for 37 cycles. For all RNA samples RT-PCR analyses were performed in at least two separate experiments. The specificity of the PCR reaction was confirmed by sequencing of individual reaction products and subsequent comparison with the published sequence for c-*kit* (Yarden et al. 1987).

^{3}H-Thymidine Incorporation Assays. The mitogenic activity of rhSCF alone or in combination with other CSFs (G-CSF, GM-CSF, M-CSF, IL-3, and EPO) was determined in a ^{3}H-thymidine incorporation assay. Myeloid leukemia cells in exponential growth phase were washed three times with

complete medium (RPMI 1640, 10% FCS, 1 m*M* L-glutamine) and then plated at a concentration of 5×10^4 cells/ml in 96-well flat-bottomed microtiter plates (200 µl/well) containing various concentrations (0–500 ng/ml) of rhSCF, alone or in combination with other CSFs. The other factors were used in concentrations known to be saturating (100 U/ml). After a culture period of 68 h at 37°C, 5% CO_2, the cells were exposed to a 4-h pulse of 0.5 µCi ^{3}H-thymidine (25 Ci/mmol; Amersham). Finally, the cells were harvested on glassfiber strips and the incorporated radioactivity measured in a scintillation counter (Packard).

Results

Receptor Expression on Myeloid Leukemic Cells. Using ^{125}I-rhSCF in chemical crosslinking and binding studies, as well as by immunostaining with the c-*kit* oncoprotein antibody YB5.B8, we found detectable levels of SCF receptors on the cell surface of 12 of the 28 tested myeloid leukemia cell lines (Table 1). Crosslinking studies demonstrated a normal-sized (150-kDa), single-class, high-affinity receptor for SCF on all positive lines. The number of SCF binding sites on these receptor-positive lines, as determined by Scatchard analysis, ranged between 1200 and 29000 per cell (Table 2). Using RT-PCR, 25 of 30 lines were positive for c-*kit* messenger (m)RNA expression. The expression of SCF binding sites depended on the presence of cytokines in the culture medium prior to the binding assay. $MO7_e$ cells had 13500 binding sites when cultured with medium alone, but only 2900 when cultured in medium containing SCF (100 ng/ml) (Table 2).

Mitogenic Activity of rhSCF on Myeloid Leukemia Cells. We tested rhSCF on 30 myeloid leukemia cell lines in proliferation assays. A significant proliferative response to rhSCF was detected in five cell lines (GM-153, acute myeloid leukemia; GM/SO, chronic myeloid leukemia; HEL and TF-1, erythroleukemia; $MO7_e$, megakaryoblastic leukemia; Table 1). Half-maximal proliferation in response to rhSCF was found at concentrations of about 10 ng/ml (cell line $MO7_e$, data not shown). The stimulation indices in the responder lines varied between 1.8 and 235.8. Synergistic activity of rhSCF with other CSFs were detected in SCF-responsive cells. In $MO7_e$ cells, SCF showed only minor synergism with IL-3 and GM-CSF in inducing proliferation. However, the proliferation of these cells in response to SCF alone was rather high (Table 3). In contrast to $MO7_e$ cells, GM/SO cells proliferated best in response to GM-CSF alone, or after stimulation with a combination of GM-CSF and SCF (Table 4). In these cells, SCF alone had only minor mitogenic activity. Interestingly, synergistic activity of SCF was also found with EPO. The erythroleukemia cell line TF-1 showed very similar biological characteristics with respect to its growth in response to GM-CSF and synergistic activities with SCF and EPO. In addition, this cell

Table 1. Proliferative responses of leukemia cells to stem cell factor

Type	Cell line	Proliferative response to rhSCF[a]	Stimulation index (rhSCF alone)	^{125}I-rhSCF crosslinking/YB5.B8 staining	c-*kit* mRNA (RT-PCR)
Acute myeloid leukemia	HL-60	−		−	+
	KG-1	−		−	+
	KG-1a	−		−	+
	RC-2A	−		−	+
	CTV-1	−		−	+
	OCI-AML-1	−			+
	OCI-AML-1a	−			+
	OCI-AML-2	−		−	+
	OCI-AML-3	−		−	+
	TK-1B	−		−	−
	PLB-985	−		+	+
	GM-153	+	1.8	+	+
Acute monoblastic leukemia	THP-1	−		−	+
	ML-2	−		−	−
Monoblastic leukemia	U-937	−		−	+
	DEL	−		−	−
Chronic myeloid leukemia	GM/SO	+	7.7	+	+
	LAMA-84	−		+	+
	EM-2	−		−	−
	EM-3	−		−	+
	GDM-1	−		+	+
	TMM	−		+	+
Erythroleukemia	TF-1	+	44.3	+	+
	KMOE	−		+	+
	K-562	−		−	+
	SPI-801	−		−	−
	SPI-802	−		+	+
	HEL	+	2.0	+	+
Basophilic leukemia	KU-812	−		+	+
Megakaryocytic leukemia	$MO7_e$	+	235.8	+	+

[a] Alone or in combination with G-CSF, GM-CSF, M-CSF, IL-3, or EPO.

Table 2. Stem cell factor binding sites on leukemia cells (Scatchard analysis)

Cell line	Type	SCF binding sites per cell	Proliferative response to SCF	Staining with YB5.B8
PLB-985	Acute myeloid	1200	–	+
K-562	Erythroleukemia	0	–	–
SPI-802	Erythroleukemia	11120	–	+
HEL	Erythroleukemia	3600	+	+
GM/SO	Chronic myeloid	29000	+	+
LAMA-84	Chronic myeloid	2800	–	+
KU-812	Basophilic	18400	–	+
$MO7_e$	Megakaryoblastic		+	+
Cultured in:				
rhSCF		2900		
medium		13500		

Table 3. Proliferation (^{3}H-thymidine uptake) of $MO7_e$ cells in response to single or combined cytokines. ^{3}H-thymidine uptake in the absence of growth factors (spontaneous proliferation) was 288 ± 47 cpm

Added factor	Stimulation index	
	Mean	Standard deviation
G-CSF	1.04	0.11
M-CSF	1.07	0.30
EPO	0.87	0.10
GM-CSF	45.07	2.65
IL-3	55.10	2.07
GM-CSF + IL-3	116.04	7.37
SCF	235.87	15.25
SCF + GM-CSF	251.25	10.94
SCF + IL-3	253.99	16.82
SCF + GM-CSF + IL-3	260.94	34.37

line also responded to IL-3 as well as to GM-CSF (data not shown). Synergistic activities between SCF, G-CSF, GM-CSF, and IL-3 were seen in the acute myeloid leukemia (AML) line GM-153 (Table 5).

Discussion

We were able to define a subset of myeloid leukemia cell lines that have receptors for SCF and respond to this factor with proliferation. The ability to grow after stimulation with SCF seemed not to correlate with a distinct

Table 4. Proliferation (^{3}H-thymidine uptake) of chronic myeloid GM/SO cells. ^{3}H-thymidine uptake in the absence of growth factors (spontaneous proliferation) was 3545 ± 906 cpm

Added factor	Stimulation index	
	Mean	Standard deviation
G-CSF	1.24	0.29
M-CSF	1.12	0.12
EPO	4.97	0.88
GM-CSF	42.90	2.94
IL-3	1.80	0.13
SCF	7.72	0.83
SCF + GM-CSF	49.78	1.07
SCF + IL-3	8.07	0.23
SCF + EPO	13.14	0.25
SCF + GM-CSF + IL-3	56.27	7.43

Table 5. Proliferation (^{3}H-thymidine uptake) of acute myeloid leukemia cells (GM-153). ^{3}H-thymidine uptake in the absence of growth factors (spontaneous proliferation) was 4328 ± 589 cpm

Added factor	Stimulation index	
	Mean	Standard deviation
G-CSF	1.40	0.15
M-CSF	1.05	0.06
GM-CSF	2.30	0.49
IL-3	3.90	0.84
SCF	2.56	0.13
SCF + G-CSF	4.11	0.37
SCF + GM-CSF	5.86	0.93
SCF + IL-3	6.75	0.28
SCF + GM-CSF + IL-3	7.56	0.58

morphological type of myeloid leukemic cells. The responding cell lines had different FAB types. Broudy et al. (1990) also found SCF receptor expression on 100% of fresh AML blast samples using Scatchard analysis, but only 7 of 20 AMLs responded to SCF. Their data and our results on cell lines and also on fresh leukemic blasts (Pietsch et al. 1992a) indicate that the proliferative response did not correlate with the number of SCF receptors on the surface of myeloid leukemia cells (Table 2). Using PCR techniques we were able to detect c-*kit* mRNA in 25 of 30 cell lines, although only 12 of 28 tested lines expressed the c-*kit* protein on the surface as judged by chemical crosslinking and immunofluorescence. This result may reflect protein expression being regulated by posttranscriptional control mechanisms, or a certain level of mRNA being necessary to lead to detectable protein expression on the cell surface. The mitogenic activity of SCF on leukemic blasts seems to be important for the clinical behavior of myeloid leukemia cells in vivo. The expression of the antigen detected by the monoclonal antibody YB5.B8, which later turned out to be the SCF receptor (Lerner et al. 1991), defined a subset of acute nonlymphoblastic leukemias with poor prognosis (Ashman et al. 1988). Using our approach to study the effects of SCF on the proliferation of AML blasts we were able to define four biological subgroups of myeloid leukemia cells in respect to their response to SCF. The *first* subgroup (16 of 28 lines) did not express SCF receptors and consequently was not able to respond to SCF. The *second* subgroup expressed SCF receptors and uses SCF as a growth factor (cell line $MO7_e$, Table 3). In this subgroup, significant synergistic activities were not detected because of the strong proliferation induced by SCF alone. However, we could not exclude synergistic activities at nonsaturating doses of the cytokines tested in this subtype of leukemias. The *third* subgroup also expressed SCF receptors but did not respond with proliferation to SCF. As an example, the cell line LAMA-84 expressed normal numbers of normal-sized, high-affinity receptors (not shown). Preliminary data showed that in LAMA-84 cells, like in responder cells, specific protein phosphorylation occurred shortly after exposure to SCF, so the signal transduction seemed not to be defective (P. Rauprich et al., unpublished observations). It is likely that these cells use SCF as a nonproliferative signal. Another possibility is that the cells are already maximally activated by the SCF present in FCS (2–5 ng/ml; K. Zsebo, unpublished results), or by endogenously produced SCF. In fact, we were able to demonstrate SCF mRNA in this line and also in about half of the tested cell lines, some of them coexpressing c-*kit* oncoprotein (Pietsch et al. 1992b). This suggests a autocrine growth stimulus via endogenously produced SCF. However, recent studies showed no elevation of SCF serum levels in patients with myeloid leukemias (T. Pietsch, unpublished results). The *fourth* subgroup of myeloid leukemia cells also expressed c-*kit* oncoprotein, but the response to SCF alone was rather moderate. However, combinations of SCF with other hematopoietic factors induced strong synergistic proliferative responses of these leukemic cells (for example, line GM-153, Table 5). This reflects the situation in the normal bone marrow, where approximately 2% of the mononucleated cells have SCF receptors (Ashman et al. 1989): the effects of SCF on normal bone marrow progenitor cells expressing receptors for SCF are barely detectable in progenitor cell assays like CFU-GM, BFU-E, or CFU-GEMM, if the factor is used alone. After combination of this factor with a lineage-restricted factor like EPO, GM-CSF, IL-3, or G-CSF, synergistic effects are seen in respect to an increase of the number and size of colonies without a change in their cellular composition (McNiece et al. 1991a).

Hypotheses about the mechanisms of SCF action include the idea that SCF helps quiescent normal stem cells to enter the cell cycle, and induce or increase the expression of specific receptors for the other lineage-specific CSFs on the surface of the progenitor cells. We also have evidence that the expression of SCF receptors is downregulated by its own ligand, as shown on the $MO7_e$ line (Table 2). When cultured in medium alone, the cells expressed significantly higher numbers of SCF receptors than cells cultured in the presence of SCF. The growth-promoting activity of SCF was most potent when it was combined with one or more CSFs. This effect can also be explained by an upregulation of the specific receptors, so that the leukemic cells become more responsive to the corresponding factors. Because expression of SCF receptors on myeloid leukemia cells defines a subset with poor prognosis, it is likely that this is due to the action of SCF. A role of SCF in lymphoblastic leukemia has also to be considered because SCF is known to synergize with IL-7 on normal lymphoblastic progenitor cells (McNiece et al. 1991b). Agents like antibodies or soluble receptors may be able to block these actions and may be future therapeutic tools. On the other hand, SCF may also be a potent synchronizing agent to bring quiescent leukemic cells into cycle and increase the susceptibility of leukemic cells to chemotherapeutic agents (Andreeff and Welte 1989). Further studies are necessary to evaluate the potential clinical use of this factor or its antagonists.

Acknowledgements. We thank Dr. Martin Hadam for FACS analyses and Anne Ohrdorf, Birgit Teichmann, and Petra Beenken for excellent technical assistance.

References

Andreeff M, Welte K (1989) Hematopoietic colony-stimulating factors. Semin Oncol 16:211–229

Ashman LK, Roberts MM, Gadd SJ, Cooper SJ, Juttner CA (1988) Expression of a 150 kDa cell surface antigen identified with monoclonal antibody YB5.B8 is associated with poor prognosis in acute non-lymphoblastic leukemia. Leuk Res 12:923–928

Ashman LK, Cambereri AC, Cole SR, Gadd SJ (1989) Functional studies on a 150-kDA cell-surface antigen expressed by haemopoietic progenitor cells, mast cells and some AML cells, using mAb YB5.B8. In: Knapp W (ed) Leucocyte typing IV. Oxford University Press, Oxford, pp 943–945

Broudy VC, Smith FO, Lin N, Zsebo K, Egrie J, Bernstein ID (1990) Recombinant human stem cell factor (rhuSCF) stimulates the growth of hematopoietic colonies from patients with acute nonlymphocytic leukemia (ANNL) by binding to a specific receptor. Blood 76 [Suppl 1]:134 (abstr)

Hadam MR (1985) Flow cytometryand surface marker phenotyping using monoclonal antibodies: a combined approach to precisely define the state of the immune system. In: Gillisen G, Theurer KE (eds) New aspects in physiological antitumor substances. Karger, Basel, pp 120–146

Kawasaki ES (1990) Amplification of RNA. In: Innis MA, Gelfand DH, Shinsky JJ, White TJ (eds) PCR protocols. Academic, San Diego, p 21

Lerner NB, Nocka KH, Cole SR, Qiu F, Strife A, Ashman LK, Besmer P (1991) Monoclonal antibody YB5.B8 identifies the human *c-kit* protein product. Blood 77:1876–1883

Martin F, Suggs S, Lu H, Langley K, Johnson M, Okino K, Morris C, McNiece I, Jacobson F, Johnson M, Parker V, Flores J, Patel A, Birkett N, Smith K, Fisher E, Erjavec H, Herrera C, Mendiaz E, Wypych J, Sachdev R, Pope JA, Zsebo K (1990) Primary structure and functional expression of rat and human stem cell factor DNAs. Cell 63:203–211

Medlock E, Yung Y, McNiece I, Langley K, Mineo Daley C, Dubbell C, Mendiaz B, Sachdev R, Smith K, Zsebo K (1990) Role of stem cell factor (SCF) in the stimulation of the mast cell lineage. Blood 76 [Suppl 1]:155 (abstr)

McNiece IK, Langley KE, Zsebo MK (1991a) Recombinant human stem cell factor synergizes with GM-CSF, G-CSF, IL-3 and Epo to stimulate human progenitor cells of the myeloid and erythroid lineages. Exp Hematol 19:226–231

McNiece IK, Langley KE, Zsebo MK (1991b) The role of stem cell factor in B-cell differentiation: synergistic interactions with IL-7. J Immunol 146:3785–3790

Oez S, Tittelbach H, Fahsold R, Schaetzl R, Bührer C, Azpodien J, Kalden JR (1990) Establishment and characterization of a granulocyte-macrophage colony-stimulating factor-dependent human myeloid cell line. Blood 76:578–582

Pietsch T, Kyas U, Ludwig W-D, Welte K (1992a) Mitogenic effect of human stem cell factor alone or in combination with G-CSF, GM-CSF, and IL-3 on fresh leukemic blasts from patients with stem cell factor receptor-positive AML. In: Freund M et al. (eds) Cytokines in hemopoiesis, oncology, and AIDS II. Springer, Berlin Heidelberg, 171–178

Pietsch T, Kyas U, Steffens U, Yakisan E, Hadam MR, Ludwig W-D, Zsebo K, Welte K (1992b) Effects of human stem cell factor (*c-kit* ligand) on proliferation of myeloid leukemia cells: Heterogeneity in response and synergy with other hematopoietic growth factors. Blood 80:1199–1206

Sambrook J, Fritsch EF, Maniatis T (1989) Molecular cloning: a laboratory manual. Cold Spring Harbor Laboratory, Cold Spring Harbor

Scatchard G (1949) The attraction of proteins for small molecules and ions. Ann NY Acad Sci 51:660

Yarden Y, Kuang W-J, Yang-Feng T, Coussens L, Munemitsu S, Dull TJ, Chen E, Schlessinger J, Francke U, Ullrich A (1987) Human protooncogene *c-kit*: a new cell surface receptor tyrosine kinase for an unidentified ligand. EMBO J 11:3341–3351

Zsebo K, Martin F, Suggs S, Wypych J, Lu H, McNiece I, Medlock E, Morris F, Sachdev R, Tung W, Birkett N, Smith K, Yuschenkoff V, Mendiaz E, Jacobson F, Langley K (1990a) Biological characterization of a unique early acting hematopoietic growth factor. Exp Hematol 18/6:703 (abstr)

Zsebo K, Williams D, Geissler E, Broudy V, Martin F, Atkins H, Hsu R-Y, Birkett N, Okino K, Murdock D, Jacobson F, Langley K, Smith K, Takeishi T, Cattanach B, Galli S, Suggs S (1990b) Stem cell factor (SCF) is encoded at the *Sl* locus of the mouse and is the ligand for the *c-kit* tyrosine kinase receptor. Cell 63:213–224

Zsebo K, Wypych J, McNiece I, Lu H, Smith K, Karkare S, Sachdev R, Yuschenkoff V, Birkett N, Williams L, Satyagal V, Tung W, Bosselman B, Mendiaz E, Langley K (1990c) Identification, purification, and biological characterization of hematopoietic stem cell factor from buffalo rat liver conditioned medium. Cell 63:195–201

Morphologic Basis for the MIC Classification in Acute Myeloid Leukemia

H. Löffler

Department of Internal Medicine II, University of Kiel, Chemnitzstraße 22, W-2300 Kiel, Fed. Rep. of Germany

Classification System

Classic morphology and cytochemistry are the basic techniques for the classification of acute myeloid leukemias (AML) according to the FAB-criteria. While the main categories existed before, the borders of the morphologic subtypes were not precisely defined. The FAB group made proposals for different categories originally including the following six subtypes: M1, M2, and M3 for granulocytic leukemia, M4 and M5 for myelomonocytic and monocytic leukemia, and M6 for erythroleukemia. After the addition of the variant form of M3 (M3v), the M4 subtype with abnormal eosinophils (M4Eo), and acute megakaryoblastic leukemia (M7) in 1985, the FAB classification consisted of ten subtypes including the variants of M5 (Bennett et al. 1985).

While the classification of the AML subtypes M1 to M6 is largely based on morphology and cytochemistry, megakaryoblastic leukemia (M7) cannot be identified with sufficient certainty without immunology or the more complicated electron-microscopic platelet peroxidase technique. Recently, the FAB-group proposed the inclusion of minimally differentiated acute myeloid leukemia (M0) into the subclassification of AML. The diagnosis of AML M0 cannot be made on morphologic grounds alone as the blasts sometimes resemble lymphoblasts or undifferentiated blasts; myeloperoxidase and Sudan Black B reactions as well as chloroacetate esterase are negative. The evidence for myeloid differentation is usually provided by the reactivity with monoclonal antibodies against the myeloid-associated antigens CD13 and CD33. B- and T-lymphoid markers are negative, and terminal deoxynucleotidyl transferase (TdT) is expressed in half of the cases (Bennett et al. 1991).

Some of the additions in 1985 were necessary since cytogenetic findings pointed to the existence of specific morphologic-cytogenetic entities. This group of AMLs include promyelocytic leukemia and its microgranular

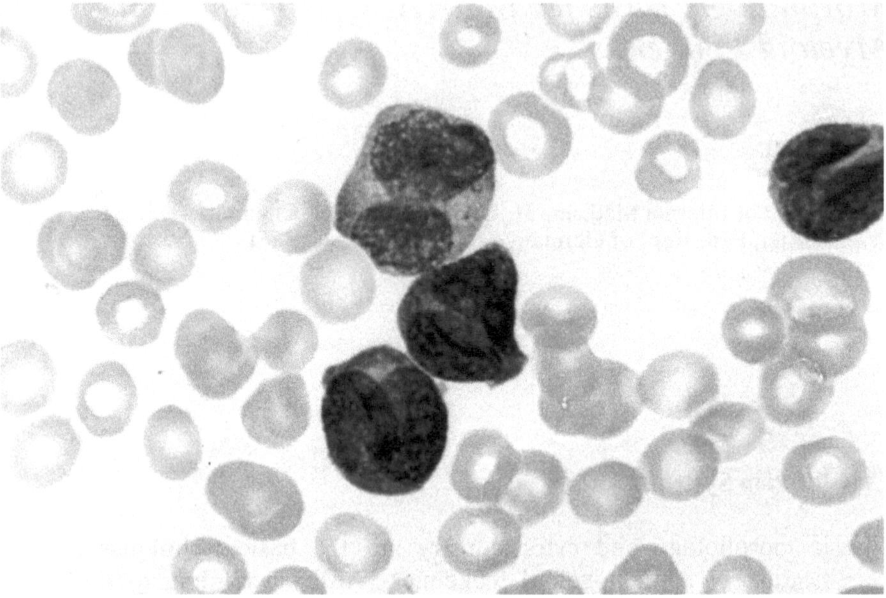

Fig. 1. Bilobed nuclei in a variant form of acute promyelocytic leukemia (M3v), with "agranular" cytoplasm. The cells were very strongly peroxidase positive, and HLA-DR antigens were not found

variant (M3 and M3v) with the typical chromosome abnormality t(15;17), a proportion of cases with the subtype M2 with t(8;21), and the myelomonocytic variant with abnormal eosinophils and the inv(16). The MIC group (Second MIC Cooperative Study Group 1988) also proposed to include a variant of M2 with basophilic maturation and the t(6;9) or t/del12 abnormalities but it has meanwhile been shown that these aberrations are not as closely correlated with morphologically defined subtypes as the previously mentioned ones. For instance, t(6;9) can be found in myelodysplasia or in AML without basophils. Nevertheless, AML with a high percentage of basophilic precursors or basophilic maturation exists and it must be separated from chronic granulocytic leukemia in blast crisis, which often has a high percentage of basophilic precursors. In addition to "acute basophilic leukemias" there exist cases with immature eosinophilic precursors which could either be included into the FAB classification as another variant of M2 or as an independent entity.

A very rare form of AML with monocytic features (M4 or M5) and conspicuous erythrophagocytosis has been shown to be associated with t(8;16); a more frequent finding in monocytic leukemias is the involvement of 11q23, the most frequent translocation in this type of leukemia being t(9;11). Until recently, changes of chromosomes 3 were thought to be associated with megakaryoblastic leukemia (M7). A new chromosome abnormality has been described with acute megakaryoblastic leukemia in infants, an association which occurs with high frequency: t(1;22) (Carroll et al. 1991; Baruchel et al. 1991).

Prerequisites for the Morphological and Cytochemical Classification

Carefully prepared films (smears) of aspirated bone marrow containing marrow particles and peripheral blood are required. In case of insufficient aspiration, bone marrow trephine biopsies and histological sections have to be prepared. If possible, both techniques should be combined, especially if there are no marrow particles aspirated. Panoptic staining (Pappenheim, Giemsa) should provide an orange staining of the erythrocytes and a clear distinction of all types of granules. In addition, a reproducible peroxidase technique (Sudan Black B gives about the same results), nonspecific esterase (α-naphthylacetate or butyrate), chloroacetatesterase, and, as an additional staining, periodic acid–Schiff stain should be applied.

From experiences with a central morphology registry and from discussions in expert meetings it is evident that the distinction of M2, M3, M3v (Fig. 1), and M1/M5 as well as the definition of M3 cause problems in daily routine. I have tried to summarize some of the distinctive features of the subtypes M2 and M3, M3v, M5a, and M5b in Table 1.

Using the definition of the FAB group it must be accepted that the percentage of peroxidase- or Sudan Black B-positive blasts is not a defining criterion for M2 or M3. There are many cases of M2 with nearly 100% peroxidase-positive blasts, while on the other hand there exist cases with a partial peroxidase deficiency in the granulocytic precursors and the mature granulocytes. M3 and M3v as a rule have very strong peroxidase in 90%–100% of the abnormal promyelocytes, and I have seen only one case with a nearly total deficiency of peroxidase and Sudan Black B in an otherwise typical M3v leukemia. Since the availability of a very potent differentiating therapy with all-*trans*-retinoic acid (tretinoin), it is essential to distinguish the AML subytpes M3 and M3v from the other AML subtypes.

Another cause of trouble for morphologic diagnosis is megakaryoblastic leukemia (M7). The morphologic spectrum ranges from lymphoblast-like cells (L2) to tumor-like cells, since some cases can show clumping of the blasts, and cytoplasmic basophilia is often prominent. With the availability of the monoclonal antibodies CD61, CD41a, and CD42b megakaryoblastic leukemia can be positively identified since cytochemistry gives only an indication and morphology alone is usually not sufficient.

At this time the MIC classification covers only a proportion of AML cases. The three most frequent and well-characterized entities, M2/t(8;21), M3/M3v/t(15;17), and M4Eo/inv(16), and the new entity M7/t(1;22) comprise about 30% of all cases with chromosome abnormalities.

Table 1. Some of the distinctive features of the AML subtypes M2, M3, M3v, M5a, and M5b

FAB type	Cell size and form	Nuclear shape	Cytoplasm	Granules	Auer rods	Peroxidase/ Sudan Black B	Esterase
M2	Hetero- geneous	Round, oval	Variable; often abundant	Fine prominent	Single	Up to 100% positive	Occasionally Golgi-zone positive
M3	Medium, oval	Reniform, irregular	Moderately abundant	Coarse red or purple	Multiple, bundles or faggots	Usually 100%, very strong	Negative, occasionally diffuse weak
M3v	Medium, irregular	Bilobed, convoluted, reniform	Scanty–moderately abundant	Sparse, fine, or agranular cytoplasm	Rare cells with bundles	Usually 100% medium strong	Negative, occasionally diffuse weak
M5a	Large, round	Round, oval	Variable; often abundant	Usually absent	0	Usually 0	Diffuse, very strong
M5b	Medium, pleomorphic	Pleomorphic, convoluted	Moderately abundant	Sparse, fine, red	Rare, single	Fine granular	Diffuse, strong

The greater part has no consistent morphologic-cytogenetic correlations, so for the time being the classic categories with the incorporation of information derived from new techniques must still form the basis for routine classification.

References

Baruchel A, Daniel MT, Schaison G, Berger R (1991) Nonrandom t(1;22) (p12-q13;q13) in acute megakaryocytic malignant proliferation. Cancer Genet Cytogenet 54:239–243

Bennett JM, Catovsky D, Daniel MT, Flandrin G, Galton DAG, Gralnick HR, Sultan C (1985) Proposed revised criteria for the classification of acute myeloid leukemia. Ann Intern Med 103:620–625

Bennett JM, Catovsky D, Daniel MT, Flandrin G, Galton DAG, Gralnick HR, Sultan C (1991) Proposal for the recognition of minimally differentiated acute myeloid leukaemia (AML-M0). Br J Haematol 78:325–329

Carroll A, Civin C, Schneider N, Dahl G, Pappo A, Bowman P, Emami A, Gross S, Alvarado C, Phillips C, Krischer J, Crist W, Head D, Gresik M, Ravindranath Y, Weinstein H (1991) The t(1;22)(p13;q13) is nonrandom and restricted to infants with acute megakaryoblastic leukemia: a Pediatric Oncology Group study. Blood 78:748–752

Second MIC Cooperative Study Group (1988) Morphologic, immunologic and cytogenetic (MIC) working classification of the acute myeloid leukaemias. Br J Haematol 68:487–494

Molecular Genetics of the t(15;17) Translocation in Acute Promyelocytic Leukemia

A. Biondi[1], A. Rambaldi[2], P.P. Pandolfi[3], M. Alcalay[3], L. Longo[3], V. Rossi[1], G. Giudici[1], F. Lo Coco[4], and P.G. Pelicci[3]

[1] Clinica Pediatrica Università Milano, H.S. Gerardo, via Donizetti 106, 20152 Monza, Italy
[2] Divisione Ematologia, Ospedali Riuniti Bergamo and Istituto Ricerche Farmacologiche M. Negri, Bergamo, Italy
[3] Clinica Medica Università di Perugia, Perugia, Italy
[4] Dipartimento di Biopatologia, Divisione Ematologia, I Università Roma, Rome, Italy

Introduction

Acute Promyelocytic Leukemia (APL) is a distinct subset of acute myeloid leukemia (AML) (FAB-M3 according to the French-American-British Cooperative Group). It is morphologically distinguished by the presence of hyper-granular leukemic blasts (Sultan et al. 1973; Bennett et al. 1976). The clinical propensity of APL patients to hemorrhage, the feature that first drew the attention to this type of acute leukemia, is thought to be due to the release of procoagulants by the granules in the malignant promyelocytes (Gralnick and Abrell 1973; Falanga et al. 1988). APL are cytogenetically distinguished by a balanced reciprocal chromosome 15;17 translocation-t(15;17) (Rowley et al. 1977; Mitelman 1988). The high frequency (70 to 100% of cases) and the tumor-type specificity of the t(15;17) suggest that chromosome break-points affect DNA sequence that might be crucial in the pathogenesis of this malignancy.

Mapping of Chromosome Breakpoints in APL

The 17q11–21 chromosome region is of particular interest because it is implicated in a number of karyotype alterations associated with various subtypes of AML (Mitelmann 1988). In particular it is the chromosomal region involved in the t(15;17) of APL (Larson et al. 1984). Several genes that are potentially relevant for the pathogenesis of AMLs have been mapped in the 17q11–21 region: the c-erbA-1 and the c-erbB-2 proto-oncogenes which encode proteins closely related to the thyroid hormone receptor, respectively (Sap et al. 1986); the gene coding for the hemopoietic myeloid specific growth factor, G-CSF (Nagata et al. 1986); the Retinoic Acid receptor-α (RAR-α) gene implicated in controlling proliferation and differentiation in several cell types including myeloid cells (Pektovich et al. 1987);

Recent Results in Cancer Research, Vol. 131

and the gene for the myeloid specific enzyme myeloperoxidase (MPO) (Weil et al. 1987). There are scarce information on either the respective position of these genes and their proximity to the breakpoints. c-erbA-1, G-CSF and c-erbB-2 have been mapped proximal to the APL breakpoint (Xu et al. 1988). By in situ hybridization we were able to demonstrate that chromosome 17 breakpoint in APLs is situated between the c-erbB-2 and RAR-α genes. We mapped the MPO gene to 17q22–23 (Donti et al. 1986), which lies far from the 17q21 APL breakpoint, as others have done (Chang et al. 1986; Longo et al. 1990a). In addition we demonstrated that the RAR-α gene and the breakpoint are located in the same cytogenetic band (17q21). Moreover Southern blot analysis of a large series of APL DNAs suggested that the c-erbB-2 locus is not directly affected by the breakpoint (Longo et al. 1990a).

The Chromosome 17 Breakpoint Lies Within the Rar-α Locus

In order to elucidate a possible involvement of the RAR-α gene in the 17 breakpoint, high molecular weight DNA was extracted from the blasts of 20 leukemia patients who met all the morphological criteria for the FAB M3 classification. 18 displayed the typical t(15;17), and two had a normal karyotype (Longo et al. 1990b). DNA were digested with the EcoRI, HindIII or BamHI restriction enzymes and hybridized to DNA probes representative of different portions of the RAR-α cDNA. As shown in Fig. 1 the K/S probe representative of the 5' end of the RAR-α p63 cDNA (kindly provided by Dr.P. Chambon) revealed additional hybridizing fragments that differed from the control DNA germline pattern with one (four cases), two (seven cases) or all three (two cases) of the restriction enzymes used. No deviation from the germline configuration was seen in any case with either the RAR-α IT or P/R cDNA probes, which contain the intermediate or the 3′ portions of the RAR-α p63 cDNA, respectively. The analysis of a large panel of normal and non-APL leukemic samples DNA, rule out the possibility that the K/S-hybridizing extra-fragments are not the consequence of genetic variation. In addition, DNA was extracted from the BM cells of two APL patients who had entered morphological remission after conventional chemotherapy. These DNAs, and DNAs extracted from blasts of the same patients before remission, were digested with the HindIII restriction enzyme, hybridized to the K/S probe, and compared. As shown in Fig. 2 the K/S extra-fragments seen in the APL blasts had disappeared in one case (No 3) and become fainter in the other (No 14).

To map the rearrangements within the RAR-α locus, the segment containing the corresponding K/S exons was isolated and characterized and APL DNAs were analyzed with genomic RAR-α probes. Fig. 3B gives a limited restriction enzyme map and the exon-intron organization of the 5' portion of the normal RAR-α locus as derived from the analysis of the K/S

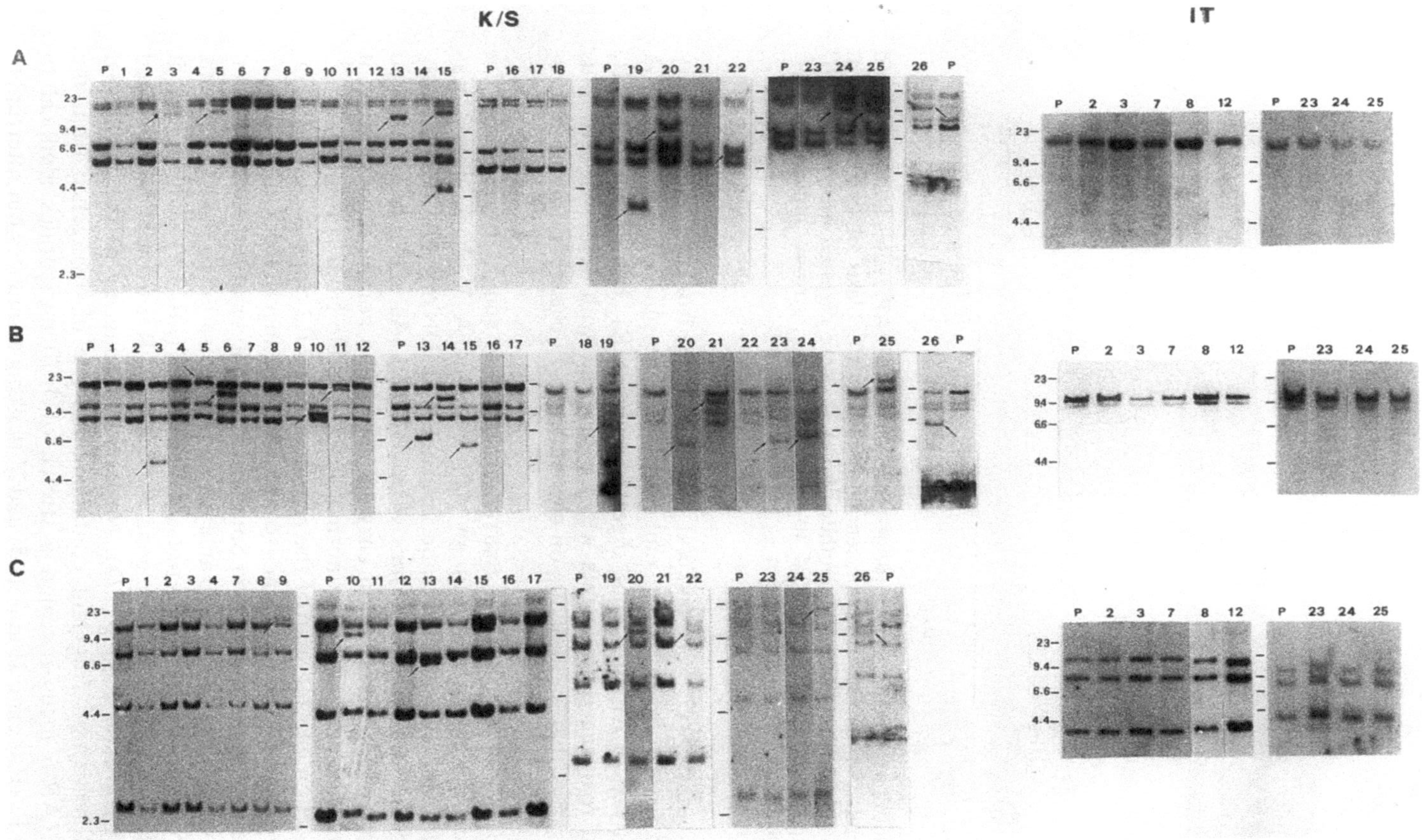

Fig. 1. Southern blot analysis of the RAR-α gene in APLs. DNAs from 20 APLs were digested with EcoRI (**A**), HindIII (**B**), or BamHI (**C**) restriction enzymes and hybridized to the K/S probe. *P*, placenta DNA. *Arrows* indicate RAR-α-rearranged bands. Molecular weight markers are indicated at the left of each panel

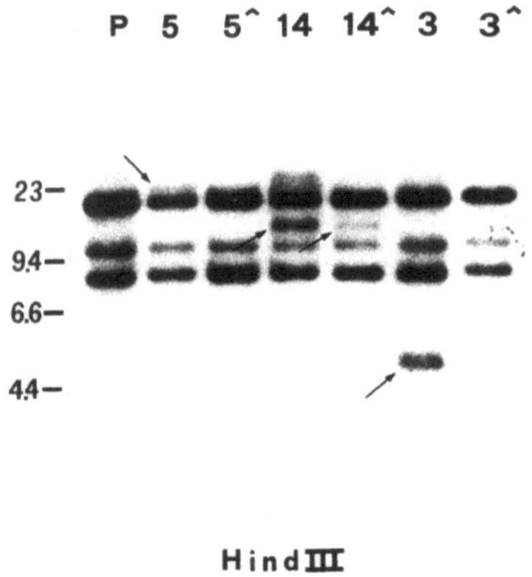

Fig. 2. Southern blot analysis of the RAR-α gene in two APL cases at diagnosis and during remission. DNAs from placenta (*P*), BM APL blasts of two patients at diagnosis (14^,3^) and after chemotherapy (14,3), were digested with the *HindIII* restriction enzyme and hybridized to the K/S probe. Arrows indicate RAR-α rearranged bands

complementary λ8C, λ2A and λa1 clones isolated from a λ phage library prepared from normal human embryonic lung fibroblast DNA. All DNA isolated from 20 APL patients, digested with EcoRI, HindIII and BamHI, displayed rearranged fragments when hybridized with H18, X5, HB thus demonstrating that breakpoints on chromosome 17 cluster in the first intron of RAR-α locus.

The origin of the RAR-α rearrangements was sought by isolating the rearranged RAR-α gene from an APL patient. A λ phage library was prepared from genomic DNA and screened with DNA probe HB (Alacaly et al. 1991). Two types of clones were obtained. As one type overlapped extensively with the restriction enzyme map of the normal RAR-α gene, it probably included part of the normal RAR-α allele from chromosome 17. The restriction enzyme map of the representative λR2 clone is shown in Fig. 3C. The second type of clones contained rearranged RAR-α sequences reminiscent of those disclosed in Southern blot analysis of total chromosomal DNA. Restriction enzyme map analysis and hybridization to RAR-α genomic and cDNA probes of one representative clone (λR13A) showed that it matched the germline RAR-α gene 3′ of the RAR-α exon II but diverged 5′ of RAR-α exon II (Fig. 3D). Nucleotide sequencing of the 2.1-kb Bgl l-BamHI restriction fragment containing the site of divergence from the normal RAR-α locus revealed a stretch of 1670 nucleotides identical to germline RAR-α exon II and its 5′ and 3′ flanking sequences but interrupted

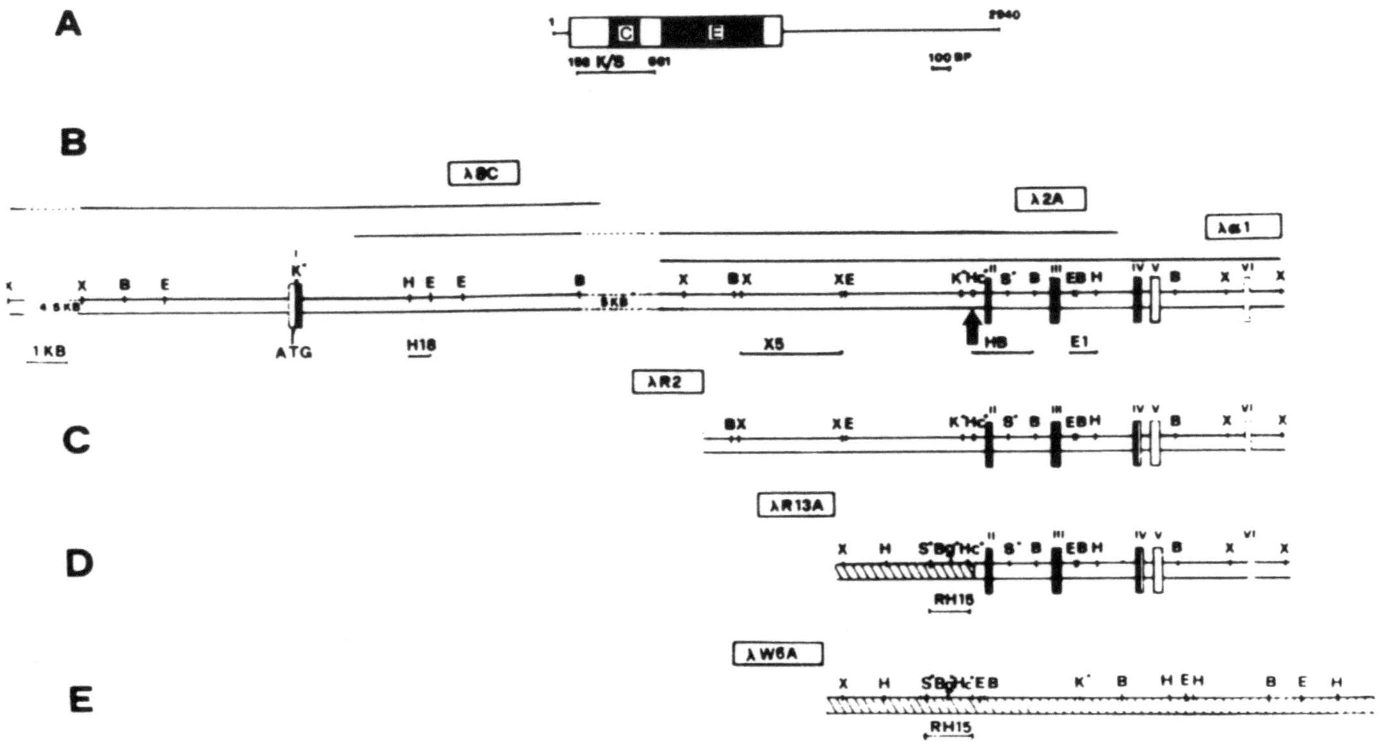

Fig. 3. Schematic representation of the RAR-α cDNA (**A**), genomic organization of the germ-line RAR-α 5' portion (**B**), the normal (**C**) and recombined (**D**) RAR-α genes from one APL patient, and the normal counterpart of the chromosome 15-derived sequences involved in the RAR-α recombination (**E**). *B*, BamHI; *E*, EcoRI; *H*, HindIII; *X*, XbaI; *I*, SmaI; K, KpnI; *Hc*, HincII; *Bg*, BglI. The dots after K,S,Hc and Bg restriction enzyme sites indicate that they were only partially mapped

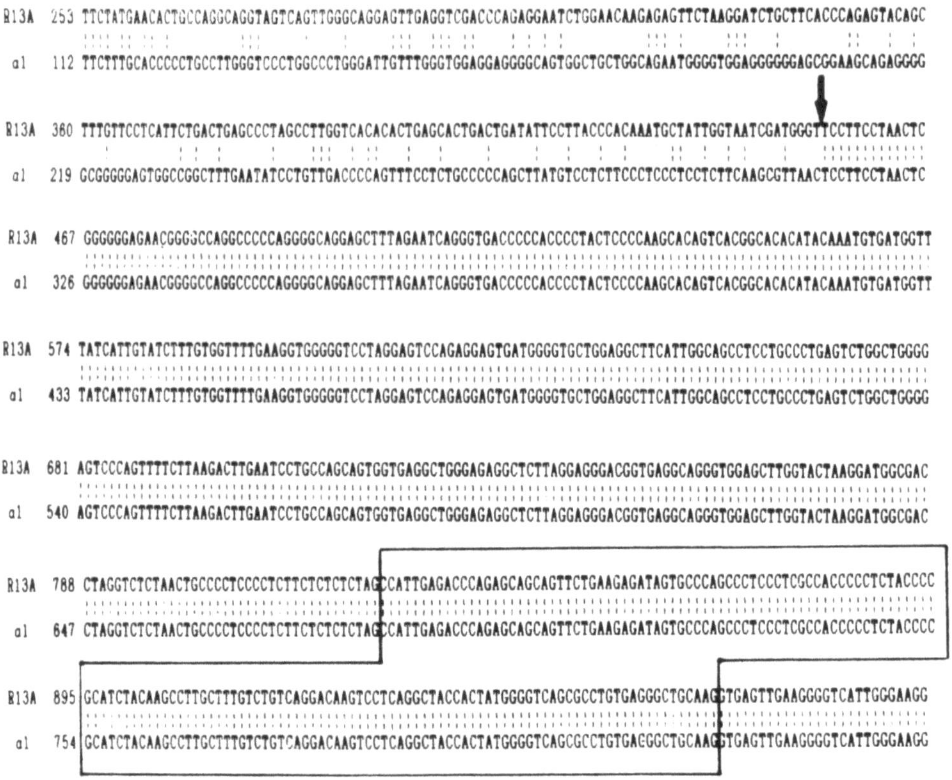

Fig. 4. Nucleotide sequencing of the chromosome 15;17 cross-over junction (λR13A) and comparison with the normal RAR-α gene (α1). The 2.7-kb KpnI-EcoRI fragment of the normal RAR-α gene (α1), which contains exons II and III, and the 2.1-kb Bgl I-BamHI fragment of the rearranged RAR-α gene (λR13A), which spans exon II and the point of divergence from the normal counterpart, were sequenced

within RAR-α intron I, 370 base pairs upstream from the splicing donor site of exon II (Fig. 4). To determine the chromosome origin of the nonhomologous RAR-α sequences in clone λR13A, human-rodent somatic cell hybrids were probed with the RH15 SmaI-HincII DNA fragment, representative of the nonhomologous sequences, in Southern blot experiments. Only hybrids containing the human chromosome 15 hybridized to the RH15. In situ hybridization of the same probe to human metaphases from normal peripheral blood lymphocytes showed that RH15 sequences map to the 15q23-q24 chromosome bands, which correspond to the APL chromosome 15 breakpoint region (Larson et al. 1984). Thus these data indicate that the λR13A clone contains one of the two break sites of the 15;17 translocation. Two other independent groups have reported the isolation of the APL translocation breakpoint and similarly demonstrated that it occurs within the RAR-α locus (Borrow et al. 1990; de Thè et al. 1990).

Having demonstrated that DNA sequences involved in chromosome 17 recombination are common to the majority of APLs, we addressed whether the type of chromosome 15 recombination, that has been cloned, is common to a II APLs. The answer was sought by isolating the normal counterpart of the chromosome 15-derived sequences, by screening a human genomic lybrary from human embryo lung fibroblasts with the RH15 probe. The restriction enzyme map of a representative RH15 complementary clone (λW6A) is shown in Fig. 3E. To map the translocation breakpoint within the isolated chromosome 15 DNA region, the RH15 DNA probe was hybridized to HindIII-digested APL DNAs. The RH15 probe hybridized to a HindIII 9-kb fragment in human germline DNA and to one rearranged fragment in 73% of APL cases analyzed. This suggest that the APL chromosome breakpoints cluster within the HindIII 9-kb RH15 homologous DNA fragment and recalls the picture seen in the chromosome 9 breakpoint cluster region in the t(9;22) of chronic myelogenous leukemias. The findings that some patients displayed the germline configuration after HindIII digestion and RH15 probe hybridization, implicate that the chromosome 15 breakpoint in a minority of APL patients lies outside tha above mentioned chromosome 15 breakpoint cluster region. The chromosome 15-specific locus involved in the t(15;17) was originally named myl and more recently renamed PML (for "promyelocytes") (de Thè et al. 1991; Kakizuka et al. 1991).

The Translocated RAR-α Portion is Aberrantly Transcribed as a Part of PML/RAR-α Fusion mRNA

To determine whether tha rearrangements of the RAR-α locus interfere with its expression pattern, Northern blot experiments were performed on RNAs extracted from APL blasts (Longo et al. 1990b). When the I/T and K/S RAR-α cDNA probes were hybridized with RNAs from non-APL leukemic cells and normal cells (granulocytes, monocytes, lymphocytes, mesothelial cells and amnion cells) only the typical 3.8 and 2.8-kb transcripts were detected (data not shown). However, when the RNAs from 8 APL cases were hybridized with the same two probes, the two typical RAR-α transcripts appeared at an intensity that varied both within and between samples in seven cases. Figure 5 shows the results on RAR-α expression pattern in APLs. All eight cases exhibited one or two RAR-α aberrant transcripts of three different sizes: 4.4 kb in three cases and 4.0 and 3.5 in five.

PML/RAR-α cDNAs were isolated by screening one APL cDNA library with a RAR-α cDNA probe (Pandolfi et al. 1991). The library was prepared from poly $(A)^+$ mRNA extracted from bone marrow blasts of the same case from which the RAR-α rearrangement shown in Fig. 3C was isolated. A total of 6×10^5 phages was screened with a RAR-α cDNA probe, and six

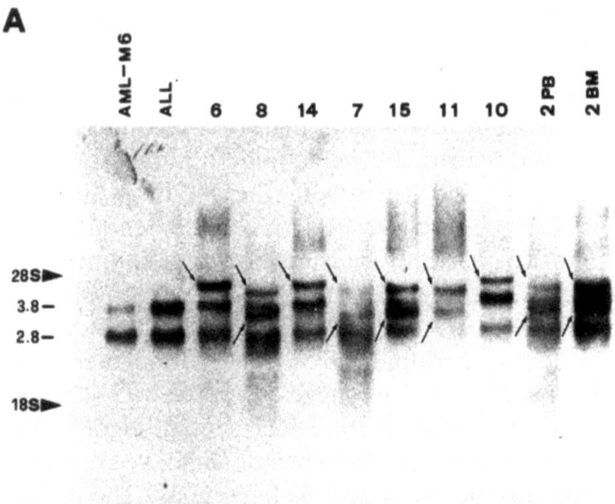

Fig. 5. RAR-α gene expression patterns in APLs. RNA samples from BM blasts of eight APLs, one AML-M6 and one ALL were analyzed by Northern blotting using th IT probe. Both PBL and BM blasts were analyzed in patient No.2. Ribosomal RNAs (28S and 18S) are given as size markers. The estimated length (3.8 and 2.8 kb) of the RAR-a typical double transcript is also given. Arrows indicate aberrant RAR-α transcripts

positive recombinants were isolated. The partial sequences identified two of the positive clones as being RAR-β and RAR-γ, two as RAR-α and two as PML/RAR-α. A partial restriction enzyme map of the two PML/RAR-α cDNAs (pLA5 and pLA6) indicated that they overlapped over a sequence of approximately 3.1 kb (Fig. 6A). The entire 3101 bp PML/RAR-α merged sequence is shown in Fig. 6B. Comparison of the PML/RAR-α sequence with the normal PML cDNA (isolated by screening a human cDNA library with a PML genomic DNA probes derived from an APL PML/RAR-α fusion gene) (Pandolfi et al. 1991) and RAR-α sequences (Giguere et al. 1987) showed that DNA region 1-1645 of the chimeric cDNA corresponds to the 85-1729 region of the PML cDNA sequence and nucleotide region 1646-3101 of the PML/RAR-α corresponds to nucleotides 281-1736 of the reported RAR-α sequence. The PML/RAR-α junction was found to be

Fig. 6a,b. DNA and primary amino acid sequence of the PML/RAR-α cDNA. **a** Schematic representation of the PML/RAR-α sequence and limited restriction map of the PML/RAR-α cDNAs. **b** The complete nucleotide sequence of the LA5 and LA6 PML/RAR-α cDNAs is shown with the predicted amino acid sequence given below the ORF. The putative initiation codon of the translation (ATG) is underlined. PML/RAR-α junction is double underlined

a

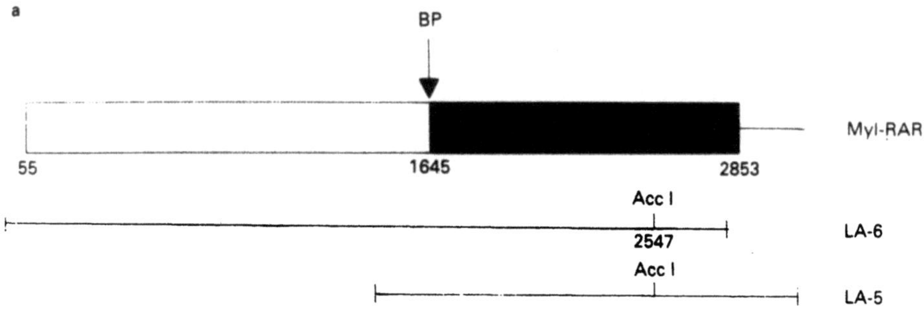

b

CCCGCCCGATCTCCGAGGCCCCAGCAGGACCCCGCCCGGCCCCAGGAGCCCACCATGCCTCCCCCCGAGACCCCCTCTGAAGGCCGCCAGCCCAGCCCCAGCCCCAGCCCTACAGAGCGA 120
MetProProProGluThrProSerGluGlyArgGlnProSerProSerProSerProThrGluArg 22

GCCCCCGCTTCGGAGGAGGAGTTCCAGTTTCTGCGCTGCCAGCAATGCCAGGCGGAAGCCAAGTGCCCGAAGCTGCTGCCTTGTCTGCACACGCTGTGCTCAGGATGCCTGGAGGCGTCG 240
AlaProAlaSerGluGluGluPheGlnPheLeuArgCysGlnGlnCysGlnAlaGluAlaLysCysProLysLeuLeuProCysLeuHisThrLeuCysSerGlyCysLeuGluAlaSer 62

GGCATGCAGTGCCCCATCTGCCAGGCGCCCTGGCCCCTAGGTGCAGACACACCCGCCCTGGATAACGTCTTTTTCGAGAGTCTGCAGCGGCGCCTGTCGGTGTACCGGCAGATTGTGGAT 360
GlyMetGlnCysProIleCysGlnAlaProTrpProLeuGlyAlaAspThrProAlaLeuAspAsnValPhePheGluSerLeuGlnArgArgLeuSerValTyrArgGlnIleValAsp 102

GCGCAGGCTGTGTGCACCCGCTGCAAAGAGTCGGCCGACTTCTGGTGCTTTGAGTGCGAGCAGCTCCTCTGCGCCAAGTGCTTCGAGGCACACCAGTGGTTCCTCAAGCACGAGGCCCGG 480
AlaGlnAlaValCysThrArgCysLysGluSerAlaAspPheTrpCysPheGluCysGluGlnLeuLeuCysAlaLysCysPheGluAlaHisGlnTrpPheLeuLysHisGluAlaArg 142

CCCCTAGCAGAGCTGCGCAACCAGTCGGTGCGTGAGTTCCTGGACGGCACCCGCAAGACCAACAACATCTTCTGCTCCAACCCCAACCACCGCACCCCTACGCTGACCAGCATCTACTGC 600
ProLeuAlaGluLeuArgAsnGlnSerValArgGluPheLeuAspGlyThrArgLysThrAsnAsnIlePheCysSerAsnProAsnHisArgThrProThrLeuThrSerIleTyrCys 182

CGAGGATGTTCCAAGTTGCTGTGCTGCTCGTGCGCGCTCCTTGACAGCAGCCACAGTGAGCTCAAGTGCGACATCAGCGCAGAGATCCAGCAGCGACAGGAGGAGCTGGACGCCATGACG 720
ArgGlyCysSerLysLeuLeuCysCysSerCysAlaLeuLeuAspSerSerHisSerGluLeuLysCysAspIleSerAlaGluIleGlnGlnArgGlnGluGluLeuAspAlaMetThr 222

CAGGCGCTGCAGGAGCAGGATAGTGCCTTTGGCGCGGTTCACGCGCAGATGCACGCGGCCGTCGGCCAGCTGGGCCGCGCGCGTGCCGAGACCGAGGAGCTGATCCGCGAGCGCGTGCGC 840
GlnAlaLeuGlnGluGlnAspSerAlaPheGlyAlaValHisAlaGlnMetHisAlaAlaValGlyGlnLeuGlyArgAlaArgAlaGluThrGluGluLeuIleArgGluArgValArg 262

CAGGTGGTAGCTCACGTGCGGGCTCAGGAGCGCGAGCTGCTGGAGGCTGTGGACGCGCGGTACCAGCGCGACTACGAGGAGATGGCCAGTCGGCTGGGCCGCCTGGATGCTGTGCTGCAG 960
GlnValValAlaHisValArgAlaGlnGluArgGluLeuLeuGluAlaValAspAlaArgTyrGlnArgAspTyrGluGluMetAlaSerArgLeuGlyArgLeuAspAlaValLeuGln 302

CGCATCCGCACGGGCAGCGCGCTGGTGCAGAGGATGAAGTGCTACGCCTCGGACCAGGAGGTGCTGGACATGCACGGTTTCCTGCGCCAGGCGCTCTGCCGCCTGCGCCAGGAGGAGCCC 1080
ArgIleArgThrGlySerAlaLeuValGlnArgMetLysCysTyrAlaSerAspGlnGluValLeuAspMetHisGlyPheLeuArgGlnAlaLeuCysArgLeuArgGlnGluGluPro 342

CAGAGCCTGCAAGCTGCCGTGCGCACCGATGGCTTCGACGAGTTCAAGGTGCGCCTGCAGGACCTCAGCTCTTGCATCACCCAGGGGAAAGATGCAGCTGTATCCAAGAAAGCCAGCCCA 1200
GlnSerLeuGlnAlaAlaValArgThrAspGlyPheAspGluPheLysValArgLeuGlnAspLeuSerSerCysIleThrGlnGlyLysAspAlaAlaValSerLysLysAlaSerPro 382

GAGGCTGCCAGCACTCCCAGGGACCCTATTGACGTTGACCTGCCCGAGGAGGCAGAGAGAGTGAAGGCCCAGGTTCAGGCCCTGGGGCTGGCTGAAGCCCAGCCTATGGCTGTGGTACAG 1320
GluAlaAlaSerThrProArgAspProIleAspValAspLeuProGluGluAlaGluArgValLysAlaGlnValGlnAlaLeuGlyLeuAlaGluAlaGlnProMetAlaValValGln 422

TCAGTGCCCGGGGCACACCCCGTGCCAGTGTACGCCTTCTCCATCAAAGGCCCTTCCTATGGAGAGGATGTCTCCAATACAACGACAGCCCAGAAGAGGAAGTGCAGCCAGACCCAGTGC 1440
SerValProGlyAlaHisProValProValTyrAlaPheSerIleLysGlyProSerTyrGlyGluAspValSerAsnThrThrThrAlaGlnLysArgLysCysSerGlnThrGlnCys 462

CCCAGGAAGGTCATCAAGATGGAGTCTGAGGAGGGGAAGGAGGCAAGGTTGGCTCGGAGCTCCCCGGAGCAGCCCAGGCCCAGCACCTCCAAGGCAGTCTCACCACCCCACCTGGATGGA 1560
ProArgLysValIleLysMetGluSerGluGluGlyLysGluAlaArgLeuAlaArgSerSerProGluGlnProArgProSerThrSerLysAlaValSerProProHisLeuAspGly 502

CCGCCTAGCCCCAGGAGCCCCGTCATAGGAAGTGAGGTCTTCCTGCCCAACAGCAACCACGTGGCCAGTGGCGCCGGGGAGGCAGCCATTGAGACCCAGAGCAGCAGTTCTGAAGAGATA 1680
ProProSerProArgSerProValIleGlySerGluValPheLeuProAsnSerAsnHisValAlaSerGlyAlaGlyGluAlaAlaIleGluThrGlnSerSerSerSerGluGluIle 542

GTGCCCAGCCCTCCCTCGCCACCCCCTCTACCCCGCATCTACAAGCCTTGCTTTGTCTGTCAGGACAAGTCCTCAGGCTACCACTATGGGGTCAGCGCCTGTGAGGGCTGCAAGGGCTTC 1800
ValProSerProProSerProProProLeuProArg'leTyrLysProCysPheValCysGlnAspLysSerSerGlyTyrHisTyrGlyValSerAlaCysGluGlyCysLysGlyPhe 582

TTCCGCCGCAGCATCCAGAAGAACATGGTGTACACGTGTCACCGGGACAAGAACTGCATCATCAACAAGGTGACCCGGAACCGCTGCCAGTACTGCCGACTGCAGAAGTGCTTTGAAGTG 1920
PheArgArgSerIleGlnLysAsnMetValTyrThrCysHisArgAspLysAsnCysIleIleAsnLysValThrArgAsnArgCysGlnTyrCysArgLeuGlnLysCysPheGluVal 622

GGCATGTCCAAGGAGTCTGTGAGAAACGACCGAAACAAGAAGAAGAAGGAGGTGCCCAAGCCCGAGTGCTCTGAGAGCTACACGCTGACGCCGGAGGTGGGGGAGCTCATTGAGAAGGTG 2040
GlyMetSerLysGluSerValArgAsnAspArgAsnLysLysLysLysGluValProLysProGluCysSerGluSerTyrThrLeuThrProGluValGlyGluLeuIleGluLysVal 662

CGCAAAGCGCACCAGGAAACCTTCCCTGCCCTCTGCCAGCTGGGCAAATACACTACGAACAACAGCTCAGAACAACGTGTCTCTCTGGACATTGACCTCTGGGACAAGTTCAGTGAACTC 2160
ArgLysAlaHisGlnGluThrPheProAlaLeuCysGlnLeuGlyLysTyrThrThrAsnAsnSerSerGluGlnArgValSerLeuAspIleAspLeuTrpAspLysPheSerGluLeu 702

TCCACCAAGTGCATCATTAATACTGTGGAGTTCGCCAAGCAGCTGTTTGGCTTCACCACCCTCACCATCGCCGACCAGATCACCCTCCTCAAGGTCGCCTGCGTGGACATCCTGATCCTG 2280
SerThrLysCysIleIleAsnThrValGluPheAlaLysGlnLeuPheGlyPheThrThrLeuThrIleAlaAspGlnIleThrLeuLeuLysValAlaCysValAspIleLeuIleLeu 742

CGGATCTGCACGCGGTACACGCCCGAGCAGGACACCATGACCTTCTCGGACGGGCTGACCCTGAACCGGACCCAGATGCACAACGCTGGCTTCGGCCCCCTCACCGACCTGGTCTTTGCC 2400
ArgIleCysThrArgTyrThrProGluGlnAspThrMetThrPheSerAspGlyLeuThrLeuAsnArgThrGlnMetHisAsnAlaGlyPheGlyProLeuThrAspLeuValPheAla 782

TTCGCCAACCAGCTGCTGCCCCTGGAGATGGATGATGCGGAGACGGGGCTGCTCAGCGCCATCTGCCTCATCTGCGGAGACCGCCAGGACCTGGAGCAGCCGGACCGGGTGGACATGCTG 2520
PheAlaAsnGlnLeuLeuProLeuGluMetAspAspAlaGluThrGlyLeuLeuSerAlaIleCysLeuIleCysGlyAspArgGlnAspLeuGluGlnProAspArgValAspMetLeu 822

CAGGAGCCGCTGCTGGAGGCGCTAAAGGTCTACGTGCGGAAGCGGAGGCCCAGCCGCCCCCACATGTTCCCCAAGATGCTAATGAAGATTACTGACCTGCGAAGCATCAGCGCCAAGGGG 2640
GlnGluProLeuLeuGluAlaLeuLysValTyrValArgLysArgArgProSerArgProHisMetPheProLysMetLeuMetLysIleThrAspLeuArgSerIleSerAlaLysGly 862

GCTGAGCGGGTGATCACGCTGAAGATGGAGATCCCGGGCTCCATGCCGCCTCTCATCCAGGAAATGTTGGAGAACTCAGAGGGCCTGGACACTCTGAGCGGACAGCCGGGGGGTGGGGGG 2760
AlaGluArgValIleThrLeuLysMetGluIleProGlySerMetProProLeuIleGlnGluMetLeuGluAsnSerGluGlyLeuAspThrLeuSerGlyGlnProGlyGlyGlyGly 902

CGGGACGGGGGTGGCCTGGCCCCCCCGCCAGGCAGCTGTAGCCCCAGCCTCAGCCCCAGCTCCAACAGAAGCAGCCCGGCCACCCACTCCCCGTGACCGCCCACGCCACATGGACACAGC 2880
ArgAspGlyGlyGlyLeuAlaProProProGlySerCysSerProSerLeuSerProSerSerAsnArgSerSerProAlaThrHisSerPro 933

CCTCGCCCTCCGCCCCGGCTTTTCTCTGCCTTTCTACCGACCATGTGACCCCGCACCAGCCCTGCCCCACCTGCCCTGCCCGGGAGTACTGGCGACCTTCCCTGGGGGACGGGGAGGGAG 3000
GAGGCAGCGACTCCTTGGACAGAGGCCTGGGCCCTCAGTGGACTGCCTGCTCCCACAGCCTGGGCTGACGTCAGAGGCCGAGGCCAGGAACTGAGTCAGGC 3101

located at nucleotide 1645/1646. The PML/RAR-α sequence contains a single open reading frame (ORF) starting at position 1 and ending at the TGA codon at position 2853. The first in-frame ATG is found at position 55. The ATG and TGA codons are those of the normal PML and RAR-α mRNAs respectively. The 2799 ORF encodes a putative protein of 933 amino acids with a predicted molecular weight of 103443 kDa and consists of the major portion of both the RAR-α and PML-coding regions. However the RAR-α A domain and the 59 carboxy-terminal amino acids of the PML putative protein were missing and the N-terminal 530 amino acid PML portion was fused to the carboxy B-F RAR-α portion.

PML/RAR-α Fusion Protein is a Transcription Factor

The capacity of the PML/RAR-α to act as a retinoid-inducible transcription factor was tested by its ability to regulate the expression of a specific Retinoic Acid (RA)-responsive reporter gene. The TRE-TK-CAT plasmid, which is made up of a previously identified palindromic RA-thyroid hormone RE linked to a tk-CAT fusion gene, was used as an RA-regulated reporter gene. Transcriptional activation was analyzed in transient plasmid vectors expressing the RAR-α or PML/RAR-α or PML proteins into Hela cells. The results obtained indicate that PML/RAR-α fusion protein may activate the transcription of a reporter gene when RA was present, but decrease it when no RA was added. Moreover, PML/RAR-α had greater ligand-independent transcriptional inhibition and ligand-dependent transcriptional activity than RAR-α.

RAR-α Gene Rearrangement as Molecular Marker for APL Clone

The definition of the DNA rearrangements involved in hematopoietic tumors has not only provided pathogenetic markers but also permitted more accurate diagnosis and monitoring of the patient response to therapy. In order to explore the feasibility to use RAR-α gene rearrangement as molecular marker to monitor the APL clone, a large panel of APLs DNA were analyzed with different genomic probes with the aim to identify the most informative ones (Biondi et al. 1991). Table 1 shows the main clinical, morphological and cytogenetic features of the patients included. As shown both M3 and M3v were included as well as pediatric and adult patients. Chromosome preparations were adequate for the analysis in 18 of the 23 cases. Sixteen patients (88%) manifested the t(15;17) translocation. Patients nos. 7 and 25 displayed an apparently normal karyotype. As shown in Table 2 by using a limited number of restriction enzymes and chromosome 15 and 17-derived probes allow the translocation breakpoints to be identified in all APL patients. The RAR-α and PML rearrangements should also allow

Table 1. Clinical and hematologic findings in 26 patients with APL

Patient N°	Age/Sex	FAB	Karyotype	WBC ($\times 10^9$/L)	DIC	Induction regimen	Outcome
1	14/F	M3	t(15;17)	1.2	YES	"3 + 7"	Death + 15M
2	8/F	$M3_v$	t(15;17)	84.3	YES	"3 + 7"	CR + 9M after Auto BMT
3	13/M	M3	t(15;17)	2.0	YES	"3 + 7"	Hemorrhagic Death + 18M
4	8/F	$M3_v$	t(15;17)	81.0	YES	NO	Hemorrhagic Death 4d
5	6/M	$M3_v$	t(15;17)	87.0	YES	"3 + 7"	Mism. BMT in 2°CR; Death
6	13/F	$M3_v$	t(15;17)	90.0	YES	"3 + 7"	CR + 12M after Auto BMT
7	47/F	$M3_v$	46; XX	172.0	YES	"3 + 7"	Hemorrhagic Death + 3d
8	27/F	M3	t(15;17)	0.4	YES	"3 + 7"	Infectious Death + 24d
9	13/F	M3	t(15;17)	4.2	YES	"3 + 7"	Hemorrhagic Death + 2M
10	8/M	M3	t(15;17)	10.2	YES	"3 + 7"	Hemorrhagic Death + 17M
11	5/M	M3	t(15;17)	7.0	YES	"3 + 7"	CR + 4M after Allo BMT
12	60/M	M3	t(15;17)	19.6	YES	"3 + 7"	Infectious Death + 19d
13	38/F	M3	t(15;17)	2.2	YES	"3 + 7"	CR + 5M
14	70/F	$M3_v$	t(15;17)	53.4	NO	"3 + 7"	Death + 14d
15	42/M	M3	t(15;17)	42.0	YES	"3 + 7"	CR + 3M
16	25/M	$M3_v$	failure	120.0	YES	"3 + 7"	CR + 12M after Allo BMT
17	48/F	M3	t(15;17)	1.2	YES	"3 + 7"	Death + 15M
18	36/M	M3	failure	28.9	YES	IDA	Death + 14M
19	67/F	M3	t(15;17)	1.9	YES	RA	Death + 20d
20	40/M	M3	N.D.	23.4	NO	IDA	CR + 2M
21	25/F	M3	failure	2.6	YES	IDA	Death + 9M
22	46/F	M3	N.D.	1.5	YES	IDA	CR + 1M
23	37/F	M3	failure	3.2	YES	IDA	CR + 3M
24	24/M	M3	failure	0.8	YES	IDA	CR + 1M
25	26/M	M3	46; XY	2.0	YES	"3 + 7"	Hemorrhagic Death + 8M
26	46/F	M3	N.D.	1.5	YES	"3 + 7"	CR + 1M

Abbreviations: DIC: disseminated intravascular coagulation; CR: complete remission; N.D.: not done; "3 + 7": anthracyclines+cytosine arabinoside and 6-Thioguanine; IDA: idarubicin; RA: retinoic acid; Auto BMT: autologous bone marrow transplantation; Allo BMT: allogeneic bone marrow transplantation.

Table 2. Rearrangement of the RAR α and PML genes in 26 patients with APL

Patient No	RAR-α						PML	
	K/S		HB		H18		RH15	
	E^	H^^	E	H	E	H	E	H
1	G*	G	G	G	G	G	G	R°
2	G	G	G	G	G	R	G	G
3	R	R	G	G	R	G	G	ND
4	G	R	G	R	G	R	R	R
5	G	G	G	R	G	R	G	G
6	G	G	G	G	R	G	G	G
7	G	R	G	R	G	R	R	R
8	G	R	G	R	G	R	G	G
9	G	G	G	R	G	G	G	R
10	R	R	R	R	G	R	R	R
11	G	R	G	R	G	R	R	R
12	R	R	G	G	R	G	G	G
13	R	R	G	G	R	G	R	R
14	R	G	G	G	R	G	R	R
15	G	G	G	G	R	G	G	R
16	R	R	R	R	G	R	R	R
17	G	R	G	R	G	G	ND	R
18	G	R	G	R	G	R	G	G
19	R	G	G	G	R	G	R	R
20	G	G	G	ND	G	G	R	R
21	R	R	G	G	R	G	R	R
22	G	G	G	G	ND	G	G	R
23	R	R	R	R	G	G	R	R
24	G	G	G	G	G	R	R	R
25	R	R	R	R	G	R	R	R
26	R	ND	R	ND	G	G	R	R

Abbreviations: G*: both alleles in germline configuration; R°: at least on allele rearranged; E^: EcoRI; H^^: Hindlll; ND: not done.

patient response to be accurately monitored during and after therapy (Lo Coco et al. 1991). Figure 7 showed the results of molecular monitoring of five APL patients who received treatment with all-trans retinoic acid. Two out of five patient, greater of 60 years old, were treated at onset of disease, whereas the other three received the same treatment at the time of first relapse. Molecular analyses were performed on bone marrow and peripheral blood samples collected at diagnosis (lane A), between the treatment days 14 and 16 (lane B), and at confirmation of complete remission (CR). As shown, in the four patient (nos 2, 3, 4 and 5) who achieved CR, Southern blot analysis demonstrated that CR in RA-treated APL patients is accompanied by the reconstitution of an apparently normal, non-clonal

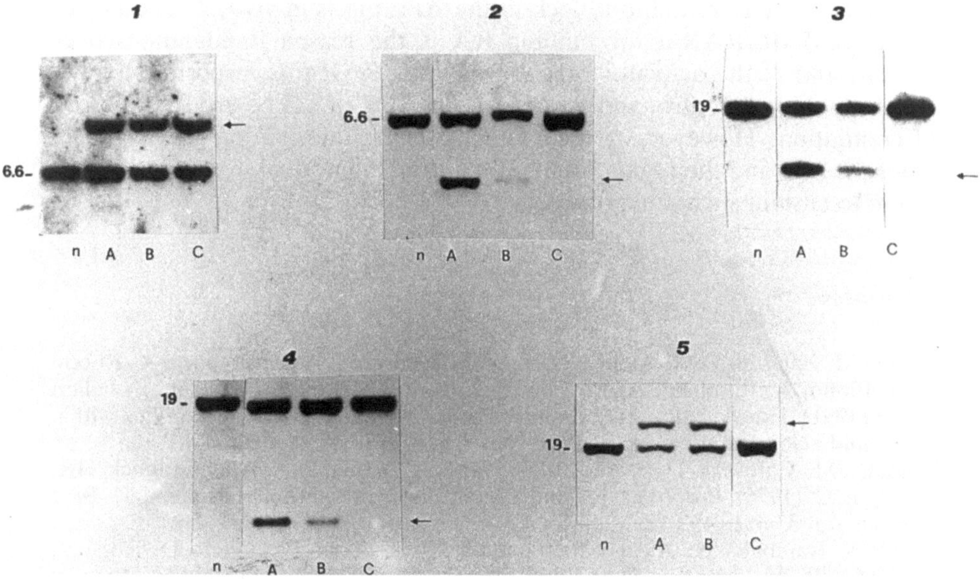

Fig. 7. DNA configuration of the RAR-α locus of five APL patients receiving treatment with all-trans retinoic acid. The H18 RAR-α probe detected rearrangements on EcoRI (pts. 1 and 2) or HindIII (pts 3,4 and 5) digestions. Lanes A, BM controls before treatment. Lanes B, intermediate controls treatment-day 14–16, performed on BM samples. Rearranged bands are indicated by *arrows*. *n*: placenta DNA

hematopoiesis. It could be argued that the limitation of DNA rearrangement analysis in monitoring patient response to therapy is that Southern blot analysis can only identify neoplastic promyelocytes when they represent at least 5% to 10% of the total cell population in the sample. However, this defect can be overcome by using the much more sensitive polymerase chain reaction (PCR) technique to identify the APL-specific RAR-α-PML fusion transcripts that are present in all APL cases.

Conclusions

One of the important question that still remains to be solved is to define the role of the PML/RAR-α protein during myeloid differentiation and possibly promyelocytic leukemogenesis. Our findings indicate that the ability of the PML/RAR-α protein to act either as a repressor or as an activator would seem to depend on the concentration of RA, and to be more potent than the activity of RAR-α. It is tempting to speculate that: 1. The repressor activity PML/RAR-α observed at low RA concentration inhibits RA-sensitive genes leading to the differentiation block in the APL blasts in vivo; 2. The higher affinity of PML/RAR-α for binding RA is the reason it dominates over RAR-α; and 3. the activator function of PML/RAR-α is resposible for the extremely high in vitro and in vivo sensitivity of APLs to RA-induced differentiation. However, at the moment scanty information are available about the role and the regulation of RA during the normal myeloid differentiation to sustain such a hypothesis.

References

Alcalay M, Zangrilli D, Pandolfi PP, Longo L, Mencarelli A, Giacomucci A, Rocchi M, Biondi A, Rambaldi A, Lo Coco F, Diverio D, Donti E, Grignani F, Pelicci PG (1991) Translocation breakpoint of acute promyelocytic leukemia lies within retinoid acid receptor α locus. Proc Natl Acad Sci USA 88:1977–1981

Bennett JM, Catovsky D, Daniel MT, Flandrin G, Galton DAG, Gralnick HR, Sultan C (1976) Proposals for the classification of the acute leukemias. Br J Haematol 33:451–458

Biondi A, Rambaldi A, Alcalay M, Pandolfi PP, Lo Coco F, Diverio D, Rossi V, Mencarelli A, Longo L, Zangrilli D, Masera G, Barbui T, Mandelli F, Grignani F, Pelicci PG (1991) RAR-α gene rearrangements as a genetic marker for diagnosis and monitoring in acute promyelocytic leukemia. Blood 77:1418–1422

Borrow J, Goddard AD, Sheer D, Solomon E. (1990) Molecular analysis of acute promyelocytic leukemia breakpoint cluster region on chromosome 17. Science 249:1577–1580

Chang KS, Trujillo JM, Cook RG, Stass SA (1986) Human myeloperoxidase gene: molecular cloning and expression in leukemic cells. Blood 68:1411–1414

de Thé H, Chomienne C, Lanotte M, Degos L, Dejean A (1990) The t(15;17) translocation of acute promyelocytic leukaemia fuses the retinoic acid receptor a gene to a novel transcrived locus. Nature 347:558-561

de Thè H, Lavau C, Marchio A, Chomienne C, Degos L, Dejean A (1991) The PML-RAR-α fusion mRNA generated by the t(15;17) translocation in acute promyelocytic leukemia encides a functionally altered RAR. Cell 66:675–684

Donti E, Montanucci A, Longo L, Mencarelli A, Pandolfi P, Tabilio A, Nanni M, Alimena G, Avanzi G, Pegoraro L, Grignai F, Pelicci PG (1986) The myeloperoxidase gene in acute promyelocytic leukemia. Science 244:823–826

Falanga A, Alessio MG, Donati MB, Barbui T (1988) A new procoagulant in acute leukemia. Blood 71:870–875

Giguere V, Ong ES, Segui P, Evans RM (1987) Identification of a receptor for the morphogen retinoic acid. Nature 330:624–629

Gralnick HR, Abrell E (1973) Studies of the procoagulant and fibrinolytic activity of promyelocytes in acute promyelocytic leukemia. Br J Haematol 24:89–99

Kakizuka A, Miller WH, Umesono K, Warrel RP Jr, Frankel SR, Murty VVVS, Dmitrovsky, Evans RM (1991) Chromosomal translocation t(15;17) in human acute promyelocytic leukemia fuses RAR-α with a novel putative transcription factori, PML. Cell 66:663–674

Larson RA, Kondo K, Vardiman JW, Butler AE, Golomb HM, Rowley JD (1984) Evidence for a 15;17 translocation in every patient with acute promyelocytic leukemia. Am J Med 76:827–841

Lo Coco F, Avvisati G, Diverio D, Petti MC, Alcalay M, Pandolfi PP, Biondi A, Rambaldi A, Moleti ML, Mandelli F, Pelicci PG (1991) Molecular evaluation of

response to all-trans retinoic therapy in patients with acute promyelocytic leukemia. Blood 8:1657–1659
Longo L, Donti E, Mencarelli A, Avanzi G, Pegoraro L, Alimena G, Tabilio A, Venti G, Grignani F, Pelicci PG (1990a) Mapping of chromosome 17 breakpoints in acute myeloid leukemia. Oncogene 5:1557–1563
Longo L, Pandolfi PP, Biondi A, Rambaldi A, Mencarelli A, Lo Coco F, Diverio D, Pegoraro L, Avanzi G, Tabilio A, Zangrilli D, Alcalay M, Donti E, Grignani F, Pelicci PG (1990b) Rearrangements and aberrant expression of the RAR-α gene in acute promyelocytic leukemias. J Exp Med 172:1571–1575
Mitelman F (1988) Catalog of chromosome aberrations in cancer, 3rd edn Liss, New York
Nagata S, Tsuchiya M, Asano S, Kaziro Y, Yamazaki T, Yamanoto O, Hirata Y, Kubota N, Oheda M, Nomura H (1986) Molecular cloning land expression of cDNA for human granulocyte colony-stimulating factor. Nature 319:415–418
Pandolfi PP, Grignani F, Alcaly M, Mencarelli A, Biondi A, Lo Coco F, Grignani F, Pelicci PG (1991) Structure and origin of the acute promyelocytic leukemia myl/RAR-α cDNA and characterization of its retinoid-binding and transactivation properties. Oncogene 6:1285–1292
Petkovich M, Brand NJ, Krust A, Chambon P (1987) A human retinoic acid receptor wich belongs to the family of nuclear receptors. Nature 330:444–450
Rowley JD, Golomb HM, Dougherty C (1977) 15/17 translocation, a consistent chromosomal change in acute promyelocytic leukemia. Lancet i:549–550
Sap J, Munoz A, Damm K, Goldberg Y, Ghysdael J, Leutz A, Beug H, Vennstrom B (1986) The c-erb-A protein is a high-affnity receptor for thyroid hormone. Nature 324:635–640
Sultan C, Heilmann-Gouaultme M, Tulliez M (1973) Relationship between blast-cell morphology and occurence of a syndrome of disseminated intravascular coagulation. Br J Haematol 24:255–259
Weil SC, Rosner GL, Reid MS, Chisholm RL, Farber NM, Spitznagel JK, Swanson MS (1987) cDNA cloning of human myeloperoxidase: decrease in myeloperoxidase mRNA upon induction of HL-60 cells. Proc Natl Acad Sci USA 84:2057–61
Xu W, Gorman PA, Rider SH, Hedge PJ, Moore G, Prichard C, Sheer D, Solomon E (1988) Construction of a genetic map of human chromosome 17 by use of chromosome-mediated gene transfer. Proc Natl Acad Sci USA 85:8563–8567

Immunophenotype of Hematologic Neoplasms with a Translocation t(8;21)

O.A. Haas[1], U. Köller[2], N. Grois[1], and H. Nowotny[3]

[1] Children's Cancer Research Institute, St. Anna Children's Hospital, Kinderspitalgasse 6, A-1090 Vienna, Austria
[2] Institute of Immunology, University Vienna, Borschkegasse 8a, A-1090 Vienna, Austria
[3] Ludwig Boltzmann Institute for Leukemia Research and Hematology, Hanusch Hospital, A-1140 Vienna, Austria

Introduction

In an attempt to combine morphologic, immunologic, and cytogenetic information, the Second MIC (morphology, immunology, cytogenetic) Cooperative Study Group (1988) has developed a new preliminary working classification for acute myeloid leukemia (AML) (1988). Despite their efforts however, the particular immunophenotypic characteristics of these proposed morphologic/cytogenetic subtypes are still poorly defined. In order to establish the immunologic marker profile of the MIC subgroup M2/t(8;21), we have immunologically phenotyped blast cells of 21 patients with this type of hematologic neoplasm. The heterogeneous clinical, hematologic, and cytogenetic features of our cases allowed us also to determine to what extent this phenotype depends on age and/or sex, whether it is modified in relapse or differs in de novo and secondary forms, and how it might be influenced by the presence of additional chromosome abnormalities.

Material and Methods

Patients. Twenty one patients (12 males and 9 females) with hematologic neoplasms and a t(8;21) diagnosed within the last 5 years in our institutions were studied. Their ages ranged from 13 to 83 years (median 42 years). According to the FAB criteria, 18 patients were morphologically classified as having M2 disease, one as having M1, one as having M4, and one as having refractory anemia with excess of blasts in transformation (RAEB-t) with myelomonocytic blast cells. Two patients had a previous history of neoplasia. Patient 16 had had breast cancer 9 years before diagnosis of leukemia and had been treated with mastectomy and irradiation therapy. Patient 20 had suffered from colon and ovarial carcinoma 12 years before diagnosis of leukemia. In addition to a history of occupational exposure to

Recent Results in Cancer Research, Vol. 131

insecticides, patient 5 had received radium therapy for ankylosing spondylitis. Patient 6 was initially diagnosed as having chronic myeloid leukemia (CML) in accelerated phase and had therefore been treated with hydroxyurea and 6-mercaptopurine in another hospital. Patients 14 and 18 were only seen at relapse.

Two patients suffered from a solid leukemic tumor deposit. While patient 15 presented with a leukemic infiltration of the maxilla at diagnosis, patient 14 developed a myelosarcoma of the stomach and urinary bladder prior to bone marrow (BM) relapse 9 months after allogeneic bone marrow transplantation (BMT).

Patients were treated according to standard polychemotherapy regimens. Subsequently, four patients (7, 10, 14, 17) underwent allogeneic BMT and three patients (1, 2, 19) autologous BMT. Complete remission was achieved in 17 patients (81%). Durations of first remission ranged from 3 to 52 months (median 11 months). Overall survival time ranged from 0.5 to 52 months (median 19 months). Eleven patients are still alive with survival times of between 11 and 52 months (median 24 months), the longest survivors being transplanted patients.

Immunologic phenotyping was performed with a panel of monoclonal antibodies and their staining pattern was assessed with a fluorescence microscope according to standard methods as previously described (Köller et al. 1989). Cytogenetic studies were performed according to standard routine cytogenetic techniques as previously described (Haas et al. 1984; Lambrou et al. 1986).

Results

The results of our immunologic and cytogenetic study are summarized in Table 1. All specimens revealed an exclusively myeloid phenotype which was basically in line with the morphologically defined maturation stage of these leukemias. Blast cells displayed CD15 (17/21 cases) and CD_w65 (20/21 cases) antigens in the majority of patients. The reaction pattern with the CD13, CD33, and CD11b monoclonal antibodies (MoAbs) was more heterogeneous. At diagnosis, the monocytic antigen CD14 was present only on a small proportion of blast cells in four patients (9, 13, 16, 21), two of whom (16, 21) were morphologically classified as having FAB M4. Terminal deoxynucleotidyl transferase (TdT) and other investigated B- and T-cell markers were negative in all instances. Although some of the patients (6, 13, 20, 21) presented with a marked granulocytic hyperplasia, resembling a CML in accelerated phase, neither erythroid nor megakaryocytic differentiation antigens were detected. Similarly, cases considered "secondary leukemias" (patients 5, 16, 20) were also negative for such components.

Phenotyping was also performed in seven patients (5, 10, 13, 14, 17, 19, 21) at relapse. CD11b, which was expressed in a small proportion of cells

Table 1. Immunologic phenotype of blast cells and cytogenetic findings in 21 patients with at (8;21)

Patient	Status	Monoclonal antibodies							Abnormalities in addition to t(8;21)(q22;q22)
		HLA-DR	CD 11b	CD 13	CD 14	CD 15	CD 33	CD w65	
1	DG	90	5	0	0	50	0	90	[20]
2	DG	90	60	40	0	30	70	90	[20]
3	DG	90	20	40	0	50	70	50	[20]
4	DG	90	50	90	5	30	80	60	[20]
5	DG	70	20	0	0	40	20	60	[20]
	RE	90	0	0	0	20	0	60	[20]
6	DG	40	0	50	0	50	50	50	−Y [20]
7	DG	50	30	0	0	80	80	90	−Y [5]
8	DG	90	10	40	0	20	90	80	−Y [17]
9	DG	90	0	50	40	0	0	30	−Y [20]
10	DG	80	30	20	0	0	10	60	−Y [20]
	RE	70	0	0	0	50	20	70	−Y [7]/−Y, t(10;22)(q22;q31) [2]/normal [12]
11	DG	90	nt	80	0	80	90	90	−Y [20]
12	DG	90	nt	20	0	70	70	90	−Y [16]/−Y, +der(21)t(8;21) [4]
13	DG	60	40	0	10	90	80	90	−Y, der(13) [16]
	RE	90	0	30	0	20	30	70	not performed
14	RE	90	0	60	0	70	60	90	−Y [4]/normal [16]
	RE	80	0	10	30	70	20	80	−Y, 1p + [17]/normal [3]
15	DG	90	20	20	0	40	30	80	del(9)(q22) [20]
16	DG	90	90	80	40	90	90	90	del(9)(q22) [18]/−Y, del(9)(q22) [2]
17	DG	90	0	10	0	10	50	80	−[5]/del(9)(q22) [5]/−X, del(9)(q22) [10]
	RE	80	0	0	0	70	20	90	−[1]/normal [15]
18	RE	90	0	80	0	15	40	70	del(9)(q22), +15,+18 [20]
19	DG	90	0	0	0	10	0	10	der(19) [21]
	RE	90	20	50	0	50	50	70	der(19),t(3;9)(q21;q34) [4]
	RE	80	nt	nt	0	50	nt	60	der(19),t(3;9)(q21;q34),t(2;5)(p16;q13) [6]/ der(19),t(3;9)(q21;q34)[4],t(2;5)(p16;q13),−10[9]
20	DG	40	nt	20	5	70	0	70	inv(2)(p21q36) [20]
21	DG	70	70	40	20	70	70	80	− [13]/del(7)(q22) [7]
	RE	70	0	70	60	30	70	80	not performed

DG, diagnosis; RE, relapse; nt, not tested; [ ], number of mitoses.
Results are expressed as the percentage of cells labeled by each antibody.

(median 30%) in 12 out of 16 cases analyzed at diagnosis, was completely lacking in six out of seven patients. Except for an augmented monocytic component in two patients (14, 21), no further immunophenotypic changes were evident. It is of interest to note that the established immunophenotype was also independent of the cytogenetic patterns recorded in the patients.

Cytogenetic investigations were performed in 19 patients at diagnosis and in two (14, 18) for the first time at first relapse. The translocation t(8;21)(p22;q22) was observed as the sole anomaly in five patients (24%), whereas karyotype evolution had already occurred in the others (76%). Loss of a sex chromosome was seen in 11 cases (6–14, 16, 17; 52%) and a deletion of the short arm of chromosome 9, del(9)(q22), was present in three patients (15–18; 14%). Other sporadic additional chromosome abnormalities included a del(7)(q22), inv(2), a 19q+, and extra chromosomes 15 and 18.

Seven cases which were originally analyzed at diagnosis were reinvestigated at relapse. While no further changes had occurred in four of them, an additional t(10;22)(q22;q31) and extra material on chromosome 1p was seen in patients 10 and 14, respectively. In patient 19 an additional t(3;9) was observed at first relapse. Further evolution of this clone during a second relapse after autologous BMT was characterized by an additional t(2;5) and monosomy 10, respectively.

Discussion

Following a suggestion of the Second MIC Cooperative Study Group, we have determined the immunologic phenotype of a representative selection of hematologic neoplasms with a t(8;21) at diagnosis and relapse. Our patients, 21 children and adults, suffered from myelodysplastic syndromes and de novo or secondary forms of acute myeloid or myelomonocytic leukemias, in some of which BM eosinophilia or a marked granulocytic hyperplasia was evident. Cytogenetically, they consisted of cases with and without karyotype evolution, the latter being mostly due to the typical loss of a sex chromosome and/or a deletion of the long arm of chromosome 9.

Despite the diverse clinical, hematologic, and cytogenetic features of the cases investigated, our analysis revealed a marker profile which, in good agreement with the morphologically defined maturation stage, was either pure myeloid or myelomonocytic. This phenotype remained basically unchanged in relapse and was not influenced by the presence of secondary karyotype abnormalities. In addition, "de novo" and "secondary" forms were indistinguishable by morphologic, cytogenetic and immunologic criteria.

All our cases were TdT negative. This is in sharp contrast to the recent report by Schachner et al. (1988), who found that 55% of AML with a t(8;21) were TdT positive. Reactivity of this nuclear antigen has been shown to depend strongly on the technique used, and false-positive results have been described, especially with heteroantisera and indirect immunofluorescence techniques (Barr et al. 1984). Our studies were performed with a monoclonal TdT reagent. Moreover, in our hands 12%–15% of all investigated AML cases are TdT positive (Schwarzinger et al. 1990; Willière et al. 1990), a figure which is in the upper quarter of published results (Bradstock et al. 1981; Jani et al. 1983).

The combination of marked granulocytic hyperplasia with a lack of hiatus leukemicus, the presence of hypogranular myeloid precursors, pseudo-Pelger-Huet abnormalities, and reduced or missing neutrophil alkaline phosphatase are encountered in some cases with a t(8;21) (patients 6, 13, 20 & 21 in this paper; Kamada et al. 1976; Kohli et al. 1988; Raskind et al. 1988; Swirsky et al. 1984) and may render such cases hematologically and clinically indistinguishable from CML. Furthermore, as also seen in one of our cases (7), Swirsky et al. (1984) have pointed out that because of the low blast cell counts in some cases a transforming myelodysplastic syndrome must be taken into differential diagnostic considerations. Thus, cytogenetic analysis remains the only reliable differential diagnostic tool in such cases. Whereas both in the acute stages of CML and in the myelodysplastic syndromes the erythropoeitic and thrombopoeitic system is commonly involved (Bettelheim et al. 1985a; Köller et al. 1992), this was not seen in any of our t(8;21) cases with a marked granulocytic hyperplasia. These findings provide further evidence that, in contrast to CML, where the genetic change affects a multipotent stem cell, the t(8;21) occurs in a late committed progenitor cell. Interestingly, Ema et al. (1990) have recently shown that, in response to granulocyte colony-stimulating factor or interleukin-3, leukemic cells with a t(8;21) differentiate in vitro into neutrophils or both neutrophils and eosinophils. The in vivo potential for differentiaton of t(8;21) blast cells, on the other hand, was elegantly affirmed by the direct demonstration of the translocated chromosomes in mature granulocytes with the help of the "premature chromosome condensation" technique (Hittelman et al. 1988).

Although the t(8;21) is considered one of the specific markers for de novo AML (Second MIC Cooperative Study Group 1988; Swirsky et al. 1984; Trujillo et al. 1979; Groupe Français de Cytogénétique Hématologique 1990), it has nevertheless been repeatedly reported in connection with carcinogen exposure, particularly chemicals, petrols, insecticides, and minerals (Mitelman et al. 1981; Fourth International Workshop on Chromosomes in Leukemia 1984), but also in secondary leukemias (Kantarjian et al. 1986; Davies et al. 1988; De Cuia et al. 1989; Knottenbelt et al. 1989). Despite the fact that secondary leukemias frequently display multilineage involvement and express the blood group H antigen (Köller et al. 1991), none of our cases with a history of carcinogen exposure (patient 5) or occurring secondary after solid tumors (patients 16, 20) displayed such a phenotype. Therefore, our findings strongly support earlier suggestions (Kantarjian et al. 1986; Davies et al. 1988) that these leukemias differ from true secondary leukemias which, cytogenetically, often have complex rearrangements and abnormalities involving chromosomes 5 and 7 (Pedersen-Bjergaard and Philip 1987). Rather, they represent second malignancies occurring coincidentally in genetically predisposed individuals. The similar, lineage-restricted phenotype indicates the involvement of the same, already myeloid determined progenitor cells in both de novo and secondary leukemias with a t(8;21). This observation obviously has important prognostic implications. Kantarjian et al. (1986) have pointed out the good response to chemotherapy obtained in patients with putative secondary leukemias and favorable cytogenetic abnormalities, such as the t(8;21).

Our analysis represents the first approach to establishing the detailed immunologic phenotypes of particular, cytogenetically defined subgroups of acute leukemia. In order to further evaluate the significance of our findings, it will be necessary to investigate other such AML subgroups. The fact that Bettelheim et al. (1985b) have reported the unexpected absence of the CD15 in acute promyelocytic leukemia (AML M3), which is exclusively associated with a t(15;17), further suggests a close relationship between specific cytogenetic changes and immunophenotypic patterns and underlines the necessity of further such studies.

Acknowledgements. We thank all clinicians involved in this study for their excellent cooperation and particularly for providing patients' material and clinical information. This work was supported by a grant from the Jubiläumsfonds der Österreichischen Nationalbank, grant no. 3838 and the Fonds zur Förderung der wissenschaftlichen Forschung, grant no. P-7777.

References

Barr R, Koekebakker M, Mahony J (1984) Demonstration of terminal desoxynucleodityl transferase in single cells by indirect immunofluorescence: II. An examination of specificity. Leuk Res 8:429–434

Bettelheim P, Lutz D, Majdic O, Paietta E, Haas O, Linkesch W, Neumann E, Lechner K, Knapp W (1985a) Cell lineage heterogeneity in blast crisis of chronic myeloid leukaemia. Br J Haematol 59:395–409

Bettelheim P, Panzer S, Majdic O, Stockinger H, Roithner A, Köller U, Meryn S, Lechner K, Knapp W (1985b) Unexpected absence of a myeloid surface antigen (3-fucosyl-*N*-acetyllactosamine) in promyelocytic leukemia. Leuk Res 9:1323–1327

Bradstock KF, Hoffbrand AV, Ganeshaguru K, Llewellin P, Patterson K, Wonke B, Prentice HG, Bennett M, Pizzolo G, Bollum FJ, Janossy G (1981) Terminal deoxynucleodityl transferase expression in acute non-lymphoid leukemia: analysis by immunofluorescence. Br J Haematol 47:133–143

Davies SV, Murray JA, Bowser-Riley SM (1988) Secondary leukemia with a translocation t(8;21)? Cancer Genet Cytogenet 31:271–274

DeCuia MR, Alimena G, Gastaldi R, Spiriti MAA, Giona G, Mancini M, Mandelli F (1989) Acute myeloblastic leukemia with t(8;21) following Philadelphia-positive acute lymphoblastic leukemia. Leukemia 3:310–313

Ema H, Kitano K, Suda T, Sato Y, Muroi K, Ohta M, Yoshida M, Sakamoto S, Eguchi M, Miura Y (1990) In vitro differentiation of leukemic cells to eosinophils in the presence of interleukin-5 in two cases of acute myeloid leukemia with the translocation *t*(8;21)(q22;q22). Blood 75:350–356

Fourth International Workshop on Chromosomes in Leukemia, 1982 (1984) The correlation of karyotype and occupational exposure to potential mutagenic and carcinogenic agents in acute non-lymphocytic leukemia. Cancer Genet Cytogenet 11:326–331

Groupe Français de Cytogénétique Hématologique (1990) Acute myelogenous leukemia with an 8;21 translocation. A report on 148 cases from the Groupe Francais de Cytogenetique Hematologique. Cancer Genet Cytogenet 44:169–179

Haas OA, Schwarzmeier JD, Nacheva E, Fischer P, Paietta E (1984) Investigations on karyotype evolution in patients with chronic myeloid leukemia (CML). Blut 48:33–43

Hittelman WN, Agbor P, Petkovic I, Andersson B, Kantarjian H, Walters R, Koller C, Beran M (1988) Detection of leukemic clone maturation in vivo by premature chromosome condensation. Blood 72:1950–1960

Jani P, Verbi W, Greaves MF, Bevan D, Bollum FJ (1983) Terminal desoxynucleodityl transferase in acute myeloid leukemia. Leuk Res 7:17–29

Kamada N, Okada K, Oguma N, Tanaka R, Mikami M, Uchino H (1976) C-G translocation in acute myelocytic leukemia with low neutrophil alkaline phosphatase activity. Cancer 37:2380–2387

Kantarjian HM, Keating MJ, Walters RS, Beran M, McLaughlin P, McCredie KB, Freireich E (1986) The association of specific "favorable" cytogenetic abnormalities with secondary leukemia. Cancer 58:924–927

Knapp W, Dörken B, Gilks WR, Rieber EP, Schmidt RE, Stein H, von dem Borne AEGKr (1989) Leucocyte typing IV. White cell differentiation antigens. Oxford University Press, Oxford

Knottenbelt E, Hallett J, Jacobs P (1989) T(8;21) translocation in myelodysplasia secondary to essential thrombocythemia. Am J Hematol 30:233–235

Kohli M, Daly H, Davison EV, Kernahan J, Reid MM (1988) Translocation t(8;21) associated with marked granulocytic hyperplasia. Cancer Genet Cytogenet 31: 193–197

Köller U, Haas OA, Ludwig WD, Bartram CR, Harbott J, Panzer-Grümayer R, Hansen-Hagge T, Ritter J, Creutzig U, Knapp W, Gadner H (1989) Phenotypic and genotypic heterogeneity in infant acute leukemia: II. Acute nonlymphoblastic leukemia. Leukemia 3:708–714

Köller U, Krieger O, Haas OA, Bettelheim P, Majdic O, Knapp W (1992) Immunological phenotyping of blood and bone marrow cells from patients with myelodysplastic syndroms (MDS). In: Schmalzl F, Mufti GJ (eds) Myelodysplastic syndromes. Springer, Berlin Heidelberg New York

Lambrou M, Novotny H, Lutz D, Schweizer D (1986) Hypo- and hypertetraploidy in a case of erythroleukemia analyzed by fluorochrome banding techniques. Cancer Genet Cytogenet 23:115–125

Mitelman F, Nilsson PG, Brandt L, Alimena G, Gastaldi R, Dallapiccola B (1981) Chromosome pattern, occupation, and clinical features in patients with acute nonlymphocytic leukemia. Cancer Genet Cytogenet 4:197–214

Pedersen-Bjergaard J, Philip P (1987) Cytogenetic characteristics of therapy-related acute nonlymphocytic leukaemia, praeleukaemia and acute myeloproliferative syndrome: correlation with clinical data for 61 consecutive cases. Br J Haematol 66:199–207

Raskind WH, Papayannopoulou T, Hammond WP (1988) T(8;21) with a phenotype of chronic myeloid leukemia. Am J Hematol 28:266–269

Schachner J, Kantarjian H, Dalton W, McCredie K, Keating M, Freireich EJ (1988) Cytogenetic association and prognostic significance of bone marrow blast cell terminal transferase in patients with acute myeloblastic leukemia. Leukemia 2:667–671

Schwarzinger I, Valent P, Köller U, Marosi C, Schneider B, Haas O, Knapp W, Lechner K, Bettelheim P (1990) Prognostic significance of surface marker expression on blasts of patients with de novo acute myeloblastic leukemia. J Clin Oncol 8:423–430

Second MIC Cooperative Study Group (1988) Morphologic, immunologic and cytogenetic (MIC) working classification of the acute myeloid leukemias. Br J Haematol 68:487–494

Swirsky DM, Li YS, Matthews JG, Flemans RJ, Rees JKH, Hayhoe FGJ (1984) 8;21 translocation in acute granulocytic leukaemia: cytological, cytochemical and clinical features. Br J Haematol 56:199–213

Trujillo JM, Cork A, Ahearn MJ, Yoouness EL, McCredie KB (1979) Hematologic and cytologic characterization of 8/21 translocation acute granulocytic leukemia. Blood 53:695–706

Willière G, Stockinger H, Köller U, Majdic O, Schnabl E, Lutz D, Bettelheim P, Knapp W (1990) Terminal deoxynucleotidyl transferase and CD7 expression in acute myeloid leukemias are not associated with a high frequency of immunoglobulin and/or T cell receptor gene rearrangement. Leukemia 4:278–281

Diagnostic and Prognostic Importance of Immunophenotyping in Adults with Acute Myeloid Leukemia

A. Orfao[1], B. Vidriales[2], M. Gonzalez[2], M.C. Lopez-Berges[2], M.C. del Cañizo[1], and J.F. San Miguel[2]

[1] Department of Cytometry. University Hospital of Salamanca, Paseo de San Vicente s/n, 37007 Salamanca, Spain
[2] Department of Hematology, University Hospital of Salamanca, 37007 Salamanca, Spain

Introduction

Acute myeloblastic leukemia (AML) is known to have highly variable clinical and biological characteristics. In recent years the availability of monoclonal antibodies (MAbs) specific for the different myeloid lineages and their differentiation stages, together with the development of new highly sensitive techniques such as flow cytometry, have both provided new insights into the biology of AML and contributed to more accurate diagnosis and classification of these leukemia patients (Ball 1990; Drexler and Minowada 1986; Goasguen and Bennett 1990; Ludwig and Thiel 1990; Neame et al. 1986; Pessano et al. 1984; San Miguel et al. 1986b; Second MIC Cooperative Group Study 1988; Van der Reijden et al. 1983). Although there is only a limited amount of data available, some studies (Ball et al. 1991; Campos et al. 1989; Geller et al. 1990; Griffin et al. 1986; San Miguel et al. 1989; Schwarzinger et al. 1990) suggest that the immunophenotype might also be of help in the prognostic evaluation of AML patients.

In this study we report our experience on immunophenotyping adult AML patients based on a series of 333 cases. First, we analyze the membrane characteristics of the myeloid blast cells, including the megakaryoblastic leukemias, and their correlation with the FAB classification, then the aberrant cases that coexpress lymphoid associated antigens will be analyzed, and, finally, the potential prognostic value of the immunological markers together with the most relevant clinical and hematological disease characteristics will be discussed. In addition, preliminary results of DNA analysis by flow cytometry and their relation to the immunophenotype will be mentioned.

Material and Methods

Patients. All 333 patients included in this study were newly diagnosed adults (age >15 years) with "de novo" AML in accordance with the FAB criteria

Recent Results in Cancer Research, Vol. 131

Table 1. Immunological markers used in the study

Reactivity	Monoclonal antibodies
Myeloid precursors	CD9 (FMC56), CD34 (3C5), anti-HLA-DR
Early myeloid	CD13 (My7), CD33 (My9, LeuM9), CD11b (Leu15)
Granulocytic	CD15 (FMC10, VIMD5, LeuM1)
Monocytic	CD14 (LeuM3, MO2, FMC17, UCHM1)
Erythroid	Antiglycophorin A, CD71 (OKT9)
Megakaryocytic	CD41 (J15, FMC24), CD42 (AN51, FMC25), CD61 (C17)
Lymphoid	TdT, CD10 (anti-cALLA), CD7 (3A1, Leu9), CD2 (OKT11, Leu5b), CD19 (Leu12), CD4 (Leu3, OKT4)

(Bennett et al. 1985a,b). Three different induction protocols that included daunorubicin and cytarabine (cytosine arabinoside), either alone (DA) or together with thioguanine (DAT) or vincristine and prednisone (DATOP), were used for the treatment of the patients. No significant differences were observed among the survival curves obtained with these protocols. Survival was measured from the time of diagnosis up to the time of death or that of closing the study; all cases, including early deaths and patients over 60 years of age, were included in the study. In the group of patients that completed a full course of chemotherapy the proportion of complete remission (CR) was 74%.

Immunological Phenotype. Samples containing more than 30% blast cells from all 333 patients were analyzed by direct or indirect immunofluorescence with an anti-terminal deoxynucleotidyl transferase (TdT) heteroantiserum (Supertechs, Bethesda, MD, USA) and a panel of monoclonal antibodies (MAbs) whose specificity has been described elsewhere (San Miguel et al. 1986b, 1988). They included markers against the different myeloid lineages, as well as several MAbs for precursor cells and other markers to exclude lymphoid lineage (Table 1). All cases were tested for at least one specific MAb for all the different cell lineage. Fluorescence positivity was analyzed either in a fluorescence microscope (Leitz, FRG) or in a FACScan flow cytometer (Becton Dickinson, San Jose, CA, USA). A cell lineage was considered to be involved when at least 15% of the blast cells were positive for one or more of the lineage related MAbs.

DNA Analysis by Flow Cytometry. DNA analysis was performed on isolated nuclei from ammonium-chloride lysed peripheral blood (PB) cells in a subgroup of 120 patients using the technique of Vindelov et al. (1983). Measurements were made within 30 min on a FACScan flow cytometer equipped with a 15-mW argon ion laser and a doublet discrimination module (Becton Dickinson) for at least 5×10^3 nuclei. The electronics of the instrument were adjusted so that the model channel for human diploid G_0/G_1 nuclei would be 200 (maximum scale 1023 channels). Analysis of cell cycle distribution was performed using the RFIT mathematical calculation model by means of the CellFit software program (Becton Dickinson). In each case, for the assessment of DNA aneuploidy a second tube with a mixture of the patient's PB and PB from a sex-matched healthy donor was run in the flow cytometer. To exclude proliferation of non-blast cells the appropiate DNA–surface antigen double staining was performed, using a modification of the Vindelov et al. (1983) technique, by previously staining with MAbs and omitting the incubation with the solution that contained trypsin.

Statistical Methods. In the present study the immunological markers were analyzed after grouping according to their cluster of differentiation (CD), for which the marker with the highest result within a particular CD was chosen. The χ^2 test (BMDP 4F software program) (Dixon 1983) was used to estimate differences among CR rates for each clinical, hematological, and immunophenotypic characteristic, and the stepwise logistic regression model (LR, BMDP program) (Dixon 1983) was employed for the subsequent multivariate analysis of CR. Survival curves were plotted according to the method of Kaplan and Meier and comparison between curves was performed using the Breslow and Mantel–Cox tests (BMDP 1L program) (Dixon 1983). A subsequent multivariate analysis including those variagbles for which there was some indication of a significant association with survival in univariate analysis ($p < 0.1$) or for which prior studies had suggested a possible association was performed by the stepwise proportional hazards regression model for censored survival data (BMDP 2L program) (Dixon 1983).

Results and Discussion

AML Immunophenotype: Correlation with the FAB Classification

The morphological and cytochemical heterogeneity of AML is widely documented and the diagnostic value of the FAB classification for these leukemias is well-established (Bennett et al. 1985a,b). However, the discrepancies among observers and the subjectivity of the FAB classification, together with the existence of unclassified cases, point to the need for other complementary diagnostic approaches. The opportunity of studying the immunophenotype of AML blast cells has provided a new objective tool for the classification of these patients (Goasguen and Bennett 1990; Neame et al. 1986; San Miguel et al. 1986b; Second MIC Cooperative Study Group 1988).

CD13 and CD33, the earliest antigens expressed during myeloid differentiation, were negative in only 13% and 10% of our AML cases, respectively. Moreover, the combination of these two markers allowed us to detect nearly all AML cases (97.3%), representing in our hands the best reagent combination for first-line diagnostic screening for AML. The M1 leukemias showed the more undifferentiated phenotype, usually lacking expression of granulocytic antigens (75% of cases being CD15 negative); in addition, nearly 25% of patients were also negative for CD13 or CD33. In the M2 patients the expression of both early myeloid (CD13 or CD33) and granulocytic markers was much higher (95% and 50%, respectively), confirming that these cases correspond to a more advanced maturational stage. Expression of monocytic antigens was detected in 9% of the M2 cases. The M3 leukemias, despite having a relative differentiated morphological appearance, were usually negative for granulocytic markers (94% of cases) and, unlike the other subtypes, were usually lacking in the HLA-DR antigen (94%). The M4 cases displayed a similar phenotype to that of the M2 but in addition to the granulocytic markers (54% of CD15 positive cases), they also expressed monocytic antigens (CD14 was positive in 53% of the patients). In a similar way to the M1 cases, the M5a leukemias displayed a very undifferentiated phenotype with low expression of monocytic antigens (28% $CD14^+$ cases). On the other hand, this marker showed a strong reactivity in the M5b patients (74% positivity), confirming the validity of the morphological differentiation proposed by the FAB group for these subtypes (Bennett et al. 1985b). As occurred in the M2 leukemias with the expression of the CD14 antigen, some M5b cases coexpressed the CD15 antigen (44%), supporting the hypothesis that both markers are transiently expressed during both granulocytic and monocytic development.

Glycophorin A is not present in early erythroid precursor cells and it only appears at the level of colony-forming units–erythroid (CFU-E). This probably explains why only 37% of the M6 leukemias tested were positive for glycophorin A. The use of other earlier erythroid markers such as CD36 and carbonic anhydrase will be necessary for the immunological diagnosis of these leukemias.

Acute megakaryoblastic leukemia was considered a rare variant of AML until MAbs against platelet glycoproteins (Plgp) were obtained, this probably being one of the fields in which the diagnostic value of the immunophenotype has proved to be most useful (Bennett et al. 1985a; San Miguel et al. 1988). In our series, the incidence of acute megakaryoblastic leukemia in patients with "de novo" AML was 8%. Upon comparing the reactivity of the megakaryocytic MAbs against the different Plgps, we observed that their overall sensitivity was, in a decreasing order, gpIIIa (CD61), gpIIb/IIIa (CD41a), gpIb/IX complex (CD42). These results support the notion that gpIIIa is the first to be expressed during megakaryoblastic maturation, immediately followed by gpIIb/IIIa, while gpIb/IX appears at a latter stage of differentiation (San Miguel et al. 1987; Vinci et al. 1984).

Based on these results, a possible model for immunological classification of AML should include the categories we have previously proposed (San Miguel et al. 1986b), with slight modifications (Table 2). Comparison of this immunological classification with the FAB criteria shows (Table 3) that

Table 2. Possible membrane immunophenotypes in AML

Phenotype	CD13/CD33	CD15	CD14	Glico	CD41/CD61	HLADR
Undifferentiated	−	−	−	−	−	+
Myeloblastic	+	−	−	−	−	+
Promyelocytic	+	±	−	−	−	−
Myelocytic	+	+	−	−	−	+
Monocytic	+	−	+	−	−	+
Myelomonocytic	+	+	+	−	−	+
Erythroid	+	±	±	+	−	+
Megakaryocytic	+	±	±	−	+	+

Table 3. FAB versus immunophenotype: distribution of AML cases

	Undifferentiated	M1	M2	M3	M4	M5a	M5b	M6	M7	Total
Undifferentiated	8	7	2			3				20
Myeloblastic	6	24	13		13	12	5	3	2	78
Promyelocytic		2	2	45		1				50
Myelocytic	3	11	19	2	8	3	2			48
Monocytic			1		10	5	16	2		34
Myelomonocytic		1	3	1	21	4	18	1		49
Erythroid			1					7		8
Megakaryocytic	8		1		5	2	4	4	3	27
Other	5	4	2		2	2	1	2	1	19
Total	30	49	44	48	59	32	46	19	6	333

there is only a partial correlation, since, with the exception of the M3 cases, which almost always (94% of cases) displayed a constant phenotype (promyelocytic), every other morphological group contains patients from more than one immunological phenotype. Nevertheless, there is a certain degree of concordance, since the myelocytic phenotype was that with the highest incidence of M2 cases, and most M4 and M5b cases belonged to the myelomonocytic or monocytic subtypes. These results indicate that at present the classification of AML is better achieved by a systematic approach that integrates morphology, cytochemistry, and immunophenotype.

AML Cases that Coexpress Lymphoid-Associated Markers

The expression of lymphoid-related markers on myeloid blast cells can occasionally be detected, being referred to as lineage infidelity, lineage promiscuity, or hybrid leukemias (Messner and Griffin 1986). The most well known example of this is the expression of TdT in AML. This marker was

Table 4. Expression of lymphoid-associated markers in AML

Marker	Cases	
	(*n*)	(%)
TdT	25/224	11
CD2	5/46	11
CD4	78/136	57
CD7	35/168	21
CD10	12/137	9
CD19	10/120	8

originally considered lymphoid specific; however, subsequent studies (Drexler and Minowada 1986; Jani et al. 1983; Janossy et al. 1980; Lo Coco et al. 1989; Parreira et al. 1988; San Miguel et al. 1986a; Schwarzinger et al. 1990; Swirzky et al. 1988) showed that it can be present in 5%–20% of AML cases. In our series the incidence of TdT-positive adult AML cases was 11%, and the presence of this marker was not associated with a particular FAB subtype or survival. Other lymphoid related markers such as CD2, CD4, CD7, CD10, and CD19 can also be expressed in a variable number of AML cases (Ball et al. 1991; Cross et al. 1988; Kaplan et al. 1989; Lo Coco et al. 1989; Mirro et al. 1985): 11%, 57%, 21%, 9%, and 8% of our patients, respectively (Table 4). It has been suggested that the expression of these antigens may be associated with immature FAB subtypes (Parreira et al. 1988). In our experience, and in accordance with some recent reports (Swirzky et al. 1988), this association was not confirmed. In addition, upon analyzing this lymphoid-related antigen expression according to the immunological classification, there was also no association with immature phenotypes. The higher incidence of $CD4^+$ AML cases supports the recent studies on normal cells that have demonstrated the expression of this antigen in both monocytic and megakaryocytic lineages.

These aberrant cases that coexpress lymphoid markers can manifest at least in two different ways (Kaplan et al. 1989; Messner and Griffin 1986). There can be two or more distinct cell subsets with different antigenic phenotypes, or there a single blast cell population can exist that coexpresses lymphoid and myeloid markers. Although the expression of lymphoid markers was usually variable with respect to intensity in the myeloid blast cells, most of the cases included in our series belonged to the latter category, as was shown by the appropriate double-staining procedures, and only 3% of these patients displayed two distinct cell populations. Besides its clinical and prognostic importance, which will be commented on below, the recognition of these aberrant cases will probably shed some light on the biological basis of leukemia. Accordingly, we have observed in a group of 120 patients in whom flow cytometric DNA analysis was performed that, of the seven (6%)

Table 5. Immunophenotype of AML cases displaying DNA aneuploidy by flow cytometry

Case	Immunophenotype
1	$CD33^+/CD13^+/HLA\text{-}DR^+/CD9^+/CD19^+$
2	$CD13^+/HLA\text{-}DR^+$
3	$TdT^+/CD33^+/CD13^+/CD11b^+/CD15^+/HLA\text{-}DR^+/CD7^+$
4	$CD33^+/CD13^+/CD11b^+/HLA\text{-}DR^+/CD19^+$
5	$CD33^+/CD13^+/CD14^+/HLA\text{-}DR^+$
6	$CD13^+/CD11b^+/HLA\text{-}DR^+/CD7^+$
7	$CD33^+/CD13^+/CD11b^+/HLA\text{-}DR^+$

cases that displayed DNA aneuploidy, four (56%) coexpressed at least one lymphoid-related marker (Table 5), indicating that quantitatively important DNA abnormalities (>5% of total DNA/nuclei) in the AML blast cells might be associated with aberrant phenotypes.

Prognostic Value of the Immunophenotype in Adult AML

Whereas in acute lymphoblastic leukemia (ALL) the prognostic value of the immunophenotype is well established, in AML the available information is still very scanty. Nevertheless, recent reports (Ball et al. 1991; Campos et al. 1989; Champlin and Gale 1987; Geller et al. 1988; Griffin et al. 1986; Mirro et al. 1985; San Miguel et al. 1989; Schwarzinger et al. 1990) suggest the existence of a relationship between the pattern of expression of several surface antigens and prognosis of AML patients. The definitive prognostic significance of these findings requires confirmation through multivariate analysis, including other well-established clinical and hematological prognostic factors. In the present series the only markers associated with a poor response and survival were the expression of the CD9 and CD14 antigens. By contrast, the presence of granulocytic markers (CD15) indicated a better outcome. However, none of these parameters retained their prognostic influence in the multivariate analysis, the most significant prognostic factors being the failure to obtain CR, advanced age, anemia, and thrombocytopenia. The prognostic value of some of these antigens has been confirmed by other groups. Thus, CD14 also displayed an adverse prognostic significance in the series of Griffin et al. (1986), supporting on immunological grounds the poorer prognosis assigned for monocytic leukemia in the FAB classification (Bennett and Begg 1981; Sultan et al. 1981). Several groups (Campos et al. 1989; Holowiecki et al. 1986; Schwarzinger et al. 1990) have reported a favorable response to therapy in patients expressing CD15 antigen, and our results confirmed that expression of CD15 is associated with higher CR rates and longer survival.

Other myeloid antigens have also been shown to have prognostic value. Thus, the expression of CD13, CD11b, and HLA-DR has been related to a poor outcome (Geller et al. 1988; Griffin et al. 1986; Schwarzinger et al. 1990). Although these findings have not been reproduced in our series, shorter survival rates were observed in $CD13^+$ cases, but differences were not statistically significant. Interestingly, in a preliminary study performed on a small number of patients, Vaughan et al. (1983) found CD34 positivity to be associated with poor prognosis; these results were later supported by Geller et al. (1988) and Campos et al. (1989), who showed that the expression of CD34 – a stem cell marker – was a significantly adverse parameter in predicting response to therapy and survival. In our series, CD34 did not appear to be able to discriminate among patients with different survival rates, although this may be due to the use in our study of a different CD34 MAb (3C5) that may show differences in the epitope recognized compared to that used in the previous studies (My10).

An even more controversial area is the prognostic significance of lymphoid cell-associated markers in AML. Of these antigens, the most widely studied is TdT. Although preliminary reports (Bradstock et al. 1981; Jani et al. 1983; Lo Coco et al. 1989; Schwarzinger et al. 1990) pointed to an adverse prognostic impact, more recent data in larger series of patients show that TdT does not influence the outcome in AML patients (Swirzky et al. 1988). In a similar way, conflicting results have been reported for other antigens such as CD2, CD7, and CD19 (Cross et al. 1988; Champlin and Gale 1987; Mirro et al. 1985). Surprisingly, in an extensive study Ball et al. (1991) found that AML patients with a $CD2^+$ and $CD19^+$ phenotype survived longer than those whose blast cells lacked the expression of lymphocyte-associated antigens on their membrane. In our experience, none of these lymphoid-associated markers significantly influenced survival.

Recently, we have performed a study in order to analyze the correlation between antigen expression and cell cycle distribution in peripheral blood blast cells from 120 adult AML patients. Interestingly, cases expressing monocytic markers (CD14) were associated with a high peripheral blood S-phase blast cell count, this parameter being, together with age, the most important independent prognostic factor in this series of patients. These findings illustrate the possible relationship between the expression of some of these antigens and other biological characteristics of the leukemic cell that may help in the understanding of the clinical heterogeneity of AML.

References

Ball ED (1990) Immunophenotyping of acute myeloid leukemia cells. Clin Lab Med 10:721–736

Ball ED, Davis RB, Griffin JD, Mayer RJ, Davey FR, Arthur DC, Wurster-Hill D, Noll W, Elghetany MT, Allen SL, Rai K, Lee EJ, Schiffer CA, Bloomfield CD

(1991) Prognostic value of lymphocyte surface markers in acute myeloid leukemia. Blood 77:2242–2250

Bennett JM, Begg CB (1981) Eastern Cooperative Oncology Group study of the cytochemistry of adult acute myeloid leukemia by correlation of subtypes with response and survival. Cancer Res 41:4833–4837

Bennett JM, Catovsky D, Daniel MT, Flandrin G, Galton DAG, Gralnick H, Sultan C (FAB group) (1985a) Criteria for the diagnosis of acute leukemia of megakaryocyte lineage. Ann Intern Med 103:460–462

Bennett JM, Catovsky D, Daniel MT, Flandrin G, Galton DAG, Gralnick H, Sultan C (FAB group) (1985b) Proposed revised criteria for the classification of AML. Ann Intern Med 103:626–629

Bradstock KF, Janossy G, Hoffbrand AV, Ganeshguni K, Llewelin P, Prentice HG, Bollum FJ (1981) Immunofluorescence and biochemical studies of terminal deoxynucleotidyl transferase in treated acute leukemia. Br J Haematol 47:121–125

Campos L, Guyotat D, Archimbaud E, Devaux Y, Treille D, Larese A, Maupas J, Gentilhomme O, Ehrsam A, Fiere D (1989) Surface marker expression in adult acute non-lymphoblastic leukemia: correlations with initial characteristics, morphology and response to therapy. Br J Haematol 72:151–166

Champlin R, Gale RP (1987) Acute myelogenous leukemia: recent advances in therapy. Blood 68:1551–1562

Cross AH, Goorha RM, Nuss R, Behm FG, Murphy SB, Kalwinsky DK, Raimondi S, Kitchingman GR, Mirro JJ (1988) Acute myeloid leukemia with T-lymphoid features: a distinct biologic and clinical entity. Blood 72:579–587

Dixon WJ (Bio-Medical Data Package) (1983) Statistical software. University of California, Berkeley

Drexler HG, Minowada J (1986) The use of monoclonal antibodies for the identification and classification of acute myeloid leukemias. Leuk Res 10:279–290

Geller RB, Zahurak M, Hurwitz CA, Burke PJ, Karp JE, Piantadosi S, Civen C (1990) Prognostic importance of immunophenotyping in adults with acute myelocytic leukaemia: the significance of the stem-cell glycoprotein CD34 (My10). Br J Haematol 76:340–347

Goasguen JE, Bennett JM (1990) Classifications of acute myeloid leukemia. Clin Lab Med 10:661–681

Griffin JD, Davis R, Nelson DA, Davey FR, Mayer RJ, Schiffer C, McIntyre OR, Bloomfield CD (1986) Use of surface marker analysis to predict outcome of adult acute myeloblastic leukemia. Blood 68:1232–1241

Holowiecki J, Lutz D, Krzemien S, Stella-Holowiecka B, Graf F, Kelenyi G, Schranz V, Callea V, Brugiatelli M, Neri A, Magyarlaki T, Ihle R, Jagoda K, Rudzka E (1986) CD15 antigen detected by VIM-D5 monoclonal antibody for prediction of ability to achieve complete remission in acute nonlymphocytic leukemia. Acta Haematol 76:16–19

Jani P, Verbi W, Greaves MF, Bevan D, Bollum F (1983) Terminal deoxynucleotidyl transferase in acute myeloid leukemia. Leuk Res 7:17–29

Janossy G, Hoffbrand AV, Greaves MF, Ganeshguru J, Pain C, Bradstock KF, Prentice HG, Kay HEM (1980) Terminal transferase enzyme assay and immunological membrane markers in the diagnosis of leukemia: a multiparameter analysis of 300 cases. Br J Haematol 44:221–226

Kaplan SS, Penchansky L, Stolc V, Contis L, Krause JR (1989) Immunophenotyping in the classification of acute leukemia in adults. Interpretation of multiple lineage reactivity. Cancer 63:1520–1527

Lo-Coco F, Pasqualetti D, Lopez M, Panzini E, Gentile A, Latagliata R, Monarca B, De Rossi G (1989) Immunophenotyping of acute myeloid leukemia: relevance of analyzing different lineage-associated markers. Blut 58:235–240

Ludwig WD, Thiel E (1990) Routine immunophenotyping of acute leukemias. Blut 60:48–50

Messner HA, Griffin JD (1986) Biology of AML, Clin Haematol 15:641–667

Mirro J, Antoun GR, Zipf TF, Melvin S, Stass S (1985) The E-rosette associated antigen of T-cells can be identified on blasts from patients with acute myeloblastic leukemia. Blood 65:363–370

Neame PB, Soamboonsrup P, Browman GP, Meyer RM, Benger A, Wilson WEC, Walker IR, Saeed N, McBride JA (1986) Classifying acute leukemia by immunophenotyping: a combined FAB-immunologic classification of AML. Blood 68:1355–1362

Parreira A, Pombo de Oliveira MS, Matutes E, Foroni L, Morilla R, Catovsky D (1988) Terminal Deoxynucleotidyl transferase positive acute myeloid leukemia: an association with immature myeloblastic leukaemia. Br J Haematol 69:219–224

Pessano S, Palumbo A, Ferrero D, Pagliardi GL, Bottero L, Kai Lai S, Meo P, Carter C, Hubbell H, Lange B, Rovera G (1984) Subpopulation heterogeneity in human acute myeloid leukemia determined by monoclonal antibodies. Blood 64:275–281

San Miguel JF, Gonzalez M, Cañizo MC, Anta JP, Portero JA, Lopez Borrasca A (1986a) TDT activity in acute myeloid leukemias defined by monoclonal antibodies. Am J Hematol 23:9–17

San Miguel JF, Gonzalez M, Cañizo MC, Anta JP, Zola H, Lopez Borrasca A (1986b) Surface marker analysis in acute myeloid leukaemia and correlation with FAB classification. Br J Haematol 64:547–560

San Miguel JF, Gonzalez M, Orfao A, Ojeda E, Cañizo MC (1987) Expression of immunologic markers in megakaryoblasts. Blood 70:1227–1228

San Miguel JF, Gonzalez M, Cañizo MC, Ojeda E, Orfao A, Moro MJ, Fisac P, Lopez Borrasca A (1988) Leukaemias with megakaryoblastic involvement: clinical, hematological and immunological characteristics. Blood 72:402–407

San Miguel JF, Ojeda E, Gonzalez M, Orfao A, Cañizo MC, Sanchez J, Lopez Borrasca A (1989) Prognostic value of immunological markers in acute myeloblastic leukemia. Leukemia 3:108–111

Schwarzinger I, Valent P, Koller U, Marosi C, Schneider B, Haas O, Knapp W, Lechner K, Bettelheim P (1990) Prognostic significance of surface marker expression on blasts of patients with de novo acute myeloblastic leukemia. J Clin Oncol 8:423–430

Second MIC Cooperative Study Group (1988) Morphologic, immunologic and cytogenetic (MIC) working classification of the acute myeloid leukemias. Report of the Workshop held in Leuven, Belgium, September 15–17, 1986. Cancer Genet Cytogenet 30:1–15

Sultan C, Deregnaucourt CS, Ko YW, Imbert M, Ricard D'Agay MF, Gouault-Heilmann M, Brun B (1981) Distribution of 250 cases of acute myeloid leukemia according to the FAB classification and response to therapy. Br J Haematol 47:545–551

Swirzky DM, Greaves MF, Gray RG, Rees JKH (1988) Terminal Deoxynucleotidyl transferase and HLA/DR expression appear unrelated to prognosis of acute myeloid leukemia. Br J Haematol 70:193–198

Van der Reijden HJ, Van Rhenen DJ, Lansdorp PM, Van't Veer MB, Langenhuijsen MMAC, Engelfriet CP, Von Dem Borne AEG (1983) A comparision of surface marker analysis and FAB classification in acute myeloid leukemia. Blood 61: 443–448

Vaughan WP, Strauss LC, Burke PJ, Skubitz KM, Schwartz JM, Karp JE, Civin CI (1983) Surphace marker phenotypes (SMP) predict response to therapy in acute non-lymphocytic leukemia (ANLL). Proceedings of the American Society of Clinical Oncology 2:183

Vinci G, Tabilio A, Deschamps JP, Van Haecke D, Henri A, Guichard J, Tetteroo P, Landsdorp PM, Hercend T, Vainchenker W, Breton Gorius J (1984) Immunological study of in vitro maturation of human megakaryocytes. Br J Haematol 56:589–595

Vindelov LL, Christensen IJ, Nissen NI (1983) A detergent-trypsin method for the preparation of nuclei for flow cytometric DNA analysis. Cytometry 3:323–327

Immunophenotype of Acute Myeloid Leukemia: Correlation with Morphological Characteristics and Therapy Response

C. Sperling[1], H. Seibt-Jung[1], W. Gassmann[2], B. Komischke[1], C. Sauerland[3], W. Hiddemann[4], H. Löffler[2], T. Büchner[5], E. Thiel[1], and W.-D. Ludwig[1]

[1] Department of Hematology/Oncology, Klinikum Steglitz, Free University Berlin, W-1000 Berlin 45, Fed. Rep. of Germany
[2] Medical Clinic II, University of Kiel, W-2300 Kiel, Fed. Rep. of Germany
[3] Institute of Medical Informatics and Biomathematics, University of Münster, W-4400 Münster, Fed. Rep. of Germany
[4] Department of Internal Medicine, University of Göttingen, W-3400 Göttingen, Fed. Rep. of Germany
[5] Department of Internal Medicine – Hematology/Oncology, University of Münster, W-4400 Münster, Fed. Rep. of Germany

Introduction

Surface antigen analysis of leukemic blast cells with monoclonal antibodies (MoAbs) has become a routine technique for evaluating patients with acute leukemia, and contributes to the diagnosis and classification of acute myeloid leukemias (AML) (Drexler et al. 1988; Bain and Catovsky 1990; Cheson et al. 1990). In particular, reactivity with MoAbs recognizing myeloid antigens can assign cases of poorly differentiated leukemia to the myeloid lineage (FAB M0) (Lee et al. 1987; Bennett et al. 1991), and MoAbs reacting with platelet glycoproteins and immature erythroid cells are used to diagnose megakaryoblastic leukemia (FAB M7) and erythroleukemia (FAB M6) (Bennett et al. 1985; San Miguel et al. 1987). Moreover, immunophenotyping identifies acute leukemias with both myeloid and lymphoid features, an interesting subgroup of as yet unknown prognostic significance (Cross et al. 1988; Kaplan et al. 1989; Ludwig et al. 1990; Catovsky et al. 1991).

Some reports indicate that morphological characteristics correlate with surface antigen expression; thus immunophenotyping may corroborate standard morphological and cytochemical classification (Browman et al. 1986; Neame et al. 1986; Drexler 1987; Del Cañizo et al. 1987). In addition, some authors even found significant differences in the rates of complete remission (CR), remission duration, and survival in immunologically defined subgroups of AML patients (Bradstock et al. 1981; Jani et al. 1983; Griffin et al. 1986; Holowiecki et al. 1987; Lo Coco et al. 1989a; Borowitz et al. 1989; San Miguel et al. 1989; Merle-Beral et al. 1989; Campos et al. 1989; Geller et al. 1990; Schwarzinger et al. 1990; Ball et al. 1991). These results are in part conflicting, and comparison and interpretation of some studies

Recent Results in Cancer Research, Vol. 131

are hampered by relatively small or inhomogeneous patient populations, short follow-ups, and differences in methodology.

The aim of the present study was to investigate the immunophenotype and its relation to morphology and treatment results in a relatively homogeneous AML patient population treated with a standardized therapy. We prospectively analyzed the surface antigen expression of leukemic blasts from 239 adult patients enrolled in the AML Cooperative Group (AMLCG) studies with *de novo* AML at primary diagnosis and report on the correlation with morphological characteristics and therapy response.

Material and Methods

Patients. During the period from January 1985 to December 1990, we analyzed the immunophenotype of blast cells from 239 patients treated at 24 different institutions in Germany according to the protocols of the multicenter AMLCG studies (Büchner et al. 1990, 1991). Induction therapy in the 1986 study consisted of one (patients ≥60 years of age) or two (patients <60 years of age) cycles of intensive polychemotherapy including cytarabine (ara-C), daunorubicin, and thioguanine (TAD 9) and high-dose ara-C combined with mitoxantrone (HAM). Patients 60 years or older received a second cycle only when they had a significant leukemic population in their bone marrow on day 16 after initiation of therapy. Induction was followed by consolidation (TAD 9) and maintenance therapy. 223 of the patients were enrolled in the 1986 study and of these patients 207 could be evaluated with respect to therapy response.

Morphological Classification. The FAB subtype was available in 218 patients. Slides from 118 patients were reviewed by H. Löffler, Kiel, and classified according to the FAB criteria using light microscopy and cytochemical stains (Bennett et al. 1976, 1985). In the remaining 100 cases, patients were classified at the center where they were treated.

Immunophenotyping. Immunophenotyping was carried out in a single laboratory. Pretreatment heparinized bone-marrow samples or peripheral blood containing more than 80% blast cells were analyzed with an indirect immunofluorescence technique as previously described (Ludwig et al. 1988). Briefly, after isolation using standard Ficoll-Hypaque density gradient centrifugation and incubation with MoAb and fluorescein isothiocyanate (FITC)-labeled goat $F(ab')_2$ anti-mouse IgG + IgM, fluorescence of cells was evaluated using a fluorescence microscope (Zeiss) or by flow cytometry with a FACScan (Becton Dickinson). 10% heat-inactivated goat serum was added during the incubations to inhibit nonspecific antibody binding. A sample was regarded as positive when more than 20% of the cells showed MoAb binding compared to appropriate controls. Immunophenotyping was done with a panel of commercially available MoAbs reacting with myeloid (My7/CD13, My9/CD33, VIM-2/CD_w65, VIM-D5/CD15, UCHM1/CD14, J15/CD41, glycophorin A/not clustered), lymphoid (OKT11/CD2, Leu9/CD7, Leu3a/CD4, HD37/CD19) and progenitor (HPCA1/CD34, J5/CD10, OKIa1/HLA-DR) cells. For staining of the intranuclear enzyme terminal deoxynucleotidyl transferase (TdT), cytospin preparations fixed in cold methanol were incubated with rabbit anti-calf TdT antiserum, and then incubated with FITC-conjugated goat anti-rabbit IgG. When more than 10% of the cells were stained a sample was regarded as positive.

Statistical Methods. The significance of differences in the rate of complete remission (CR) between groups of patients was tested with the χ^2 test. Remission duration (CCR) is the time from the date of complete remission until relapse; survival was measured from the entry of the study until death. Both CCR and survival were analyzed using the product limit method (Kaplan and Meier 1958), and significance of differences in CCR or survival was tested with the log-rank test. Patients undergoing allogeneic bone marrow transplantation were censored at time of the transplantation. Both SAS and SPSS statistical software was applied.

Results

Antigen Expression. Expression of panmyeloid antigens (CD13, CD33, CD_w65) ranged from 75% to 88%. Less than 3% of the cell samples did not express any of these antigens; expression of only one was found in 13% and of only two in 29%. All three panmyeloid antigens were expressed in 55% of samples. Up to 24% of all cases showed an aberrant expression of lymphoid – mainly T-cell-lineage-associated – markers, whereas expression of B-cell markers (CD19) was found in less than 3%. In our series, we did not find any AML with CD10 expression. The incidence of TdT^+ AML was 19%; less than half of all cases expressed the non-lineage-restricted progenitor cell antigen CD34 and on more than 80% HLA-DR could be found (see Fig. 1).

Immunophenotype and Morphological Subtype. The incidence of FAB subtypes was similar to that in other series (M1, 18.8%; M2, 27.5%; M3, 5.5%; M4, 27.1%; M5, 16.1%; M6, 4.6%; M7, 0.5%). As expected, the expression of several of the antigens studied was not distributed equally among the morphological subtypes. Both CD_w65 and CD15 were less positive in myeloblastic leukemia without maturation (FAB M1) than in the M2 subtype, reflecting the association of these antigens with more mature granulocytic cells in normal hematopoietic development (Fig. 2a). CD14 and CD4 were typically expressed in AML with monocytic differentiation (Fig. 2b). CD7 and, to a lesser extent, TdT showed preferential expression

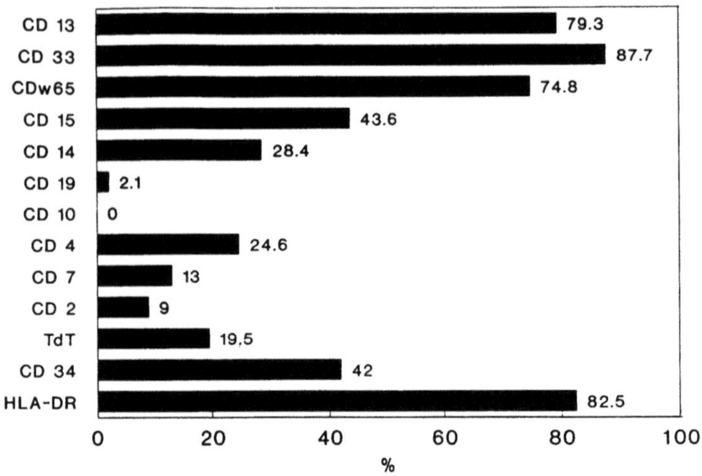

Fig. 1. Expression of myeloid, lymphoid, and non-lineage-restricted antigens in 239 patients with AML (percent of positive cases)

in immature AML, predominantly of the FAB M1 subtype, but TdT was expressed in a considerable number of myelomonocytic and monocytic leukemias as well (Fig. 2c). In the FAB M3 subtype, we could confirm the well-known absence of HLA-DR antigen characteristic of promyelocytic leukemia (data not shown). In addition, the leukemic promyelocytes mostly did not express the CD15 antigen (Fig. 2a), which is expressed on promyelocytes in normal hematopoiesis.

Immunophenotype and Treatment Outcome. 207 of the patients were evaluated with respect to treatment results, 126 of them (60.9%) achieving CR. The only antigens showing a statistically significant correlation with CR were CD15 and CD_w65 with remission rates of 68.7% vs 54.5% (P = 0.049) and 65.6% vs 44.9% (P = 0.010) for $CD15^+/CD15^-$ and CD_w65^+/CD_w65^- AML, respectively (Table 1). No correlation with the CR rate was found for any of the other antigens, including CD13, CD34, and TdT, for which an adverse effect on remission rate has been described.

The higher remission rates for $CD15^+$ and CD_w65^+ did not imply a longer CCR or survival for these patients. Life-table analysis after a median follow-up of 35 months showed that the only antigens with a significant effect on CCR were CD7 and TdT. In our series, CCR was significantly shorter with $CD7^+$ AML than with $CD7^-$ AML (P = 0.0037; Fig. 3a). A similar though weaker effect on CCR could be demonstrated for TdT positivity (P = 0.028; Fig. 3b). Survival was shorter with TdT positivity (P = 0.043); this is in contrast to CD7 expression, where it was similar in positive and negative cases despite the significantly shorter CCR for

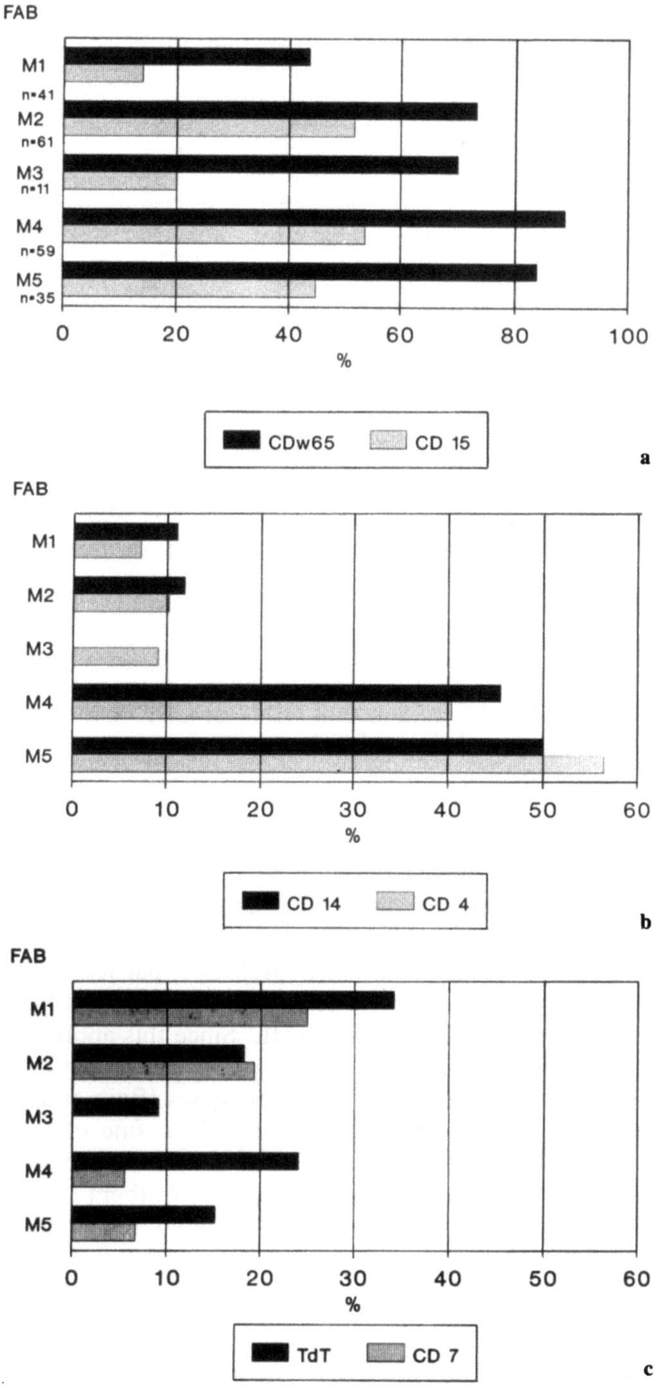

Fig. 2a–c. Expression of selected antigens in AML patients with different morphological FAB subtypes. **a** CD_w65 and CD15, **b** CD14 and CD4, **c** TdT and CD7

Table 1. Antigen expression and rate of complete remission (CR) after induction therapy

	Antigen positive		Antigen negative		
	CR rate		CR rate		
Antigen	(%)	(*n*)	(%)	(*n*)	P^a
CD7	70.8	17/24	58.4	97/166	ns
CD2	75.0	9/12	60.4	84/139	ns
CD4	65.8	25/38	57.8	70/121	ns
CD13	60.4	87/144	63.2	24/38	ns
CD33	62.1	105/169	48.1	13/27	ns
CD_w65	65.6	99/151	44.9	22/49	0.010
CD15	68.7	57/83	54.5	55/101	0.049
CD14	66.0	35/53	57.9	81/140	ns
CD34	56.8	42/74	62.6	62/99	ns
HLA-DR	63.7	107/168	45.2	14/31	ns
TdT	52.5	21/40	62.7	101/161	ns

[a] χ^2 test.

$CD7^+$ AML. An influence of CD13 or CD34 expression on CCR or survival was not detected (e.g., CD13, Fig. 3c).

Discussion

There is no doubt about the importance of immunophenotyping as a supplement to standard morphology in the differential diagnosis of acute leukemia. Analysis of surface markers is particular valuable in cases where light microscopy and cytochemistry alone do not differentiate between acute lymphoblastic leukemia and AML. Since this applies to about 10%–20% of all leukemias, it has thus become possible to make this important distinction in about 98%–99% of all leukemia cases (Bain and Catovsky 1990). In our series, more than 97% expressed at least one of the panmyeloid antigens CD13, CD33, and CD_w65. The fact that 13% expressed only one of the panmyeloid antigens and 29% only two of them indicates that at least three panmyeloid antigens should be included in a panel for AML immuno-

Fig. 3a–c. Duration of complete remission after successful induction therapy for acute myeloid leukemia in patients with **a** $CD7^+$ vs $CD7^-$ ($P = 0.0037$), **b** TdT^+ vs TdT^- ($P = 0.028$), and **c** $CD13^+$ vs $CD13^-$ AML ($P = 0.71$). Kaplan-Meier plot, P values from log-rank test

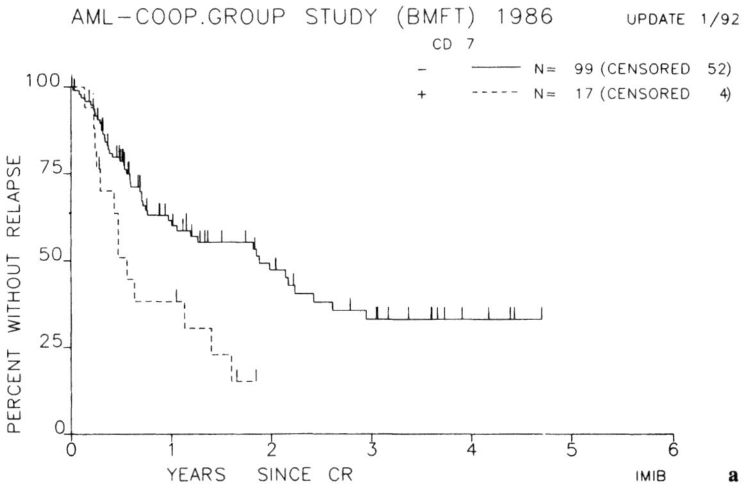
AML-COOP.GROUP STUDY (BMFT) 1986
UPDATE 1/92
CD 7
- N= 99 (CENSORED 52)
+ N= 17 (CENSORED 4)
PERCENT WITHOUT RELAPSE
100
75
50
25
0
0
1
2
3
4
5
6
YEARS SINCE CR
IMIB

a

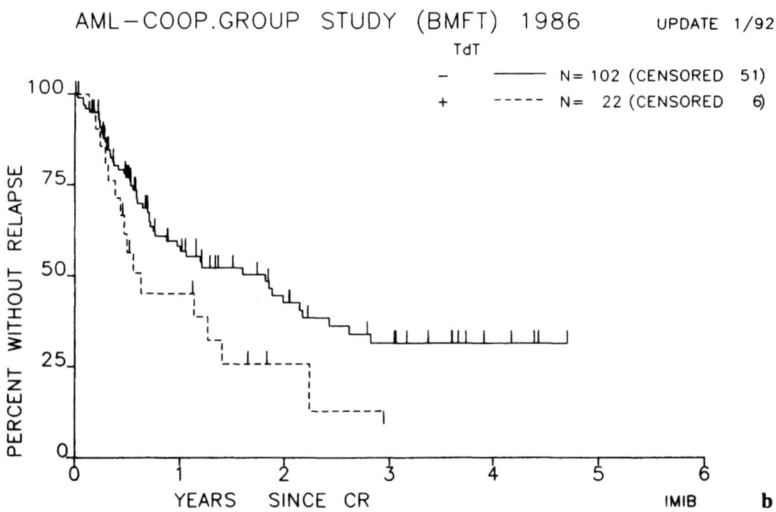
AML-COOP.GROUP STUDY (BMFT) 1986
UPDATE 1/92
TdT
- N= 102 (CENSORED 51)
+ N= 22 (CENSORED 6)
PERCENT WITHOUT RELAPSE
100
75
50
25
0
0
1
2
3
4
5
6
YEARS SINCE CR
IMIB

b

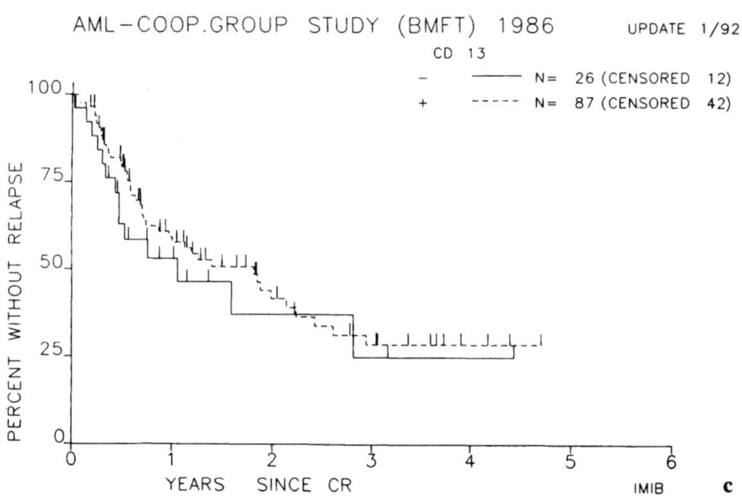
AML-COOP.GROUP STUDY (BMFT) 1986
UPDATE 1/92
CD 13
- N= 26 (CENSORED 12)
+ N= 87 (CENSORED 42)
PERCENT WITHOUT RELAPSE
100
75
50
25
0
0
1
2
3
4
5
6
YEARS SINCE CR
IMIB

c

phenotyping. Although the FAB subtypes show typical marker profiles, a direct conclusion as to the morphological subtype cannot be drawn from the immunophenotype. Cases with identical antigen expression may belong to different FAB types, and different immunophenotypes are found in the same FAB subtypes. On the other hand, the expression (or nonexpression) of markers can support FAB subtype diagnosis (for example HLA-DR^-/$CD15^-$ in FAB M3 and M3v, $CD14^+$ in M4/M5).

Certain morphological characteristics (Zittoun et al. 1984), specific cytogenetic aberrations (Keating et al. 1988), and expression of several antigens have all been considered to define prognostically relevant subgroups of AML patients. Antigens reported to be of prognostic significance include myeloid (CD13, CD15), lymphoid (CD7, CD2), and non-lineage-restricted (CD34, HLA-DR) markers and TdT. Our study did not confirm earlier reports on the prognostic implications of CD13 expression (Griffin et al. 1986; Schwarzinger et al. 1990). In our series, treatment results were identical whether the marker was positive or negative. Two myeloid markers – CD15 and CD_w65 – were associated with higher CR rates; other studies have reported this for CD15 (Holowiecki et al. 1987; Campos et al. 1989; Schwarzinger et al. 1990). Several authors have reported coexpression of the T-cell-associated antigens CD2 and CD7 and the intranuclear enzyme TdT in AML cells, but the prognostic significance of these findings remains unclear. A recent study (Ball et al. 1991) demonstrated higher remission rates as well as a longer CCR and survival for patients with $CD2^+$ AML than for those with $CD2^-$ AML. Although the CR and CCR (data not shown) were superior with $CD2^+$ AML in our series as well, the difference was not significant, probably because of the small patient group. Expression of CD7 in otherwise typical AML is characterized by cell immaturity and the leukemic cell may be related to a multipotential progenitor cell (Lo Coco et al. 1989b; Zutter et al. 1990). CD7 expression had the strongest adverse effect on the CCR among the antigens tested. Poor outcome for $CD7^+$ AML is supported by other reports (Jensen et al. 1991). One possible explanation is provided by the observation that CD7 expression may be associated with poor-prognosis cytogenetic features such as aberrations of chromosome 5 (Lutz et al. 1990). Several reports analyzing the prognostic implications of TdT positivity in AML have yielded conflicting results. While most of the studies considered TdT positivity as an adverse factor (Bradstock et al. 1981; Jani et al. 1983; Lo Coco et al. 1989a; Schwarzinger et al. 1990), some could not demonstrate any influence (Swirsky et al. 1988; Gucalp et al. 1991) and even a favorable clinical course of TdT^+ AML has been reported (Skoog et al. 1984). Our own results suggest a moderate but statistically significant shorter CCR and survival in TdT^+ AML. We did not find any influence of CD34 expression on remission rate, CCR, or survival, in contrast to earlier reports (Geller et al. 1990).

The association of morphological features with specific cytogenetic abnormalities is well known and forms the basis for the MIC classification of AML

(Second MIC Cooperative Study Group 1988). Several reports (Paietta et al. 1987; Adriaansen et al. 1988; Schachner et al. 1988; Lutz et al. 1990) and our own preliminary data (Sperling et al. 1991) suggest that specific chromosomal aberrations may be correlated with surface antigen expression as well; thus, combining morphology, immunology, and cytogenetics might help in refining the present classification. Such an integrated approach might allow us to better define biologically and clinically relevant subgroups of AML patients.

Acknowledgments. We thank all participants of the AMLCG studies for their cooperation.

References

Adriaansen HJ, van Dongen JJM, Hooijkaas H, Hählen H, van't Veer MB, Löwenberg B, Hagemeijer A (1988) Translocation (6;9) may be associated with a specific TdT-positive immunological phenotype in ANLL. Leukemia 2:136–140

Bain B, Catovsky D (1990) Current concerns in haematology 2: classification of acute leukaemia. J Clin Pathol 43:882–887

Ball ED, Davis RB, Griffin JD, Mayer RJ, Davey FR, Arthur DC, Wurster-Hill D, Noll W, Elghetany MT, Allen SL, Rai K, Lee EJ, Schiffer CA, Bloomfield CD (1991) Prognostic value of lymphocyte surface markers in acute myeloid leukemia. Blood 77:2242–2250

Bennett JM, Catovsky D, Daniel MT, Flandrin G, Galton DAG, Gralnick HR, Sultan C (1976) Proposals for the classification of the acute leukaemias. Br J Haematol 33:451–458

Bennett JM, Catovsky D, Daniel MT, Flandrin G, Galton DAG, Gralnick HR, Sultan C (1985) Criteria for the diagnosis of acute leukemia of megakaryocytic lineage (M7). Ann Intern Med 103:460–462

Bennett JM, Catovsky D, Daniel MT, Flandrin G, Galton DAG, Gralnick HR, Sultan C (1991) Proposal for the recognition of minimally differentiated acute myeloid leukaemia (AML-M0). Br J Haematol 78:325–329

Borowitz MJ, Gockerman JP, Moore JO, Civin CI, Page SO, Robertson J, Bigner SH (1989) Clinicopathologic and cytogenetic features of CD34 (My 10)-positive acute nonlymphocytic leukemia. Am J Clin Pathol 91:265–270

Bradstock KF, Hoffbrand AV, Ganeshaguru K, Llewellin P, Patterson K, Wonke B, Prentice G, Bennett M, Pizzolo G, Bollum FJ, Janossy G (1981) Terminal deoxynucleotidyl transferase expression in acute non-lymphoid leukaemia: an analysis by immunofluorescence. Br J Haematol 47:133–143

Browman GP, Neame PB, Soamboonsrup P (1986) The contribution of cytochemistry and immunophenotyping to the reproducibility of the FAB classification in acute leukemia. Blood 68:900–905

Büchner T, Hiddemann W, Blasius S, Koch P, Maschmeyer G, Tirier C, Sodomann H, Kuse R, Thiel E, Ludwig WD, Seibt-Jung H, Gassmann W, Löffler H, Aul C, Heyll A, Mertelsmann R, Anders CH, Nowrousian MR, Straif K, Hossfeld D, Becker K, Ho A, Fülle HH, Hellriegel KP, König HJ, Lengfelder E, Siegert W, Bartels H, Schwammborn J, Donhuijsen-Ant R, Vaupel HA, König E, Planker M, Emmerich R, Middelhoff G, Mainzer K, Urbanitz D, Zurborn KH, Köppler H, Nowicki L, Augener W, Karow J, Schroeder M, Eimermacher H, Fuchs R, Balleisen L, Schmitz-Hübner U, Leimer L, Heitzelmann KH, Lathan B, Meuthen I,

Baldus M, Michels-Giermann R, Fuhr HG, Sauerland MC, Heinicke A (1990) Adult AML: the role of chemotherapy intensity and duration. Two studies of the AML Cooperative Group. In: Büchner T, Schellong G, Hiddemann W, Ritter J (eds) Acute leukemias II. Springer, Berlin Heidelberg New York, pp 261–266 (Haematology and blood transfusion, vol 33)

Büchner T, Hiddemann W, Löffler G, Gassmann W, Maschmeyer G, Heit W, Hossfeld D, Weh H, Ludwig WD, Thiel E, Nowrousian M, Aul C, Lengfelder E, Lathan B, Mainzer K, Urbanitz D, Emmerich B, Middelhoff G, Donhuijsen-Ant HR, Hellriegel H-P, Heinicke A (1991) Improved cure rate by very early intensification combined with prolonged maintenance chemotherapy in patients with acute myeloid leukemia: data from the AML cooperative group. Semin Hematol 28:76–79

Campos L, Guyotat D, Archimbaud E, Devaux Y, Treille D, Larese A, Maupas J, Gentilhomme O, Ehrsam A, Fiere D (1989) Surface marker expression in adult acute myeloid leukaemia: correlations with initial characteristics, morphology and response to therapy. Br J Haematol 72:161–166

Catovsky D, Matutes E, Buccheri V, Shetty V, Hanslip J, Yoshida N, Morilla R (1991) A classification of acute leukemia for the 1990s. Ann Hematol 62:16–21

Cheson BD, Cassileth PA, Head DR, Schiffer CA, Bennett JM, Bloomfield CD, Brunning R, Gale RP, Grever MR, Keating MJ, Sawitsky, Stass S, Weinstein H, Woods WG (1990) Report of the National Cancer Institute-sponsored workshop on definitions of diagnosis and response in acute myeloid leukemia. J Clin Oncol 8:813–819

Cross AH, Goorha RM, Nuss R, Behm FG, Murphy SB, Kalwinsky DK, Raimondi S, Kitchingman GR, Mirro J (1988) Acute myeloid leukemia with T-lymphoid features: a distinct biologic and clinical entity. Blood 72:579–587

Del Cañizo MC, San Miguel JF, Gonzalez M, Anta JP, Orfao A, Lopez-Borrasca A (1987) Discrepancies between morphologic, cytochemical and immunologic characteristics in acute myeloblastic leukemia. Am J Clin Pathol 88:38–42

Drexler HG (1987) Classification of acute myeloid leukemias – a comparison of FAB and immunophenotyping. Leukemia 1:697–705

Drexler HG, Gignac SM, Minowada J (1988) Routine immunophenotyping of acute leukaemias. Blut 57:327–339

Geller R, Zahurak M, Hurwitz CA, Burke PJ, Karp JE, Piantadosi S, Civin CI (1990) Prognostic importance of immunophenotyping in adults with acute myelocytic leukaemia: the significance of the stem-cell glycoprotein CD34 (My 10). Br J Haematol 76:340–347

Griffin JD, Davis R, Nelson DA, Davey FR, Mayer RJ, Schiffer C, Mclntyre OR, Bloomfield CD (1986) Use of surface marker analysis to predict outcome of adult acute myeloblastic leukemia. Blood 68:1232–1241

Gucalp R, Paietta E, Weinberg V, Papenhausen P, Dutcher P, Wiernik PH (1991) Terminal transferase expression in acute myeloid leukaemia: biology and prognosis. Br J Haematol 77:48–54

Holowiecki J, Lutz D, Krzemien S, Graf F, Keleney G, Brugiatelli M, Callea V, Holowiecka B, Jagoda K, Ihle R, Krč I (1987) Expression of CD-15 antigen on leukemic cells – a new prognostic factor for ability to achieve complete remission and for survival in ANLL. In: Büchner T, Schellong G, Hiddemann W, Urbanitz D, Ritter J (eds) Acute leukemias. Springer, Berlin Heidelberg New York, pp 361–364 (Haematology and blood transfusion, vol 30)

Jani P, Verbi W, Greaves MF, Bevan D, Bollum F (1983) Terminal deoxynucleotidyl transferase in acute myeloid leukaemia. Leuk Res 7:17–29

Jensen AW, Hokland M, Jørgensen H, Justesen J, Ellegaard J, Hokland P (1991) Solitary expression of CD7 among T-cell antigens in acute myeloid leukemia:

identification of a group of patients with similar T-cell receptor β and γ rearrangements and course of disease suggestive of poor prognosis. Blood 78:1292–1300
Kaplan EL, Meier P (1958) Nonparametric estimation from incomplete observations. J Am Stat Assoc 53:457–481
Kaplan SS, Penchansky L, Stolc V, Contis L, Krause JR (1989) Immunophenotyping in the classification of acute leukemia in adults. Interpretation of multiple lineage reactivity. Cancer 63:1520–1527
Keating MJ, Smith TL, Kantarjian H, Cork A, Walters R, Trujillo JM, McCredie KB, Gehan EA, Freireich EJ (1988) Cytogenetic pattern in acute myelogenous leukemia: a major determinant of outcome. Leukemia 2:403–412
Lee EJ, Pollak A, Leavitt RD, Testa JR, Schiffer CA (1987) Minimally differentiated acute nonlymphocytic leukemia: a distinct entity. Blood 70:1400–1406
Lo Coco F, Lopez M, Pasqualetti D, Montefusco E, Cafolla A, Monarca B, Sgadari C, De Rossi G (1989a) Terminal tranferase positive acute myeloid leukemia: immunophenotypic characterization and response to induction therapy. Hematol Oncol 7:167–174
Lo Coco F, De Rossi G, Pasqualetti D, Lopez M, Diverio D, Latagliata R, Fenu S, Mandelli F (1989b) CD7 positive acute myeloid leukaemia: a subtype associated with cell immaturity. Br J Haematol 73:480–485
Ludwig WD, Bartram CR, Ritter J, Raghavachar A, Hiddemann W, Heil G, Harbott J, Seibt-Jung H, Teichmann J, Riehm H (1988) Ambiguous phenotypes and genotypes in 16 children with acute leukemia as characterized by multiparameter analysis. Blood 71:1518–1528
Ludwig WD, Thiel E, Köller U, Bartram CR, Harbott J, Teichmann JV, Seibt-Jung H, Creutzig U, Ritter J, Riehm H (1990) Incidence and clinical implications of acute hybrid leukemia in childhood. In: Büchner T, Schellong G, Hiddemann W, Ritter J (eds) Acute leukemias II. Springer, Berlin Heidelberg New York, pp 516–522 (Haematology and blood transfusion, vol 33)
Lutz D, Kasparu H, Nowotny H, Weber E, Krieger O, Köller U, Tüchler H, Knapp W (1990) Association of GP40/CD7 + acute myeloblastic leukemia and chromosome 5 aberrations. In: Büchner T, Schellong G, Hiddemann W, Ritter J (eds) Acute leukemias II. Springer, Berlin Heidelberg New York, pp 141–144 (Haematology and blood transfusion, vol 33)
Merle-Beral H, Nguyen Cong Duc L, Leblond V, Boucheix C, Michel A, Chastang C, Debré P (1989) Diagnostic and prognostic significance of myelomonocytic cell surface antigens in acute myeloid leukaemia. Br J Haematol 73:323–330
Neame PB, Soamboonsrup P, Browman GP, Meyer RM, Benger A, Wilson WEC, Walker IR, Saeed N, McBride JA (1986) Classifying acute leukemia by immunophenotyping: a combined FAB-immunologic classification of AML. Blood 68:1355–1362
Paietta E, Papenhausen P, Gucalp R, Reed J, Wiernik PH (1987) The 5q-deletion: correlation of breakpoints with the immunophenotype of leukemic blast cells. Leukemia 1:822–824
San Miguel JF, Gonzalez M, Orfao A, Ojeda E, Cañizo MC (1987) Expression of immunological markers in megakaryoblasts. Blood 70:1227–1228
San Miguel JF, Ojeda E, Gonzalez M, Orfao A, Cañizo MC, Sanchez J, Lopez-Borrasca A (1989) Prognostic value of immunological markers in acute myeloblastic leukemia. Leukemia 3:108–111
Schachner J, Kantarjian H, Dalton W, McCredie K, Keating M, Freireich EJ (1988) Cytogenetic association and prognostic significance of bone marrow blast cell terminal transferase in patients with acute myeloblastic leukemia. Leukemia 2:667–671
Schwarzinger, I, Valent P, Köller U, Marosi C, Schneider B, Haas O, Knapp W, Lechner K, Bettelheim P (1990) Prognostic significance of surface marker

expression on blasts of patients with de novo acute myeloblastic leukemia. J Clin Oncol 8:423–430

Second MIC Cooperative Study Group (1988) Morphologic, immunologic and cytogenetic (MIC) working classification of acute myeloid leukaemias. Br J Haematol 68:487–494

Skoog L, Öst A, Biberfeld P, Christensson B, Hast R, Lagerlöf B, Nordenskjöld B, Reizenstein P (1984) Prognostic significance of terminal transferase activity and glucorticoid receptor levels in acute myeloid leukemia. Br J Cancer 50:443–449

Sperling C, Ludwig WD, Seibt-Jung H, Haase D, Becher R, Gassmann W, Schmidt C, Böttcher S, Sauerland C, Gramatzki M, Fonatsch C, Hiddemann W, Löffler H, Büchner T, Thiel E (1991) Immunophenotype of acute myeloid leukemia (AML): correlation with morphology, cytogenetic features and response to therapy. Onkologie 14 [Suppl 2]:158 (abstr)

Swirsky DM, Greaves MF, Gray RG, Rees JKH (1988) Terminal deoxynucleotidyl transferase and HLA-DR expression appear unrelated to prognosis of acute myeloid leukemia. B J Haematol 70:193–198

Zittoun R, Cadiou M, Bayle C, Suciu S, Solbu G, Hayat M (1984) Prognostic value of cytologic parameters in acute myelogenous leukemia. Cancer 53:1526–1532

Zutter MM, Martin J, Hanke D, Kidd PG (1990) CD7 + acute non-lymphocytic leukemia: evidence for an early multipotential progenitor. Leuk Res 14:23–26

Multiparameter Analysis of Blast Cells in Patients with Acute Leukemia Following a Primary Myelodysplastic Syndrome

J.F. San Miguel[1], J.M. Hernandez[1], R. Gonzalez[2], M. Gonzalez[1], I. Sanchez[2], A. Orfao[3], M.C. del Cañizo[1], and A. Lopez-Borrasca[1]

[1] Department of Hematology, University Hospital of Salamanca, Paseo de San Vicente s/n, 37007 Salamanca, Spain
[2] Molecular Genetic Unit, Department of Medicine, University of Salamanca, 37007 Salamanca, Spain
[3] Department of Cytometry, University of Salamanca, 37007 Salamanca, Spain

Introduction

The blast cells in acute leukemia following myelodysplastic syndrome (MDS) have classically been assumed to be of myeloid lineage (Tricot et al. 1985). However, our previous preliminary data (San Miguel et al. 1986b) as well as several case reports have shown that other cell lineages, including the lymphoid, may occasionally be involved in these leukemias (Barton et al. 1980; Berneman et al. 1985; Eridani et al. 1985). Moreover, to the best of our knowledge the only broad molecular genetic study in MDS patients is that reported by Wainscoat et al. (1988), showing an absence of immunoglobulin (Ig) and T-cell receptor (TCR) gene rearrangement. However, the appearance of new cell clones in the acute transformation of MDS may induce molecular changes that so far have not been analyzed.

In order to obtain more insight into the nature of blast cells in patients with acute transformation of a previous primary MDS, we have performed a combined multiparameter analysis including morphologic, immunophenotypic, and molecular genetic investigations.

Material and Methods

Patients and Morphology. Fifty patients with an overt acute leukemia (⩾30% blast cells) following a previous primary MDS were included in the study. The median number of blast cells in the specimens analyzed was 65%. The initial diagnosis of the MDS according to the FAB criteria (Bennett et al. 1982) was: refractory anemia (RA), 11 cases; RA with ring sideroblasts (RAS), 7 cases; RA with excess of blasts (RAEB), 18 cases; RAEB in transformation (RAEBt), 9 cases; and chronic myelomonocytic leukemia (CMML), 5 cases. Bone marrow (BM) and peripheral blood (PB) smears

Recent Results in Cancer Research, Vol. 131

were stained with May–Grünwald–Giemsa (MGG) and specific cytochemical methods.

Immunologic Markers. Phenotypic analysis of the blast cells obtained at the moment of diagnosis of acute transformation was performed in all 50 patients as previously described (San Miguel et al. 1988, 1991). The panel of monoclonal antibodies (MAbs) used included: CD33 (My9), CD13 (My7), CD15 (FMC10); CD14 (LeuM3), CD41 (J15), CD61 (C17), CD42a (FMC25), CD42b (AN51), antiglycophorin A (LICR LON.R10), anti-HLA-DR (GRB1), CD9 (FMC56), CD19 (Leu12), CD20 (B1); CD7 (3A1), CD10 (J5), and terminal deoxynucleotidyl transferase (TdT). The presence of mixed-lineage immunophenotypes was assessed by appropriate individual double stainings. For the assessment of lineages, a minimum of 15% blast cells positive for one or more of the specific MAbs was required.

DNA Analysis. DNA from blood and bone marrow mononuclear cells obtained from 19 unselected acute leukemias following a previous MDS was prepared using standard proteinase K digestion, phenol/chloroform extraction, and ethanol precipitation methods. Ten-microgram samples were digested with appropriate restriction enzymes, size-fractionated by electrophoresis in 0.8% agarose gels, and transferred to nylon membranes. All blots were hybridized overnight with^{32} P-labeled DNA probes and washed twice for 30 min at 65°C in 0.1% standard saline citrate (SSC) and 0.1% sodium dodecylsulfate SDS. Ig gene analysis was carried out using genomic probes: an Ig heavy-chain joining (J_H) region probe (6 kilobases, kb, *Bam*HI–*Hin*dIII fragment) and a 2.5-kb *Eco*RI–*Eco*RI probe derived from the Ck region (Hieter et al. 1980). TCR β-chain gene rearrangement was detected using a 770-base pair (bp) complementary (c)DNA constant region probe (M131B10BB1). The configuration of the TCRγ genes was analyzed by use of the H60 probe, a 0.77-kb *Eco*RI–*Hin*dIII fragment containing J_γ 1.3 segments that hybridizes to both J_γ 1.3 and J_γ 2.3 gene segments (Lefranc and Rabitts 1985). TCRδ gene rearrangements were detected with J_δ16 (a 1.5-kb *Sac*I fragment), which recognizes J_δ 1 sequences, and the J_δ 2 probe R21XH (a 2.3-kb *Hin*dIII–*Eco*RI fragment) (Boehm et al. 1988; Baer et al. 1988). Two probes were used to identify M-*bcr* breakpoint locations: a 0.6-kb fragment, corresponding to a *Pst*I-*Bgl*II fragment hybridizing intron sequences located between M-*bcr* exons 3 and 4, designated the 3′-M-*bcr* probe; and a 5′-M-*bcr* probe corresponding to a *Bgl*II–*Hin*dIII fragment containing exon 1 and all sequences comprising subregion 0, designated the 3′-M-*bcr* probe.

Results

The immunophenotypic analysis showed that the blast cells in most leukemic transformations of MDS – 44 out of the 50 (88%) – had a myeloid phenotype. Nevertheless, in six cases a hybrid (lymphoid–myeloid) phenotype was detected (Table 1). Within the myeloid transformations four major phenotypical subgroups could be recognized: myeloblastic (MB), positivity for only CD13/CD33; granulocytic (GR), CD15 positive; monocytic (MO), expression of CD14 either alone or in combination with CD15; and megakaryocytic (MK), CD41 and CD61 positive. The distribution of these myeloid phenotypes was 30%, 9%, 47%, and 14% of cases, respectively (Table 1). In all megakaryocytic transformations, megakaryoblasts coexisted with other myeloid components. Erythroid transformations were not detected by immunological markers (glycophorin A). Double staining showed that the six hybrid cases corresponded to bilineal leukemias in which, together with the lymphoid component, different myeloid lineages were involved. The lymphoid cells consistently displayed an early B phenotype (TdT^+, $CD19^+$, $CD10^-$). Overall, a good correlation between the immunophenotypic and morphological classifications of blast cells was observed. Based on morphological criteria, the existence of mixed leukemias involving either the lymphoid or megakaryocytic lineages was also suspected; nevertheless, a classical granulocytic and/or monocytic leukemia was the most common morphological transformation in these patients (Fig. 1). The distribution of the immunophenotypic subgroups of acute leukemias according to the previous FAB diagnosis of the MDS is shown in Table 1. A significantly higher incidence of monocytic transformations was observed among RA, RAS, and CMML ($p = 0.0006$), while the myeloblastic and megakaryocytic phenotypes predominated in the RAEB and RAEBt subtypes ($p = 0.009$). The presence of a lymphoid component was detected in all MDS subgroups except CMML (Table 1).

Overall, 10 out of the 19 (52%) leukemias following a MDS studied showed rearrangements of Ig or TCR genes. The IgH gene was rearranged in one out of three hybrid transformations analyzed (Table 2). A second case showing IgH gene rearrangement corresponded to a transformation of a CMML with a granulomonocytic phenotype (Table 2). Both cases had concomitant rearrangements of TCRγ or TCRδ genes, but none of them displayed Igκ gene rearrangement. The TCRβ locus was in germline configuration in all cases. Rearrangement of the TCRγ locus was detected in four out of 19 cases, all corresponding to a previous RAEB or RAEBt. The TCRδ locus was rearranged in seven cases, being the only rearranged gene in five of them (Table 2). Regarding the immunophenotypic distribution, all three hybrid leukemias included in our study displayed the TCRδ gene in germline configuration, while this gene was rearranged in two out of the three megakaryoblastic leukemias (Table 2). Analysis of the M-*bcr* region in these 19 patients showed a germline configuration in all cases.

Discussion

The present study shows that although the granulomonocytic lineage is the most commonly involved in acute leukemias following a previous MDS, all

Table 1. Immunophenotype of acute leukemias following MDS

	Myeloblastic ($CD13^+/CD33^+$)	Granulocytic ($CD15^+$)	Monocytic ($CD14^+$)	Megakaryocytic ($CD41^+/CD61^+$)	Hybrid (lymphoid–myeloid)
RA ($n = 11$)	2[a]	0	7	1	1
RAS ($n = 7$)	0	0	5[a]	0	2
RAEB ($n = 18$)	7	3[a]	3	3	2
RAEBt ($n = 9$)	4	1	1	2	1
CMML ($n = 5$)	1	0	4	0	0
Total ($n = 50$)	14	4	20	6	6

[a] One case TdT^+, $CD19^-$.
$p = 0.0006$: $CD14^+$ in RA/RAS/CMML vs RAEB/RAEBt.
$p = 0.009$: $CD13^+$ and $CD41^+/CD61^+$ in RAEB/RAEBt vs RA/RAS/CMML.

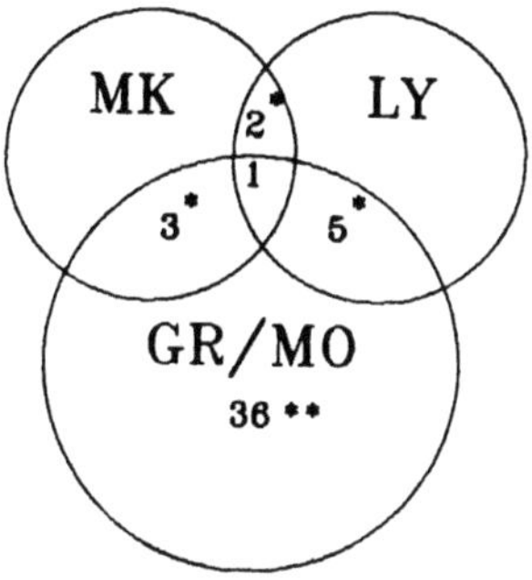

Fig. 1. Morphological cell lineages in acute leukemia following MDS. *MK*, megakaryocytic; *LY*, lymphoid; *GR/MO*, granulomonocytic. *One or **two cases with an erythroid component. Two cases were undifferentiated morphologically

Table 2. Acute leukemia following a primary MDS: summary of molecular and immunophenotypic analysis of the IgH, Tβ, Tγ, and Tδ gene rearrangements

Previous MDS diagnosis	IgH	Igκ	TCRβ	TCRγ	TCRδ	Immunophenotype
CMML	R	G	G	G	R	Granulomonocytic
RAEB	R	G	G	R	G	Hybrid
RAEB	G	G	G	R	R	Megakaryocytic
RAEB	G	G	G	R	G	Granulomonocytic
RAEBt	G	G	G	R	G	Myeloblastic
CMML	G	G	G	G	R	Granulomonocytic
RAEB	G	G	G	G	R	Megakaryocytic
RAS	G	G	G	G	R	Granulomonocytic
RA	G	G	G	G	R	Myeloblastic
RAEB	G	G	G	G	R	Granulomonocytic

The remaining nine patients showed a germline gene configuration in all genes with the following immunophenotypic distribution: four granulomonocytic, two myeloblastic, one megakaryocytic, and two hybrid. The FAB distribution of these nine cases was as follows: RA, 3; RAS, 2; RAEB, 1; RAEBt, 1; CMML, 2.
R, Rearranged; G, germinal.

cell lineages, including the megakaryocytic and lymphoid, may be involved in these patients, pointing to a pluripotential stem cell origin. The incidence of megakaryocytic transformations in the present series (12%) was slightly higher than that reported in de novo AML (8%) (San Miguel et al. 1986a) but lower than that found in blood cells of myeloproliferative disorders (31% – 35%) (Griffin et al. 1983). Moreover, in MDS, other myeloid blast cells were present, together with megakaryoblasts, similar to the picture found in AML and blast crisis of chronic myeloid leukemias (Bettelheim et al. 1985; San Miguel et al. 1985). In six cases, lymphoblasts coexisting with other myeloid components (hybrid leukemias) were detected. Interestingly, the lymphoblasts always displayed an early B phenotype (TdT^+, $CD19^+$, $CD10^-$) that differed from that found in the lymphoblastic transformations of CML, which are generally $CD10^+$ (Griffin et al. 1983; Bettelheim et al.

1985). There was a very low incidence of erythroid transformations in the present series: five cases detected by morphological criteria. This is outstanding, particularly if it is considered that abnormalities of the erythroid precursors are one of the most common features of MDS.

One interesting finding of our study is that certain types of MDS are associated with a significantly higher incidence of specific acute leukemia phenotypes. Thus, in RA, RAS, and CMML the granulomonocytic immunophenotypes predominate, while the myeloblastic and megakaryoblastic transformations were significantly more frequent among the RAEB and RAEBt. This finding may suggest a certain preferential cell lineage commitment according to the type of MDS.

The configuration of Ig and TCR genes in a series of MDS in chronic phase has recently been investigated, showing that these genes are consistently in germline configuration (Wainscoat et al. 1988). However, transformation to acute leukemia implies the appearance of new blast cell populations, as has been demonstrated by morphological and immunophenotypic analysis (San Miguel et al. 1986b). We have analyzed the Ig and TCR gene organization in 19 unselected acute leukemias following a MDS. Our results show that 52% of cases had undergone rearrangement in some of the rearranging genes. All rearrangements were detected with more than one restriction enzyme, ruling out the possibility of polymorphism. TCRγ and TCRδ were the most frequently rearranged genes, although, interestingly, only one case showed simultaneous TCRγ and TCRδ gene rearrangement. The TCRβ gene was in germline configuration in all cases. These results are different from those reported for B precursor ALL, where the association of TCRγ and TCRδ gene rearrangements is frequent and TCRβ gene rearrangement are not an unfrequent event (Van Dongen and Wolvers-Tettero 1991). Two cases displaying IgH gene reorganization also showed concomitant TCRγ and TCRδ gene rearrangement, respectively. Only one of these cases showed a B-lymphoid component. Furthermore, two other bilineal transformations that displayed an early B-cell phenotype ($CD19^+$, $CD10^-$) were in germline configuration. The absence of a correlation between gene rearrangement and the immunophenotype, as well as the presence of the Igκ locus in germline configuration, suggests that the gene rearrangements in these cases are not related to the direction of the hematopoietic differentiation in neoplastic cells. These results suggest that the detection of Ig and/or TCR gene rearrangements in cases of acute leukemia following a MDS cannot be considered as a consequence of cell lineage commitment of the neoplastic target cell, and it is possible to speculate that in these cases the leukemic cell might have originated from an uncommitted precursor that retained recombinase activity. The presence of the Philadelphia chromosome has been reported in rare cases of MDS (Roth et al. 1980; Berrebi et al. 1985) and in an isolated case of RAEBt (Smadja et al. 1989). Our results show a consistent germline configuration of the M-*bcr* region in all 19 cases, so the above-mentioned cases should be considered exceptional.

Acknowledgement. This work was supported by grants from the Fondo de Investigaciones Sanitarias de la Seguridad Social (no. 89/0651-2).

References

Baer R, Boehm T, Yssel H, Spits H, Rabbitts TH (1988) Complex rearrangements within the human Jδ-Cδ/Jα-Cα locus and aberrant recombination between Jα segments. EMBO J 7:1661

Barton JC, Conrad ME, Parmley RT (1980) Acute lymphoblastic leukaemia in idiopathic refractory sideroblastic anemia: evidence for a common lymphoid and myeloid progenitor cell. Am J Hematol 9:109

Bennet JM, Catovsky D, Daniel MT, Flandrin G, Galton DAG, Gralnisk HR, Sultan C, The France-American-British (FAB) Group (1982) Proposals for the classification of the myelodysplastic syndromes. Br J Haematol 51:189

Berneman ZN, Van Bocktaele D, de Meyer P, Van der Planken M, Vertessen F, de Block R, Peetermans ME (1985) A myelodysplastic syndrome preceding acute lymphoblastic leukaemia. Br J Haematol 60:353

Berrebi A, Bruck R, Shtalrid M, Chemke J (1985) Philadelphia chromosome in idiopathic acquired sideroblastic anemia. Acta Haematol (Basel) 72:343

Bettelheim P, Lutz D, Majdic O, Paietta E, Haas O, Linkesch W, Neumann E, Lechner K, Knapp W (1985) Cell lineage heterogenity in blast crisis of chronic myeloid leukaemia. Br J Haematol 59:395

Boehm T, Baer R, Lavenir I, Forster A, Waters JJ, Nacheva E, Rabbitts TH (1988) The mechanism of chromosomal translocation t(11;14) involving T-cell receptor C δ locus on human chromosome 14q11 and a transcribed region of chromosome 11p15. EMBO J 7:385

Eridani S, Chan LC, Halil O, Pearson TC (1985) Acute biphenotypic leukaemia (myeloid and null-ALL type) supervening in a myelodysplastic syndrome. Br J Haematol 61:525

Griffin JD, Todd III RF, Ritz J, Nadler LM, Canellos GP, Rosenthal D, Gallivan M, Beveridge RP, Weinstein H, Karp D, Schlossman SF (1983) Differentiation patterns in the blastic phase of chronic myeloid leukemia. Blood 61:85

Hieter H, Max EE, Seidman JG, Maizel JV, Leder P (1980) Cloned human and mouse kappa immunoglobulin constant and J region, genes conserved homology and functional segments. Cell 22:197–207

Lefranc MP, Rabbitts TH (1985) Two tandemly organized human genes encoding the T-cell γ constant-region sequences show multiple rearrangement in different T-cell type. Nature 316:464

Roth DG, Richman CM, Rowley JD (1980) Chronic myelodysplastic syndrome (preleukemia) with the Philadelphia chromomosome. Blood 56:262

San Miguel JF, Tavares de Castro J, Matutes E, Rodriguez B, Polli N, Zola H, McMichael AJ, Bollum FJ, Thompson DS, Goldman JM, Catovsky D (1985) Characterization of blast cells in chronic granulocytic leukaemia in transformation, acute myelofibrosis and undifferentiated leukemias. Br J Haematol 59:297

San Miguel JF, González M, Cañizo MC, Anta JP, Zola H, López Borrasca A (1986a) Surface marker analysis in acute myeloid leukaemia and correlation with FAB classification. Br J Haematol 64:547

San Miguel JF, González M, Cañizo MC, Anta JP, Hernández J, Ortega F, López Borrasaca A (1986b) The nature of blast cells in myelodysplastic syndromes evolving to acute leukaemia. Blut 52:357

San Miguel JF, González M, Cañizo MC, López-Borrasca A (1986c) Myelodysplastic syndrome evolving to a mixed myeloid-lymphoid leukaemia. Hematol Oncol 4:175

San Miguel JF, González M, Cañizo MC, Ojeda E, Orfao A, C Caballero MD, Moro MJ, Fisac P, López-Borrasca A (1988) Leukemias with megakaryoblastic involvement: Clinical, hematologic and immunologic characteristics. Blood 72:402

San Miguel JF, Hernández JM, González-Sarmiento R, González M, Sánchez I, Orfao A, Cañizo MC, López-Borrasca A (1991) Acute leukemia following a primary myelodysplastic syndrome: immunophenotypic, genotypic and clinical characteristics. Blood 78

Smadja N, Krulik M, Hagemeijer A, van der Plas D, González G, de Gramont A (1989) Cytogenetic and molecular studies of the Philadelphia translocation t(9;22) observed in a patient with myelodysplastic syndrome. Leukemia 3:236

Tricot G, Boogaerts MA, de Wolf-Peeters C, Van den Berghe H, Verwilghen RL (1985) The myelodysplastic syndromes: different evolution patterns based on sequential morphological and cytogenetic investigations. Br J Haematol 59:659

Van Dongen JJM, Wolvers-Tettero ILM (1991) Analysis of immunoglobulin and T cell receptor genes: II. Possibilities and limitations in the diagnosis and management of lymphoproliferative diseases and related disorders. Clin Chim Acta 198:93

Wainscoat JS, Fey MF, Pilkington S, Summers C, Oscier DG (1988) Absence of immunoglobulin and T-cell receptor gene rearrangements in myelodysplastic syndromes and acute nonlymphocytic leukemias. Am J Hematol 28:95

Subject Index

MIX
Papier aus verantwortungsvollen Quellen
Paper from responsible sources
FSC® C105338

If you have any concerns about our products,
you can contact us on
ProductSafety@springernature.com

In case Publisher is established outside the EU,
the EU authorized representative is:
Springer Nature Customer Service Center GmbH
Europaplatz 3, 69115 Heidelberg, Germany

Printed by Libri Plureos GmbH
in Hamburg, Germany